158 Anaesthesiologie und Intensivmedizin
Anaesthesiology and Intensive Care Medicine

vormals „Anaesthesiologie und Wiederbelebung“
begründet von R. Frey, F. Kern und O. Mayrhofer

Neue Aspekte in der Regionalanaesthesie 3

Plexus- und Epiduralanaesthesie: Technik und Komplikationen, Opiate epidural, intrathekal

Herausgegeben von H. J. Wüst, M. d'Arcy Stanton-Hicks und M. Zindler

Mit 113 Abbildungen und 67 Tabellen

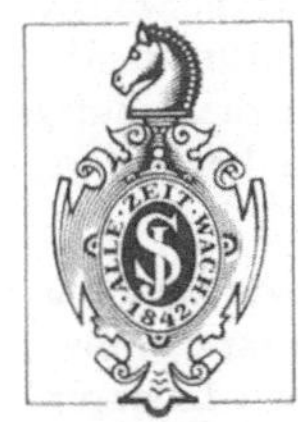

Springer-Verlag
Berlin Heidelberg New York Tokyo 1984

PD Dr. H. J. Wüst
Prof. Dr. M. Zindler
Inst. f. Anaesthesiologie,
Med. Einrichtungen d. Univ.,
Moorenstr. 5,
4000 Düsseldorf

Prof. M. d'Arcy Stanton-Hicks
Dept. of Anesthesia,
University Hospital,
Denver/Colorado
USA

CIP-Kurztitelaufnahme der Deutschen Bibliothek
Neue Aspekte in der Regionalanaesthesie / hrsg. von H. J. Wüst ... – Berlin; Heidelberg; New York; Tokyo: Springer, 1984. Teilw. mit d. Erscheinungsorten: Berlin, Heidelberg, New York. NE: Wüst, Hans-Joachim [Hrsg.]. 3. Plexus- und Epiduralanaesthesie: Technik und Komplikationen, Opiate epidural, intrathekal. – 1984. (Anaesthesiologie und Intensivmedizin; 158)

ISBN-13: 978-3-540-13023-9 e-ISBN-13: 978-3-642-69453-0
DOI:10.1007/ 978-3-642-69453-0

NE: GT

Satz: Elsner & Behrens GmbH, Oftersheim

2119/3140-543210

Vorwort

Untersuchungen der letzten Jahre haben gezeigt, daß im Vergleich zur Allgemeinnarkose die verschiedenen Verfahren der Regionalanaesthesie perioperativ einen günstigeren Einfluß auf Atmung, Kreislauf und operationsbedingte Streßreaktionen haben. Diese Vorteile, die besonders für Risikopatienten von Bedeutung sind, setzen eine sorgfältige Technik und Überwachung voraus.

Hierüber und über Maßnahmen zur Vermeidung von Komplikationen bei einer Regionalanaesthesie wurde von 26 Experten auf dem 3. Internationalen Symposium in Düsseldorf diskutiert.

In diesem Band sind 29 Vorträge zusammengefaßt, die zu den drei Themenkreisen

1. Techniken der Epidural- und Plexusanaesthesie,
2. mögliche Ursachen von Komplikationen bei Plexus- und rückenmarksnahen Leitungsanaesthesien, sowie
3. Wirkung und Gefahren der epidural bzw. intrathekal verabreichten Opiate gehalten wurden.

Unter dem Blickwinkel der Sicherheit für den Patienten wurden die Technik und die für die Blockaden verwendeten Materialien und Medikamente, insbesondere epidural verabreichte Opiate, kritisch beurteilt und Verbesserungsvorschläge erarbeitet.

Damit kann sich der klinisch tätige Anaesthesist schnell und umfassend über Aspekte der Leitungsanaesthesie informieren, die bisher in der Literatur nur wenig berücksichtigt wurden.

Dieser Band ergänzt den heutigen Erkenntnisstand über die Regionalanaesthesie, der in den beiden früheren Bänden dieser Serie dargestellt wurde.

Den Erfolg dieses Symposiums verdanken wir wiederum den informativen interessanten Beiträgen der Referenten und Diskussionsteilnehmer sowie der großzügigen Unterstützung durch die Firmen Astra Chemicals und Braun Melsungen.

Düsseldorf, im Oktober 1982

Priv.-Doz. H. J. Wüst,
Prof. M. d'Arcy Stanton-Hicks,
Prof. M. Zindler

Inhalt

Autorenverzeichnis

Abel, J., Dr. med. vet., Institut für Toxikologie der Universität, Universitätsstr. 1, D-4000 Düsseldorf

Aldrete, J. A., MD, MS Prof., Department of Anesthesiology Medical School, University of Alabama, Birmingham, Alabama 35294, USA

Alibert, F., MD, Department of Anaesthesia, Centre hospitalier region et universitaire, 1 Rue de Germont, Hôpital Charles-Nicolle, F-76038 Cedex-Rouen

Asbjørn, J., MD, Department of Anaesthesiology, Holsterbro Hospital, DK-7500 Holsterbro

Bergmann, H., Prof. Dr. med., Vorstand des Institutes für Anaesthesiologie des Allg. öffentl. Krankenhauses der Stadt Linz und Leiter des Ludwig-Boltzmann Institutes für Experimentelle Anaesthesiologie und Intensivmedizinische Forschung – Wien – Linz, A-4020 Linz

Bormann von, B., Dr. med., Institut für Anaesthesiologie der Freien Universität Klinikum Steglitz, Hindenburgdamm 30, D-1000 Berlin 45

Börner, V., Dr. med., Abteilung für Anaesthesiologie und Intensivmedizin, Justus-Liebig-Universität, Klinikstr. 29, D-6300 Gießen

Borst, R. H., Prof. Dr. med., Chefarzt der Anaesthesieabteilung des Krankenhauses Aalen, D-7080 Aalen

Brandt, M. R., MD, Department of Anaesthesia, Holsterbro, DK-7500 Holsterbro

Breulmann, M., Dr. med., Institut für Anaesthesiologie der Medizinischen Einrichtungen der Universität, Moorenstr. 5, D-4000 Düsseldorf

Christensen, P., MD, Department of Anaesthesiology Odense Sygehus, DK-5000 Odense

Clavier, E., Department of Neuroradiology, Centre hospitalier region et universitaire, 1 Rue de Germont, Hôpital Charles-Nicolle, F-76038 Cedex-Rouen

Clergue, F., MD, Department of Anaesthesiology, Hôpital de la Pitié, 83 Bd de l'Hôpital, F-75013 Paris

Crawford, J. S., FFA RCS FRCOG Consultant Anaesthetist, Birmingham Maternity Hospital, GB-Birmingham

Dennhardt, R., Prof. Dr. med., Oberarzt am Institut für Anaesthesiologie am Klinikum der Freien Universität Steglitz, Hindenburgdamm 30, D-1000 Berlin 45

Devaux, C. B., MD, Consultant of pain clinic, Centre hospitalier region ct universitaire, 1 Rue de Germont, Hôpital Charles-Nicolle, F-76038 Cedex-Rouen

Ekmekci, N., Dr. med., Abteilung für Anaesthesiologie des Kreiskrankenhauses Aalen, D-7080 Aalen

Falke, F. K., Prof. Dr. med., Oberarzt am Institut für Anaesthesiologie der Medizinischen Einrichtungen der Universität, Moorenstr. 5, D-4000 Düsseldorf

Fleischer, H., Dr. med., Abteilung für Anaesthesiologie des Kreiskrankenhauses Aalen, D-7080 Aalen

Freye, E., Priv.-Doz., Abteilung für Zentrale Diagnostik der Universitätskliniken Essen, Hufelandstr. 55, D-4300 Essen 1

Ghesquieres, F., MD, Department of Anaesthesia, Hôpital de la Pitié, 83 Bd de l'Hôpital, F-75013 Paris

Gips, H., Dr. med., Zentrum für Frauenheilkunde und Geburtshilfe der Justus-Liebig-Universität, Klinikstr. 29, D-6300 Gießen

Haag, W., Dr. med., Institut für Anaesthesiologie der Medizinischen Einrichtungen der Universität, Moorenstr. 5, D-4000 Düsseldorf

Hack, G., Priv.-Doz., Anaesthesie-Abt., Krankenhaus Singen, D-7700 Singen

Harari, A., MD, Department of Anaesthesia, Hôpital de la Pitié, 123 Bd Port Royal, F-75674 Paris-Cedex 14

Hartung, E., Dr. med., Oberarzt am Institut für Anaesthesiologie der Medizinischen Einrichtungen der Universität, Moorenstr. 5, D-4000 Düsseldorf

Hartung, H. J., Dr. med., Institut für Anaesthesiologie und Reanimation am Klinikum Mannheim der Universität Heidelberg, Postfach 23, D-6800 Mannheim

Hartvig, P., MD, Hospital Pharmacy, Akademiska Sjukhuset, S-75014 Uppsala 14

Hempelmann, G., Prof. Dr. med., Leiter der Abteilung für Anaesthesiologie und Intensivmedizin Justus-Liebig-Universität, Klinikstr. 29, D-6300 Gießen

Hettenbach, A., Dr. med., Institut für Anaesthesiologie und Reanimation am Klinikum Mannheim der Universität Heidelberg, Postfach 23, D-6800 Mannheim

Hort, W., Prof. Dr. med., Direktor des Pathologischen Institutes der Medizinischen Einrichtungen der Universität, Moorenstr. 5, D-4000 Düsseldorf

Jensen, V. Ø., MD, Department Gynecology, Holsterbro Hospital, DK-7500 Holsterbro

Karzel, K., Prof. Dr. med., Institut für Pharmakologie und Toxikologie der Rheinischen Friedrich-Wilhelms-Universität, D-5300 Bonn

Kehlet, H., MD, Ass. Chief Surgeon, Surgical Department, Kommunehospitalet, Øster Farimagsgade 5, DK-1399 Copenhagen

Klose, K., Priv.-Doz., Oberarzt am Institut für Anaesthesiologie und Reanimation am Klinikum Mannheim der Universität Heidelberg, Postfach 23, D-6800 Mannheim

Lanz, E., Priv.-Doz., Oberarzt am Institut für Anaesthesiologie der Universität Mainz, Langenbeckstr. 1, D-6500 Mainz

Lorentz, A., Dr. med., Institut für Anaesthesiologie und Reanimation am Klinikum Mannheim der Universität Heidelberg, Postfach 23, D-6800 Mannheim

Louis, C., Dr. med., Institut für Anaesthesiologie der Medizinischen Einrichtungen der Universität, Moorenstr. 5, D-4000 Düsseldorf

Lutz, H., Prof. Dr. med., Direktor des Institutes für Anaesthesiologie und Reanimation am Klinikum Mannheim der Universität Heidelberg, Postfach 23, D-6800 Mannheim

Møller, I. W., MD, Department of Anaesthesiology, Rigshospitalet, 9 Blegdamsvej, DK-2100 Copenhagen

Müller, H., Dr. med., Abteilung für Anaesthesiologie und Intensivmedizin Justus-Liebig-Universität, Klinikstr. 29, D-6300 Gießen

Osswald, P.-M., Dr. med., Oberarzt am Institut für Anaesthesiologie und Reanimation am Klinikum Mannheim der Universität Heidelberg, Postfach 23, D-6800 Mannheim

Rem, J., MD, Department of Anaesthesiology, Rigshospitalet, 9 Blegdamsvej, DK-2100 Copenhagen

Rieß, W., Dr. med., Institut für Anaesthesiologie der Universität Mainz, Langenbeckstr. 1, D-6500 Mainz

Rosenbauer, K. A., Prof. Dr. med., Direktor des Anatomischen Institutes III. der Universität, Universitätsstr., D-4000 Düsseldorf

Schielke, S., Dr. med., Abteilung für Anaesthesiologie des Kreiskrankenhauses Aalen, D-7080 Aalen

Schier, R., Dr. med., Institut für Anaesthesiologie der Medizinischen Einrichtungen der Universität, Moorenstr. 5, D-4000 Düsseldorf

Schulte-Steinberg, O. H., Dr. med., Dietrichweide 7, D-8135 Säckingen

Selander, D., MD, Department of Anaesthesia, Västra: Frölunda Hospital, S-42122 Västra: Frölunda

Sommer, U., Dr. med., Institut für Anaesthesiologie der Universität Mainz, Langenbeckstr. 1, D-6500 Mainz

Stanton-Hicks, d'Arcy M., MD, Prof. and Vice Chairman, Dept. of Anesthesiology, Univ. of Colorado, Health Sciences Center, 4200 East 9 Avenue, Denver, Colorado 80262, USA

Steenberge van, A., Dr., Department Anaesthesiology II Veiertjeslaan, B-1800 Overijse

Stehle, R., Dr. med., Abteilung für Anaesthesiologie des Kreiskrankenhauses Aalen, D-7080 Aalen

Steinhoff, H., Priv.-Doz., Oberarzt am Institut für Anaesthesiologie der Medizinischen Einrichtungen der Universität, Moorenstr. 5, D-4000 Düsseldorf

Stoyanov, M., Dr. med., Abteilung für Anaesthesiologie und Intensivmedizin Justus-Liebig-Universität, Klinikstr. 29, D-6300 Gießen

Tamsen, A., MD, Department of Anaesthesiology, Akademiska Sjukhuset, S-75014 Uppsala 14

Tessier, C., Department of Anaesthesia, Centre Hospitalier region et universitaire, 1 Rue de Germont, Hôpital Charles-Nicolle, F-76038 Cedex Rouen

Theiss, D., Dr. med., Institut für Anaesthesiologie der Universität Mainz, Langenbeckstr. 1, D-6500 Mainz

Thiebot, J., Prof., Chief Department of Neuroradiology, Centre hospitaliere region et universitaire, 1 Rue de Germant, Hôpital Charles-Nicolle, F-76038 Cedex Rouen

Thiessen, F. M. M., Institut für Anaesthesiologie der Medizinischen Einrichtungen der Universität, Moorenstr. 5, D-4000 Düsseldorf

Tung, A. S., MD, Department of Anesthesiology School of Medicine University of Pittsburgh, Pittsburgh, Pennsylvania 15261, USA

Ungemach, J., Dr. med., Institut für Anaesthesiologie und Reanimation am Klinikum Mannheim der Universität Heidelberg, Postfach 23, D-6800 Mannheim

Vester-Andersen, T., MD, Department of Anaesthesia, Rigshospitalet, 9 Blegdamsvej, DK-2100 Copenhagen

Viars, P., Prof. and Chairman, Départment d'Anesthésie, Hôpital de la Pitié, 83 Bd de l'Hôpital, F-75013 Paris

Wechsler, W., Prof. und Direktor des Institutes für Neuropathologie der Universität, Universitätsstr., D-4000 Düsseldorf

Wiest, W., Dr. med., Institut für Anaesthesiologie und Reanimation am Klinikum Mannheim der Universität Heidelberg, Postfach 23, D-6800 Mannheim

Winnie, A. P., MD, Prof. and Chairman, Department of Anesthesiology, University of Illinois, 1740 West Tayler Street, Chicago, Illinois 60612, USA

Wüst, H. J., Priv.-Doz., Oberarzt am Institut für Anaesthesiologie der Medizinischen Einrichtungen der Universität, Moorenstr. 5, D-4000 Düsseldorf

Yaksh, T., MD, Consultant in Neurosurgery Research, Mayo Clinic, Rochester, Minnesota 55905, USA

Zarén, B., MD, Department of Anaesthesiology, Akademiska Sjukhuset, S-75014 Uppsala

Zindler, M., Prof. Dr. med., Direktor des Institutes für Anaesthesiologie der Medizinischen Einrichtungen der Universität, Moorenstr. 5, D-4000 Düsseldorf

I Techniken der Regionalanaesthesie: Plexus- und Epiduralanaesthesie

Vorsitz: H. Bergmann, Linz und H. Steinhoff, Düsseldorf

Plexus anesthesia: Interscalene, Subclavian and Axillary Perivascular Techniques

A. P. Winnie

The single-injection techniques developed to provide anesthesia for the upper extremities are based on the fact that all of the nerves to the arm are contained in a tubular sheath of fascia. [8, 9, 11] The anterior scalene muscle arises from the anterior tubercles of the transverse processes of the third, fourth, fifth, and sixth cervical vertebrae and inserts on the scalene tubercle of the first rib, separating the subclavian vein from the subclavian artery, which lies posterior to this insertion. The middle scalene muscle arises from the posterior tubercles of the transverse processes of the lower six cervical vertebrae. Its insertion is separated from that of the anterior scalene muscle by the subclavian groove, through which the artery passes. Thus, since the roots of the nerves comprising the brachial plexus travel in the groove between the anterior and posterior tubercles of the transverse processes of the cervical vertebrae, they emerge from the "gutters" of the cervical processes to descend toward the first rib between the two walls of fascia covering the anterior and middle scalene muscles (i.e., they enter the interscalene space). As the roots pass down through this space, they converge to form the trunks of the brachial plexus, which together with the subclavian artery invaginate the scalene fascia to form a subclavian perivascular sheath, which in turn becomes the axillary sheath as it passes under the clavicle.

The important concept in terms of block anesthesia for upper-extremity surgery is that of a continuous, fascia-enclosed space extending from the cervical transverse processes to several centimeters beyond the axilla, or from the roots of the brachial plexus to the great nerves of the upper arm. The existence of such a continuous perineural and perivascular space renders brachial plexus block simple. Just as with peridural techniques, the space may be entered at any level. The volume of anesthetic injected at that level determines the extent of anesthesia. Thus, the technique should be determined on the basis of the surgical site, the required level of anesthesia, and the physical status and habitus of the patient, rather than on the basis of the anesthetist's bias or training. There are three convenient levels at which the brachial plexus may be blocked. Each technique is named for that portion of the compartment into which the injection is made.

Axillary Perivascular Technique

This technique of axillary block utilizes a single injection of local anesthetic as high in the axillary perivascular space as possible to minimize the amount of solution necessary to reach

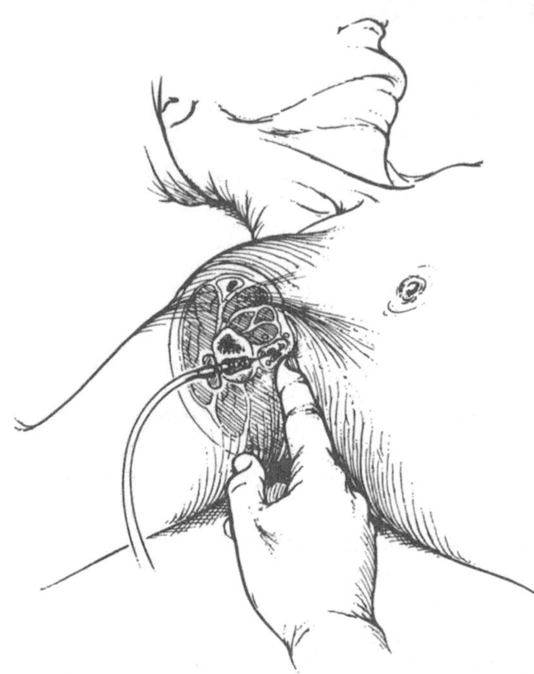

Fig. 1. Axillary perivascular brachial plexus block as carried out by the author [14]. A single injection is made superiorly tangential to the arterial pulse in a proximal direction to promote cephalad flow. The palpating finger collapses the vein and rolls it inferiorly during insertion of the needle to minimize the possibility of venipuncture. During the injection, the finger is placed distal to the needle and digital pressure is applied to prevent retrograde flow

the musculocutaneous and axillary nerves [13]. The patient is placed in the supine position with the arm abducted at about 90° and the forearm fixed and externally rotated so that the dorsum of the hand lies on the table next to the patient's head (Fig. 1). The axillary artery is palpated and followed proximally to the point where it disappears under the pectoralis major muscle. At this point, with the index finger directly over the pulse, a 1.5-inch, 21-gauge, short bevel needle is inserted just above the finger tip toward the apex of the axilla, so that it forms a 10° to 20° angle with the artery as it is advanced. The artery is thus approached gradually until the definite "click" caused by the penetration of the axillary sheath is encountered. Paresthesias are not sought, but if one is elicited, the needle is advanced no further. The tip of the needle should be superiorly tangential to the arterial wall 1 to 1.5 inches above the most proximal point of palpable pulsation (Fig. 2). Following aspiration, 20 to 40 ml of anesthetic is injected slowly, with repeated aspiration for blood intermittent during the injection. The total dose depends on the patient's size, sex, age, and the level of anesthesia desired.

Volume-anesthesia relationships with this technique have been determined radiographically after the various volumes of local anesthetic mixed with radiopaque dye were injected into the axillary perivascular space (Figs. 3, 4, 9, 10, 13, 14). An injection of 20 ml anesthetic solution is insufficient to consistently reach the level of the coracoid process at which the musculocutaneous and axillary nerves leave the sheath (Fig. 3). If anesthesia in the distribution of the nerves and relaxation of the powerful flexors of the forearm are essential, 30 to 40 ml is necessary to assure blockade (Fig. 4). Two to three milliliters of anesthetic is retained in the syringe and deposited subcutaneously outside the sheath but over the artery as the needle is being withdrawn (Fig. 5) to block the intercostobrachial nerve, which runs just superficial to the sheath and innervates the upper inner aspect of the arm.

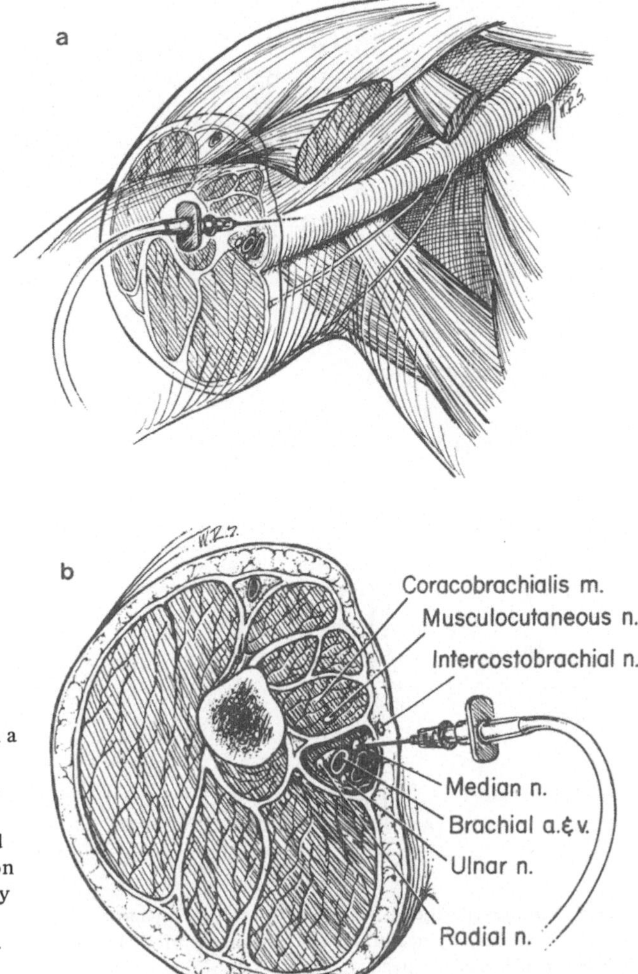

Fig. 2. a Frontal view of the axilla with a needle properly placed for an axillary perivascular block. Note that the direction of the needle and the position of the needle tip promote cephalad spread of the injection solution. **b** Cross section of the upper arm with a needle properly placed for axillary perivascular block. Note that the tip of the needle lies tangential to the artery and vein

If an increased volume of anesthetic to reach the musculocutaneous and axillary nerves cannot be used because of pre-existing disease, a low volume technique may be used whereby 10 ml local anesthetic is injected into the axillary perivascular compartment and the musculocutaneous nerve is blocked separately by reinserting the needle superior to the entire neurovascular bundle and injecting 5 ml into the substance of the coracobrachialis muscle (Fig. 6). It is not necessary to obtain paresthesias of this nerve (unless the onset of anesthesia must be immediate), for the fascia of the muscle confines the injected solution and renders blockade almost certain.

The axillary perivascular technique has certain distinct advantages and disadvantages. Inadvertent block of the phrenic, vagus, and recurrent laryngeal nerves and of the stellate ganglion is virtually impossible, as is pneumothorax and subarachnoid or epidural injection. These features also make it possible to utilize this technique for bilateral brachial block without fear of respiratory embarrassment. An additional advantage, at least from the patient's point of view, is the fact that it is not necessary to elicit parethesias. However, this technique

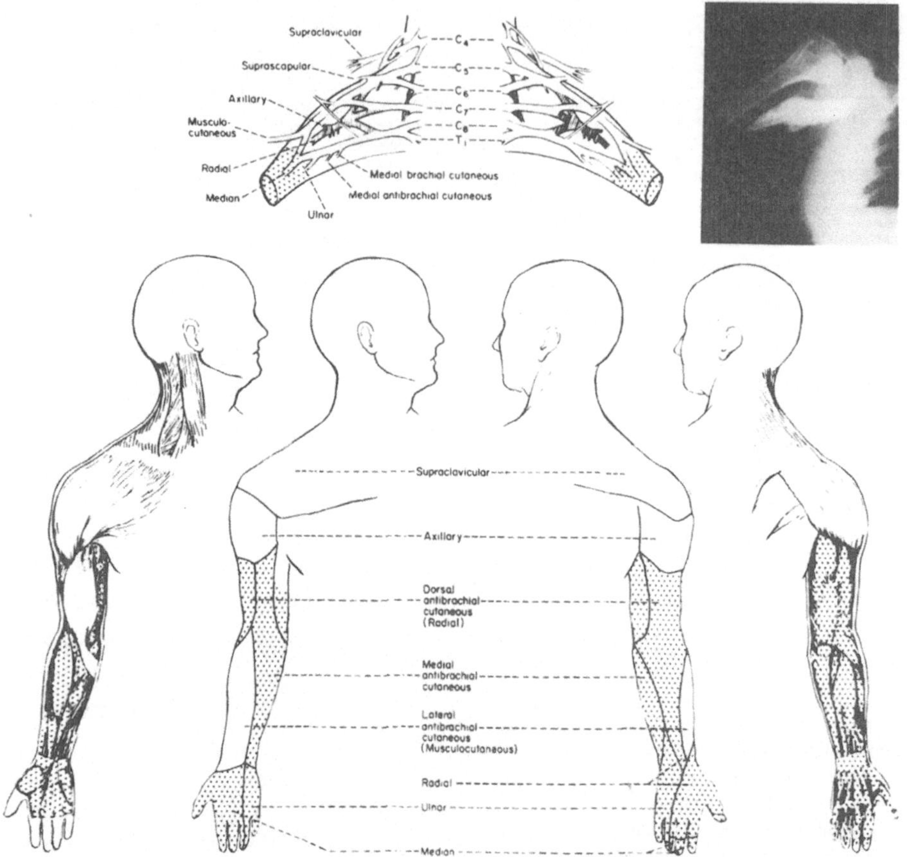

Fig. 3. Volume-anesthesia relationships after an injection of 20 ml anesthetic solution into the axillary sheath. Note the absence of sensory and motor block in the distribution of the musculocutaneous nerve when this volume is utilized

cannot be used when the patient is unable to abduct the arm to expose the axilla. In addition, larger volumes of anesthetic are required than for subclavian perivascular and interscalene techniques. Puncture of the artery or vein is possible and, though vigorous digital massage usually avoids hematoma formation, it is usually of no clinical significance when it does occur. The chance of intravenous injection is minimized by compressing the vein and displacing it slightly downward with the index finger, by using a single injection superior to the vessels, and by repeatedly aspirating before and during the injection. Intravenous injection, should it occur, will result in excitation and convulsions, depending on the volume of anesthetic that entered the vein. This complication usually requires only ventilation with oxygen [4]; however, if this is not effective, diazepam will prevent or terminate a convulsion [3]. The use of barbiturates should be avoided for the sequelae to intravenous injection are usually self-limited and of short duration. Intra-arterial injection, although theoretically possible, has never been described. However, if during insertion of the needle, the artery is penetrated, it is best to advance the needle until no blood returns and to make the injection deep to the

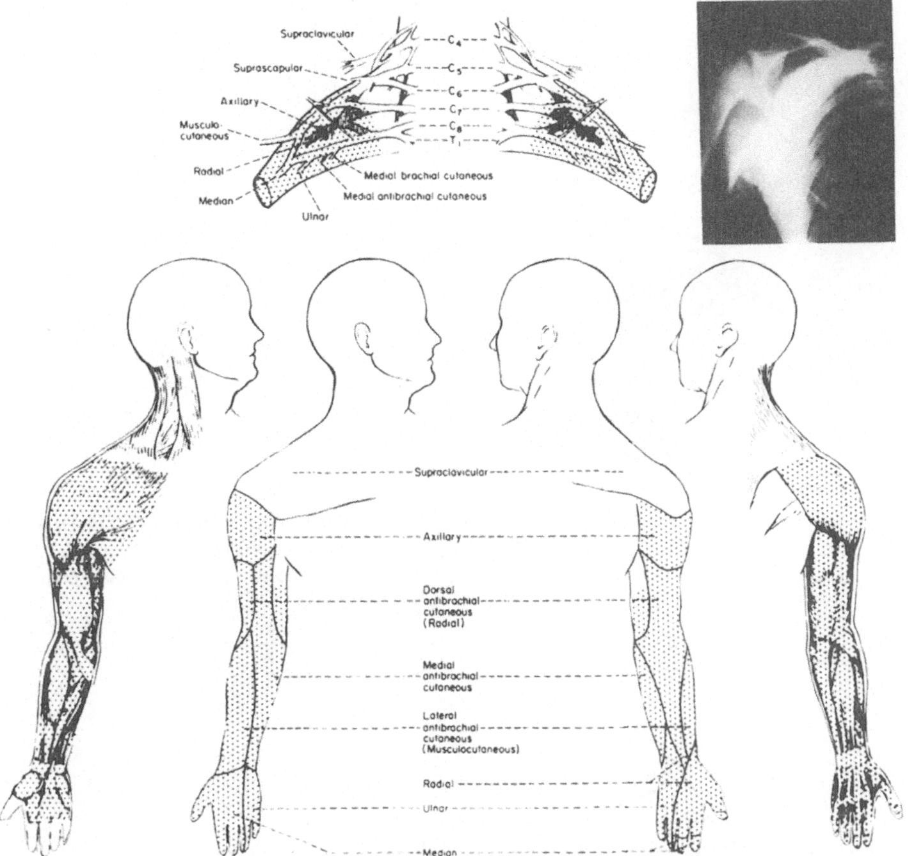

Fig. 4. Volume-anesthesia relationships after an injection of 40 ml anesthetic solution into the axillary sheath. All elements of the brachial plexus are blocked by this volume

artery. If the needle is withdrawn and redirected after penetrating the artery, the injection will be made with blood already in the sheath, enhancing the possibility of spotty or incomplete anesthesia.

The axillary perivascular technique is contraindicated with infection or malignancy in the involved extremities. Though the technique is easy to learn, it is very difficult to perform in the obese or in individuals in whom the axillary artery can not be precisely located.

Subclavian Perivascular Technique

There are several features of traditional "supraclavicular block" techniques that can be criticized on an anatomical basis alone [16]. The site of insertion of the needle is usually 1 cm above the midpoint of the clavicle. This point frequently does not lie over the first rib as de-

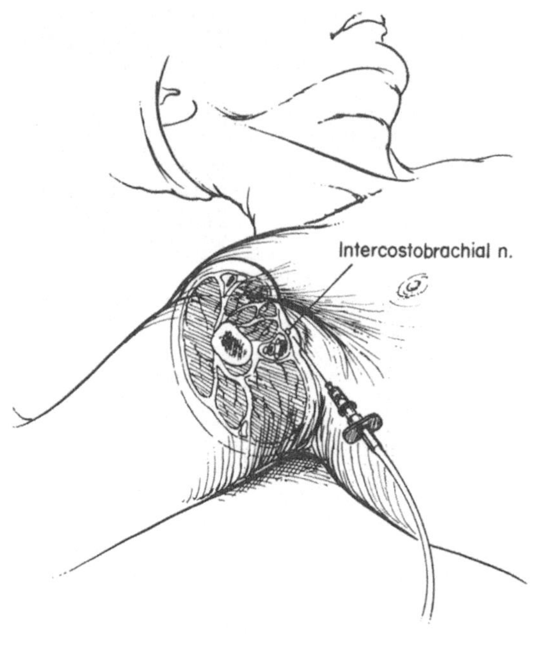

Fig. 5. The intercostobrachial nerve is blocked by depositing 2 ml local anesthetic subcutaneously just superficial to the arterial pulse

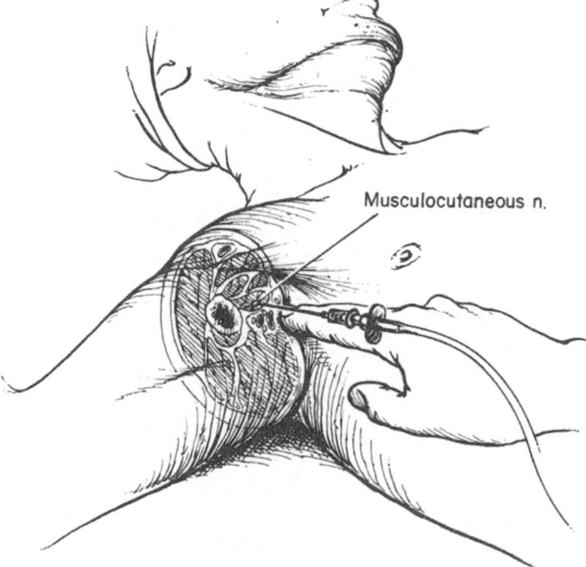

Fig. 6. The musculocutaneous nerve may be blocked separately to minimize the volume required with the axillary technique by injecting into the substance of the coracobrachialis muscle

scribed. Since the rib is said to act as a "backstop" protecting the cupola of the lung from penetration by the exploring needle, it is remarkable that the incidence of pneumothorax is not even higher than the 0.5% to 6% reported [10]. The direction of needle insertion is conventionally described as "mesiad, caudad, and dorsad." Consideration of the anatomy of the "brachial plexus" sheath presented above seems to make this illogical. Since the subclavian perivascular space is bounded by the anterior and middle scalene muscle, it is deep but very

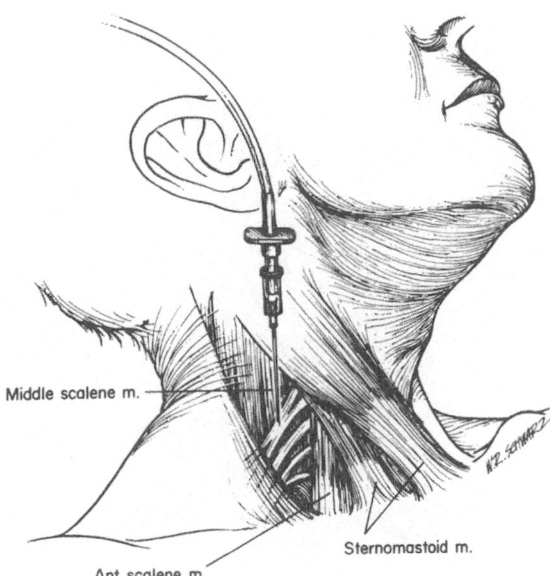

Fig. 7. The subclavian perivascular technique of brachial plexus block [17]

narrow in its anterior-posterior dimension. Thus, the direction of needle insertion advocated in the "supraclavicular techniques" results in the needle crossing the space at its narrowest diameter. Therefore, even the slightest movement during injection may cause the needle to leave the space, a possibility which is increased by multiple injections. Finally, the needle is usually "walked along the rib" to obtain consecutive paresthesias of various distributions, with an injection of anesthetic being made each time a paresthesia is elicited. This also appears to be quite illogical, as the trunks lie on top of each other vertically as they cross the first rib, not one behind the other horizontally as depicted in even the most recent texts [5, 9]. As a result, the classic techniques result in the use of large volumes of anesthetic solution, of which only a small amount may actually be within the sheath, while the remainder may be at the phrenic, vagus, or recurrent laryngeal nerves or, worse still, in the cupola of the lung. It is no wonder that Adriani wrote, "when (we) use the supraclavicular route, (we) do so with a certain amount of fear and trepidation" [1].

Applying the perivascular concept to the supraclavicular approach obviates the undesirable features of the classic techniques. The patient is placed in the dorsal recumbent position with the head turned somewhat to the side opposite that to be injected. He is told to reach for his knee (to lower the clavicle) and then to relax the arm and shoulder completely. He is then asked to elevate his head slightly to bring the clavicular head of the sternocleidomastoid muscle into prominence. The anesthetist then places his index finger behind the muscle on the anterior surface of the anterior scalene muscle. When the patient relaxes, the anesthetist rolls his palpating finger laterally across the belly of the anterior scalene muscle until the groove between anterior and middle scalene muscles is palpated. The finger is moved inferiorly in this groove until the pulse of the subclavian artery is palpated where it emerges from between the scalene muscles. With the finger still on the artery, a 1.5-inch, 21-gauge needle is inserted above this point and is directed caudad but not mesiad or dorsad (Fig. 7). The direction of insertion is such that the needle will be dorsally tangential to the subclavian artery in the

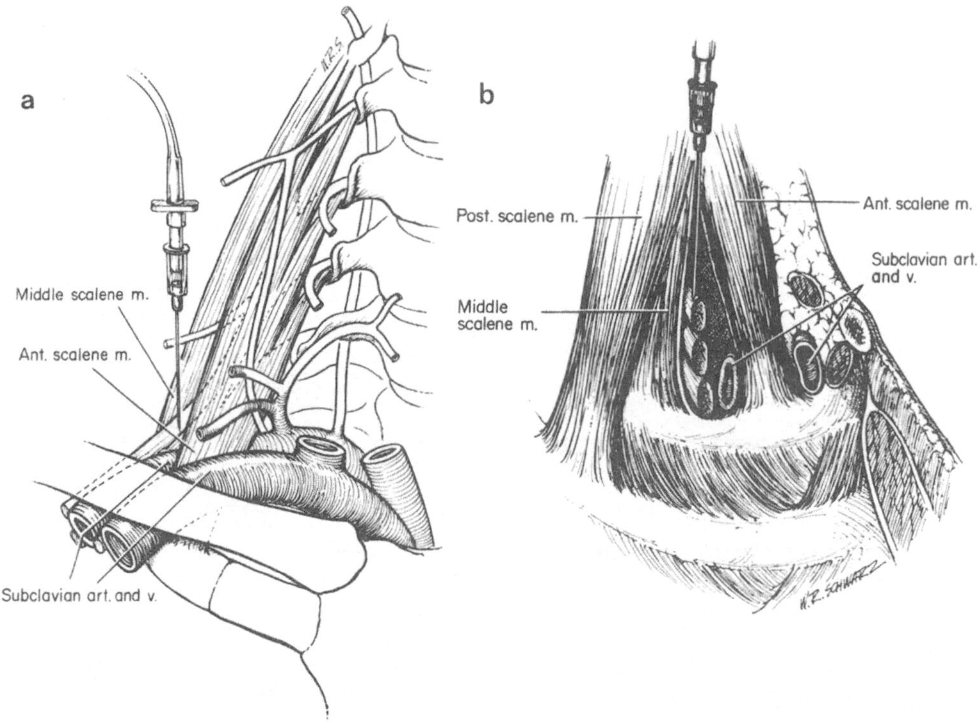

Fig. 8. a Frontal section showing a needle properly placed for a subclavian perivascular block. Note the directly caudad direction of the needle. **b** Sagittal section showing that the caudad direction of the needle places it in the longest axis of the subclavian perivascular space. Note also that the properly placed needle lies closer to the middle scalene muscle than to the anterior scalene

longest dimension of the interscalene space (Fig. 8a). The needle is advanced slowly (Fig. 8b) and, if the superior trunk is not encountered, the middle will be; if the middle trunk is not encountered, the inferior will be. If none of the three are encountered, the needle will impinge on the first rib. This is rare, however, and a paresthesia is usually evoked after advancing the needle a short distance. It is essential that the paresthesia be to the arm, forearm, or hand and not just to the shoulder, for the suprascapular nerve may be encountered outside the sheath. During the injection of the local anesthetic, a "pressure paresthesia" similar to that experienced when anesthetic solution is injected rapidly into the caudal canal offers further evidence that the needle is properly placed.

The relationship between volume injected and extent of anesthesia has been demonstrated by injecting local anesthetic mixed with radiopaque dye into the sheath at this level. It has been determined that 20 ml dye injected into the subclavian perivascular space extends from the level of the roots to the cords of the brachial plexus (Fig. 9). Hence, the anesthesia provided by this volume of anesthetic in the subclavian perivascular space results in motor and sensory loss almost identical to that produced by 40 ml in the axillary perivascular space. An X-ray taken after an injection of 40 ml dye into the subclavian perivascular space shows it spreading to a higher (and lower) level, so that when this volume of anesthetic is used clinically, anesthesia of the cervical as well as brachial plexus results (Fig. 10). Of

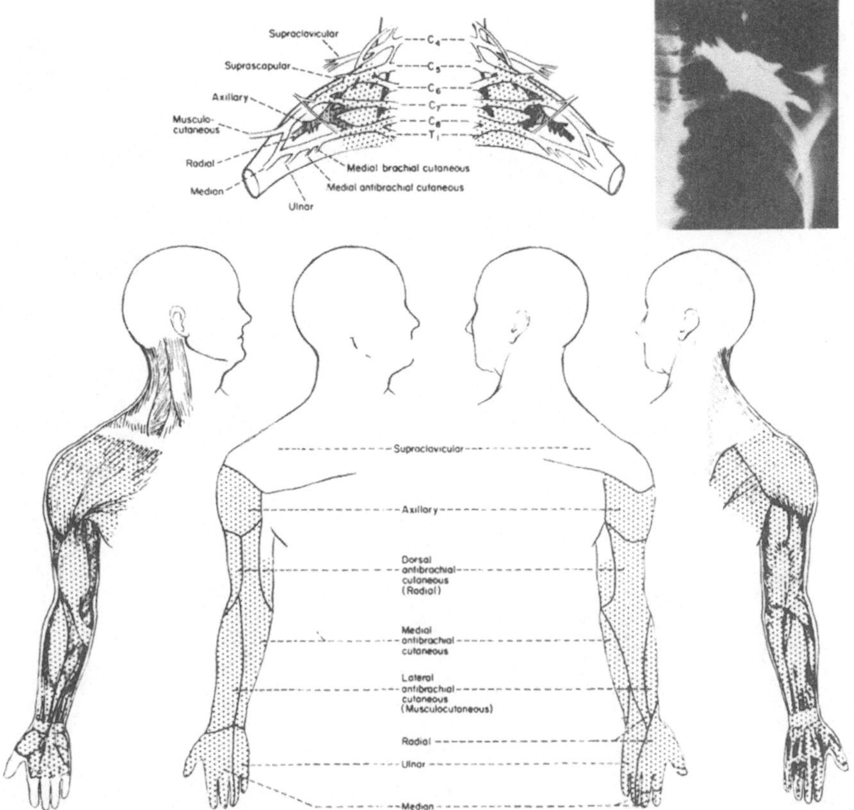

Fig. 9. Volume-anesthesia relationships after an injection of 20 ml anesthetic solution into the subclavian perivascular space. Note that the extent of anesthesia is identical to that achieved with 40 ml injected into the axillary perivascular space

course, the intercostobrachial nerve must be blocked separately if a tourniquet is to be used, just as with other techniques (see Fig. 5).

The technique of needle insertion, the use of a short needle, and the use of a single injection not only improve the incidence of satisfactory results, but also minimize the possibility of pneumothorax. Since the needle is placed parallel to the borders of the scalene muscles and since these muscles insert on the first rib, the position of the rib and vessel are located more precisely with this than with other techniques. In most cases, paresthesias are obtained before the rib has been contacted. Advantages of this technique include the ability to achieve a high level of anesthesia with a relatively small volume of anesthetic. In addition, the block may be accomplished without moving a painful extremity or shoulder. Intravenous injection is most unlikely and inadvertent subarachnoid or epidural injection virtually impossible. While it usually may be employed in the presence of injections of the hand and arm, it possibly should not be used where lesions of the neck (or chest) result in scalene adenopathy. Pneumothorax and phrenic and recurrent laryngeal block are not impossible; however, if the technique is carried out precisely as described, the possibility is extremely remote. To be perfectly safe, bilateral block should be staggered or accomplished with the axillary tech-

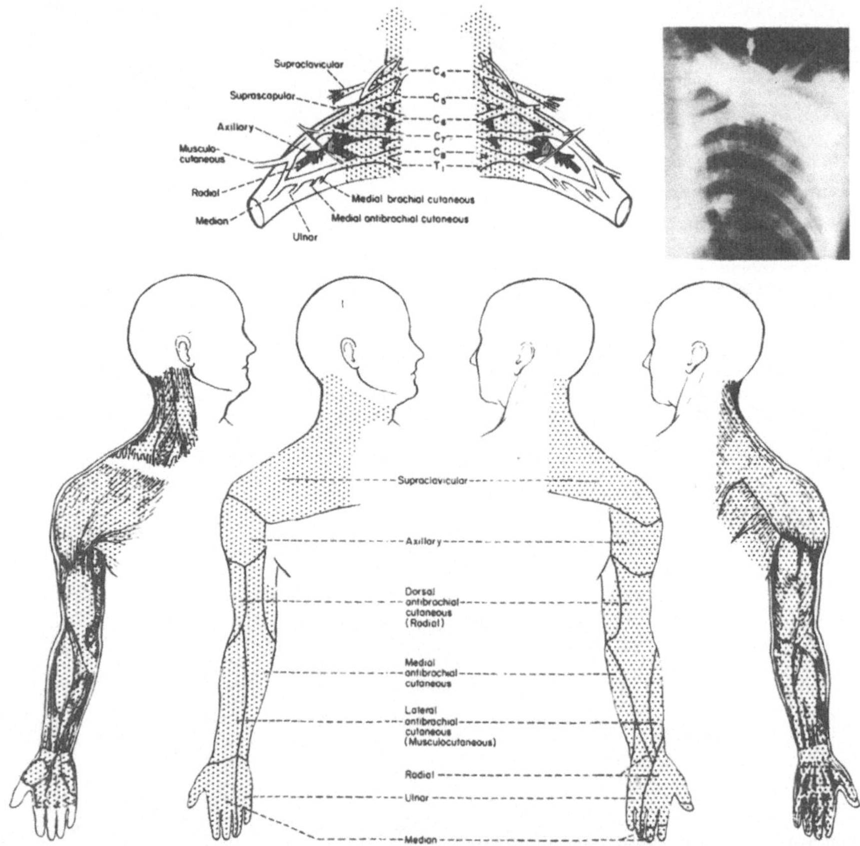

Fig. 10. Volume-anesthesia relationships after an injection of 40 ml anesthetic solution into the subclavian perivascular space. The *arrow* indicates the passage of solution upwards to involve the cervical plexus

nique on one side and subclavian on the other. A minor disadvantage lies in the need to elicit paresthesias. While this may be less pleasant for the patient, it almost guarantees anesthesia. The subclavian perivascular technique can be accomplished without evoking paresthesias, but this requires a great deal of experience and, in our experience, results in a 15% failure rate.

Interscalene Technique

It was pointed out earlier that as the roots of the brachial plexus emerge from their grooved transverse processes, they enter the interscalene space formed by the fascia covering the anterior and middle scalene muscles. Since most of this space lies above the subclavian artery and the cupola of the lung, it is an ideal point, at least from the point of view of safety, to perform a brachial block [14].

The patient is placed in a position similar to that used for the subclavian perivascular technique. The interscalene groove is identified in an identical manner. The level of the sixth

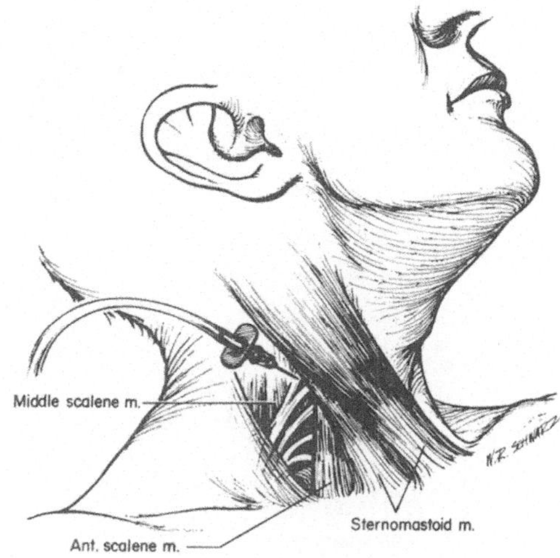

Fig. 11. Interscalene technique of brachial plexus block [15]

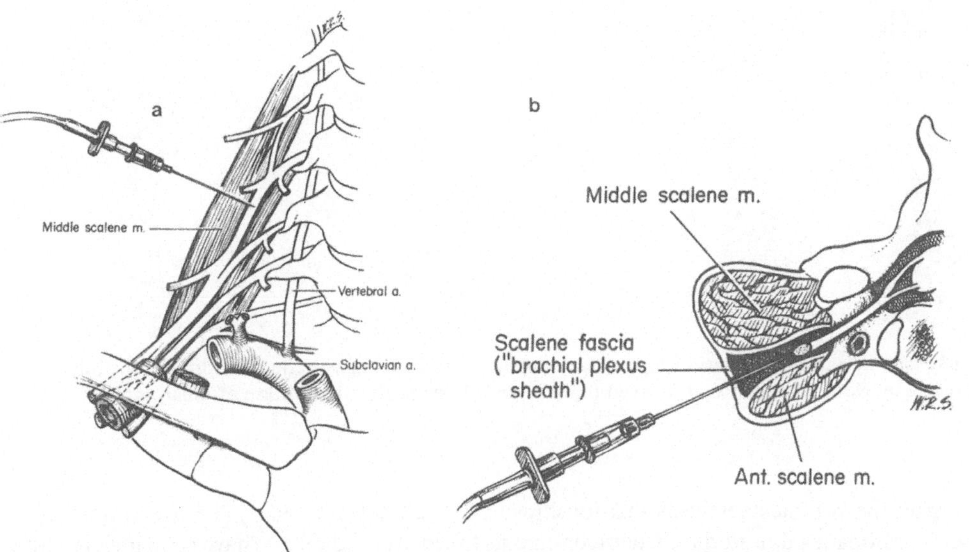

Fig. 12. a Frontal view showing a needle properly placed for an interscalene brachial plexus block. Note the slight caudad direction of the needle which is crucial to prevent a needle which has missed the roots of the plexus from entering the vertebral vessels or the epidural or subarachnoid spaces. **b** Cross-sectional view showing a needle properly placed for an interscalene brachial plexus block. Note the slight dorsad direction of needle

cervical vetebra is determined by extending a line from the cricoid cartilage laterally to the interscalene groove and, at this point, a 1.5-inch, 22-gauge needle is inserted into the groove perpendicular to the skin in all planes (Fig. 11). The direction of injection is thus slightly caudad (Fig. 12a) and dorsad as well as mesiad (Fig. 12b). The needle is advanced until a paresthesia is elicited or the transverse process is encountered. Once a paresthesia has been evoked the desired volume of anesthetic is injected.

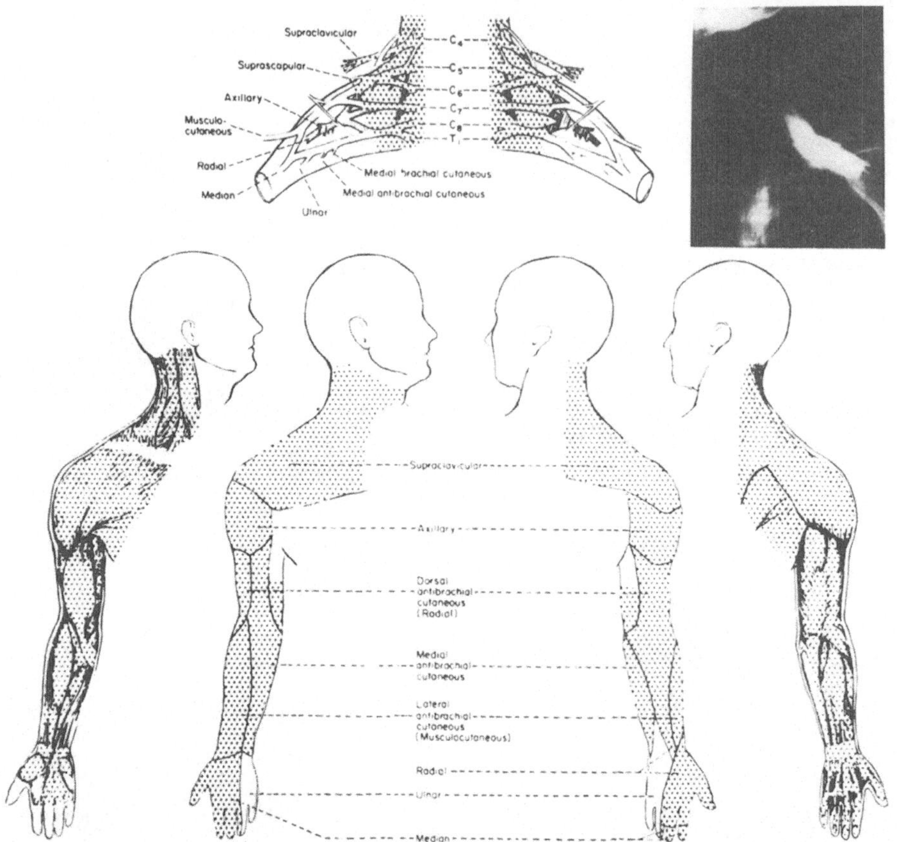

Fig. 13. Volume-anesthesia relationships after an injection of 20 ml anesthetic solution into the interscalene space. Note the absence or delayed onset of anesthesia in the distribution of ulnar nerve

Again the volume-anesthesia relationships have been determined by the use of local anesthetic-radiopaque dye studies. Roentgenograms taken after 20 ml dye have been injected into the interscalene space show the dye to be slightly higher than the same volume injected into the subclavian perivascular space. Hence, 20 ml anesthetic injected into the interscalene space results in anesthesia of the lower cervical plexus as well as the brachial plexus. Blockade of the ulnar nerve is often delayed and is occasionally absent with this volume of solution (Fig. 13). The fibers that become ulnar nerves are contained in the inferior trunk, which is frequently trapped between the subclavian artery and the first rib. Hence diffusion inferiorly to this level may be impaired or, at least, delayed.

After injection of 40 ml dye by this technique, X-rays show the interscalene space filled from the transverse processes of the upper cervical vertebrae to the coracoid process and beyond. Thus, this volume of anesthetic injected into the interscalene space results in anesthesia of both the cervical and brachial plexuses (Fig. 14).

If it is desirable to limit the volume of anesthetic and the increased volume is utilized only to facilitate ulnar block, a lesser volume may be injected into the sheath and the ulnar

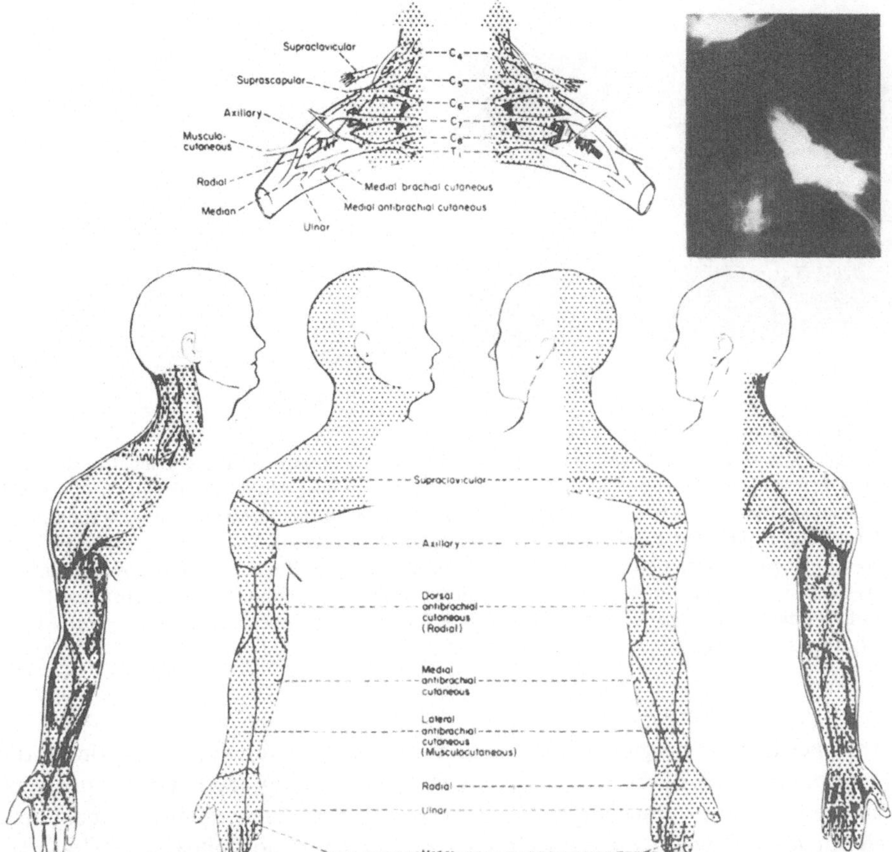

Fig. 14. Volume-anesthesia relationships after an injection of 40 ml anesthetic solution into the interscalene space. The *arrow* indicates that this volume spills cephalad and blocks the cervical as well as brachial plexus

nerve blocked at the elbow by a separate injection. The nerve is palpated midway between the medial epicondyle of the humerus and the olecranon, with the patient's arm flexed. A 25-gauge needle is inserted in the direction of the nerve and, when a paresthesia to the little finger is elicited, 5 ml anesthetic is injected. If a tourniquet is to be used, as with the other techniques, the intercostobrachial nerve must be blocked separately as described previously (Fig. 5).

The interscalene technique is particularly easy to perform in the obese, where the other techniques may be difficult, and in children or intoxicated adults, where cooperation is impossible. It is ideal for manipulations of and procedures on the upper arm and shoulder where a high level of anesthesia is obtained with a relatively small volume. Pneumothorax is impossible and this technique can be used in the presence of infection or malignancy of the arm or chest. The disadvantage of slow onset of ulnar blockade is easy to offset by increasing the volume or by blocking that nerve separately. Subarachnoid or epidural injection as well as vertebral artery injection is theoretically possible and several cases have been reported [7, 12]. The slight caudad direction of the needle, if carefully observed, should pre-

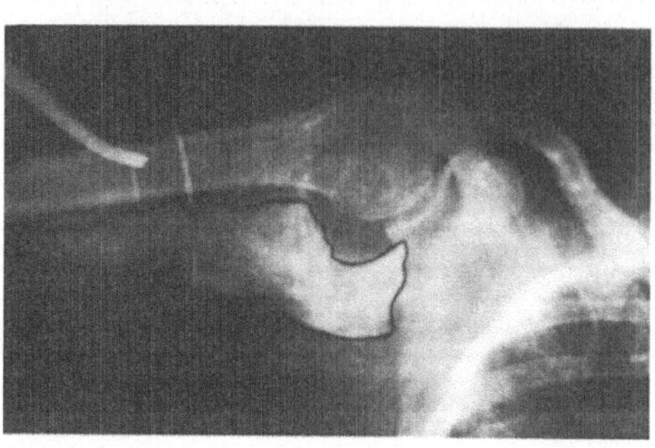

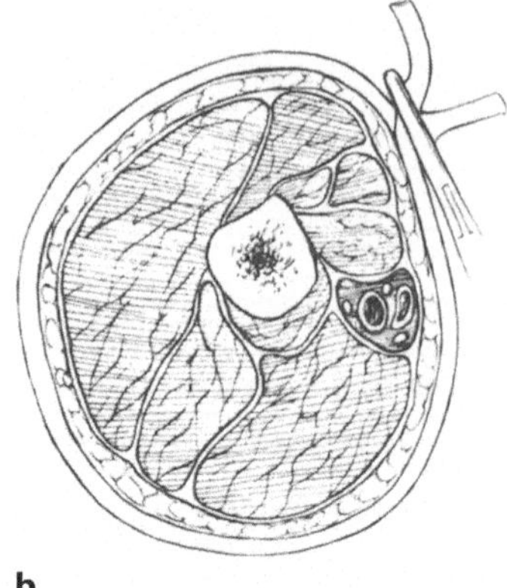

a b

Fig. 15a, b. X rays taken following injection of radiopaque dye into the axillary sheath using the technique of Eriksson and Skarby [6], wherein a tourniquet is applied behind the needle "to prevent retrograde flow of anesthetic down the sheath." (A small amount of dye has been added to the tourniquet to render it radiopaque.) The tourniquet is not able to block retrograde flow (when a sufficient volume is injected to reach it). Because the neurovascular bundle is deeply situated in the groove between the coracobrachialis muscle and the long head of the triceps, note that the humeral head obstructs the central flow of the injected anesthetic, since Eriksson and Skarby's technique calls for injection to be made more distally than that in Fig. 2

vent the needle from progressing very far between the transverse processes, preventing these complications. Block of the phrenic, vagus, and recurrent laryngeal nerves is not seen if the technique is performed precisely as outlined. Nonetheless, bilateral block should be staggered or combined with axillary block to avoid the remote possibility of respiratory embarrassment. Naturally, the technique should not be used where there is infection in or trauma to the neck.

Factors Influencing Distribution of Local Anesthetic [18]

The preceding paragraphs have emphasized the importance of the fascia-enclosed space that envelops the various components of the brachial plexus from the cervical transverse processes to the junction of the upper and middle thirds of the upper arm. Just as with peridural techniques, the extent of anesthesia following a block will depend primarily upon the level at which the anesthetic was injected (i.e., the technique used) and the volume that was injected at that level. However, there are other factors, perhaps less important but nonetheless significant, which can and do influence the volume-anesthesia relationships with two of the three techniques described.

In 1961, when calculating mathematically that 42 ml would be necessary to fill a "cylinder" of the dimensions of the axillary sheath sufficient to block the musculocutaneous nerve, de Jong assumed that the injected anesthetic solution would flow both up and down the sheath from the point of injection [2]. Obviously, that portion which flows down the

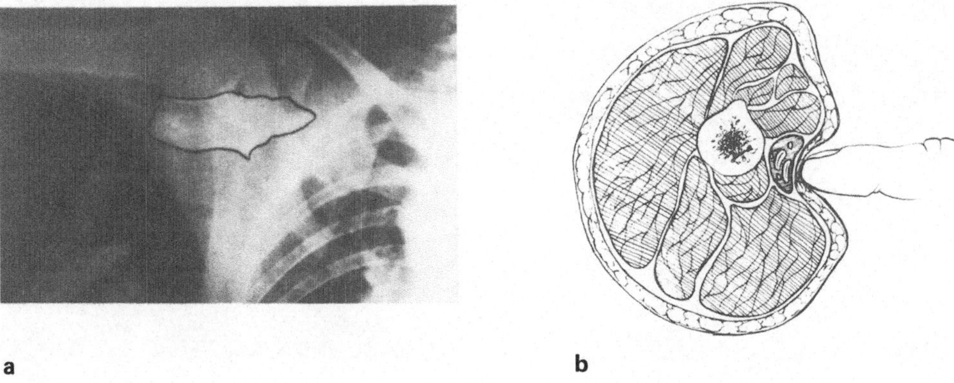

Fig. 16a, b. X rays taken following injection of radiopaque dye into the axillary sheath with the needle as high in the axilla as possible, with the needle directed centrally, and with firm digital pressure applied just behind the needle. Digital pressure is effective in blocking peripheral flow and enhancing central flow because the finger fits *between* the muscles and selectively and completely occludes the neurovascular bundle

sheath is wasted, at least in terms of the volume-anesthesia relationships. To prevent this wasteful retrograde flow, Eriksson placed a tight rubber tourniquet distal to the site of injection just prior to performing the block [6]. However, because the impact of the tourniquet is absorbed by the muscles above and below the neurovascular bundle, injected solution is free to pass through the tourniquet unobstructed (Fig. 15a, b). In addition, the major reason flow occurs in both directions with Eriksson's technique (and others) is that the injection is made perpendicular to the long axis of the neurovascular bundle and below the humeral head. If the injection is made in the direction in which the anesthetist wishes the anesthetic to flow and as high in the axilla as possible, as is done in the author's technique (Fig. 16a, b), most of the injected solution will move centrad with minimal retrograde flow. Where little retrograde flow is, it can be completely blocked by applying firm digital pressure immediately distal to the needle during the injection. Actually, the main anatomical obstruction to the central flow of anesthetic solutions injected into the axillary sheath is provided by the head of the humerus. Dye injections and X-rays have again documented that humeralhead obstruction to flow is maximal with the arm abducted to 90° (or more) and decreases until it is nonexistent as the arm is brought down to the side. Thus, if one wishes to provide the maximal level possible with any volume, not only should digital pressure be applied immediately distal to the needle during the injection, but this pressure should be maintained following the injection as well as after removal of the needle. The arm should be brought down to the side as quickly as possible upon completion of the block.

A similar maneuver is useful to minimize the volume necessary in performing an interscalene brachial plexus block. As pointed out earlier, with lower volumes of anesthetic this technique may provide delayed or incomplete anesthesia of the ulnar nerve, while with larger volumes part or all of the cervical plexus will be blocked. Thus, if cervical plexus anesthesia

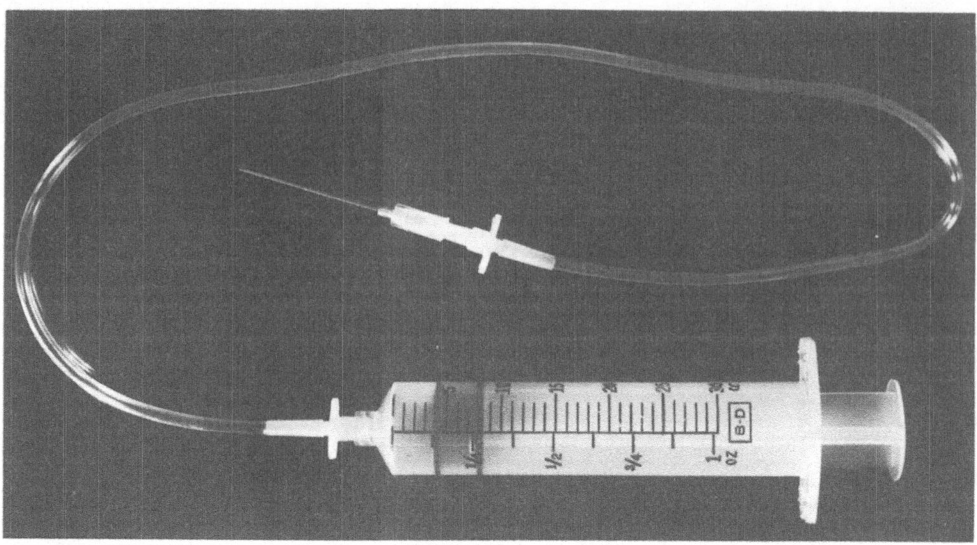

Fig. 17. The "immobile needle": The needle should have a short bevel to allow perception of the penetration of fascial planes and a translucent hub to allow instantaneous recognition of blood. The interposition of flexible tubing between the needle and the syringe allows manipulation of the syringe (refilling, etc.) without movement of the needle

is not desirable or necessary for the anticipated procedure, firm digital pressure applied just above the needle during the injection into the interscalene space prevents unnecessary cephaled spread of the anesthetic solution and promotes caudad spread, facilitating blockade of the elusive ulnar fibers in the inferior trunk.

Other factors which quite obviously alter volume-anesthesia relationships are height, age, and sex. The basic volume-anesthesia relationships described earlier are the result of studies done on healthy adult males. Our experience has shown height to be the single most important factor in determining the correct volume for either sex and at any age. This is not surprising, since it is well known that the distance from finger tip to finger tip closely approximates height. It follows then that the height should be related to the length of the "sheath" of the brachial plexus. Thus, half the height (in inches) indicates approximately the proper volume of anesthetic in an adult. The calculated volume naturally must be increased or decreased if high or low anesthesia is desired, and the concentration should be decreased somewhat in patients of poor physical status or in infants and children [14]. This rule of thumb is only a rough guide. No rule replaces the clinical judgement obtained through experience.

In the final analysis, success with any nerve block and most certainly with the perivascular techniques, depends on the precise placement and stabilization of the needle during the injection. Movement may dislodge the tip of the needle from the desired fascial plane and result in incomplete anesthesia. We developed a simple and inexpensive technique which allows complete immobilization of the needle throughout the entire performance of all nerve blocks. A small-bore disposable intravenous extension tubing is interposed between the needle and the syringe containing the anesthetic solution [15]. After the entire system has been filled with anesthetic solution, the extension tubing is clamped off and the needle is properly placed for the desired nerve-block procedure. Upon obtaining a paresthesia or after entering the proper fascial plane, the tubing is unclamped and aspiration is accomplished by an assistant (or with the anesthetist's free hand) without movement of the needle, after which the anesthetic is then injected (Fig. 17). If the syringe must be refilled and reattached, this may be done without moving the needle because of the flexibility of the extension tubing. If care is not taken to fill the extension tubing completely with anesthetic agent, several milliliters of air may be injected during performance of the block. This is not serious, but if the subclavian perivascular or interscalene techniques have been used, the presence of this subcutaneous air may lead to the mistaken impression that a pneumothorax has been produced.

This "immobile needle" has been used in thousands of nerve blocks and has unquestionably enabled us to avoid many failures or partial blocks, particularly in cases where removal of the syringe proves to be mechanically difficult or awkward.

Discussion and Conclusions

While single-injection techniques have overcome most of the objections to regional anesthesia, an equally important factor making plexus anesthesia acceptable is the advances which have been made in the area of local anesthetics. Given a group of local anesthetic agents which are capable of providing adequate anesthesia, the limiting factor has frequently been duration of action at both ends of the spectrum. Anesthetic agents are now available that are capable of providing good surgical anesthesia from about 20 min to 12 h, depending upon the concentration, addition of vasoconstrictors, and site of injection. Thus, if the anesthetist wishes to provide anesthesia for 20 min, he may choose chloroprocaine or procaine; for a 1- to 1.5 h procedure, he may choose lidocaine; for procedures lasting 2 to 2.5 h, he may choose mepivacaine; and for procedures lasting 4 to 6 h, he may add tetracaine to mepivacaine or lidocaine, with or without epinephrine. If the anesthesia and analgesia must persist for 8 to 12 h, the anesthetist may use bupivacaine. With such a wide variety of available agents, regional anesthesia is equally appropriate for outpatient surgery, where one wishes the anesthesia to be terminated rapidly upon completion of the surgical procedure, or in the hospitalized patient, where it is desirable for anesthesia to persist well into the postoperative period.

In summary, the usefulness of regional anesthesia has been extended tremendously by the recent development of single-injection techniques of brachial plexus block. These techniques enhance the efficacy as well as the safety of conduction anesthesia. The concomitant introduction of newer local anesthetic agents of varying durations of action has likewise added a new dimension to this form of anesthesia. It is hoped that these newer techniques of regional anesthesia and the availability of these newer agents will allow the anesthetist and surgeon to make this form of anesthesia available to the patient undergoing surgery on the extremities.

References

1. Accardo NJ, Adriani J (1949) Brachial plexus block: a simplified technic using the axillary route. South Med J 42:920
2. de Jong RH (1961) Axillary block of the brachial plexus. Anesthesiology 22:215
3. de Jong RH, Heavner JE (1971) Diazepam prevents local anesthetic seizures. Anesthesiology 34:523
4. de Jong RH, Wagman IH, Prince DA (1967) Effect of carbon dioxide on the cortical seizure threshold to lidocaine. Exp Neurol 17:221
5. Eriksson E (ed) (1969) Illustrated handbook of local anesthesia. Year Book Medical Publishers, Chicago, p 75
6. Eriksson E, Skarby HG (1962) A simplified method of axillary block. Nord Med 68:1325
7. Kumar A, Battit GE, Froese AB et al. (1971) Bilateral cervical and thoracic epidural blockade complicating interscalene brachial plexus block. Anesthesiology 35:650
8. Labat G (1923) Regional anesthesia: its technic and clinical application. Saunders, Philadelphia
9. Moore DC (1971) Regional block. 9th edn. Thomas, Springfield
10. Moore DC (1969) Complications of regional anesthesia. In: Bonica JJ (ed) Regional anesthesia. Davis, Philadelphia, p 233
11. Pitkin GP (1953) Conduction anesthesia, 2nd ed. Lippincott, Philadelphia
12. Ross S, Scarborough CD (1973) Total spinal anesthesia following brachial plexus block. Anesthesiology 39:458
13. Winnie AP (1975) Regional anesthesia. Surg Clin North Am 54:861
14. Winnie AP (1970) Interscalene brachial plexus block. Anesth Analg 49:455
15. Winnie AP (1969) An "immobile needle" for nerve blocks. Anesthesiology 31:577
16. Winnie AP, Collins VJ (1964) The subclavian perivascular technic of brachial plexus anesthesia. Anesthesiology 25:353
17. Winnie AP, Radonjic R, Akkineni SR, Durrani Z (1979) Factors influencing distrubution of local anesthetic injected into the brachial plexus sheath. Anesth Analg 58:225

Axillary Plexus Block – A Continuous Technique

T. Vester-Andersen

The concept of the neurovascular sheath is the basis of the axillary brachial plexus block and the main principle of the axillary technique is injection within the neurovascular sheath. This relies on the assumption that an injection within the sheath is followed by a free spread of anaesthetic solution which causes neural blockade of all the nerves within the sheath. The position of the needle point, the exact site of injection, is less important as long as the injection is made inside the sheath. Continuous block with an indwelling catheter is therefore quite a logical extension of the perivascular axillary block technique. Axillary plexus block with a catheter has been proposed by several investigators. Selander [1] from Gothenburg described in 1977 a simple and reliable technique with a Venflon catheter.

Successful insertion of a catheter into the neurovascular sheath requires attention to some technical details: (1) The patient has to be in supine position with the arm in "salute" or "sunbathing" position, the crucial point being the location of the axillary artery. (2) Intradermal infiltration followed by skin prick with a wide-Bore needle ensures a distinct sensation ("click") when the needle stylet and catheter perforate the neurovascular sheath. (3) Injection through a well placed catheter offers no resistance against injection and results in a characteristic swelling round the artery extending towards the axilla. (4) Detaching the syringe from the catheter will in most cases produce a slow back-drip of anaesthetic solution from the catheter.

Area of Blockade and Success Rate in Axillary Plexus Block

Reports concerning the success rate vary significantly. The term "success rate" seems to be most personal and quite incomparable as far as success is related to the possibility of performing the intended surgery and not to the completeness of neural blockade. Numerous reports deal with success rate related to different kinds of surgery and they range between 65% and 95%. Only Hollmén [3] and Selander [1] have based success rate on extent of neural blockade and both found high frequency of incomplete blocks.

A primary study [2] with 100 patients was performed to elucidate further the problem of incomplete blocks. The same catheter technique was used in all cases and regardless of weight, height, and age, all patients were given 40 ml 1% mepivacaine (Carbocain) with adrenaline. Surgical analgesia (Fig. 1), tested by pin prick, was obtained within all cutaneous

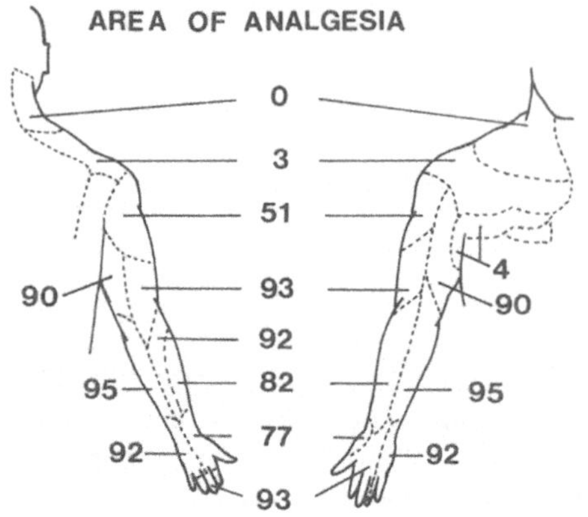

Fig. 1. Areas of analgesia in 100 perivascular axillary blocks with 40 ml 1% mepivacaine with adrenaline. Numbers indicate success rate (%) for each cutaneous nerve

nerves of the upper extremity in more than 90%, except from the lateral cutaneous nerve of the forearm (82%) and the radial nerve (77%).

Incomplete blocks, that means blocks with missing analgesia in one or several dermatomes, were found in 39%. In order to explain this high incidence of incomplete blocks, a detailed analysis of the results was undertaken. Neither variables concerning the patients' age, height, and weight nor minor variables in technique, such as paresthesias, puncture of blood vessel, cranial or caudal position of the catheter, could explain why some blocks were incomplete.

Dose of Local Anesthetic and Blockade

What can be done against the high frequency of incomplete blocks? In the course of time, several technical sophistications have been introduced but most of them with little effect. One of the most persistent, proposed by E. Eriksson, was to place a tourniquet round the upper arm to prevent a distal spread of anesthetic solution, but unfortunately this procedure did not prevent incomplete blocks.

In several ways, the perivascular brachial plexus block resembles the epidural block. The spread of anesthetic solution within the space (epidural or perivascular) determines the blockade. Nearly 20 years ago, Winnie [4] suggested that the area of analgesia depended on the dose of local anesthetic. The injected dose of local anesthetic may be increased in two ways: (1) By an increase of volume (ml) and (2) by an increase of amount (mg).

For the purpose of investigating the dose relationship we made two studies. In the first study [5], 150 patients participated. They were all given the same amount of local anesthetic (400 mg mepivacaine with adrenaline), but in different volumes. Group I received 20 ml, group II 40 ml, and group III 80 ml. In the second study [6], 90 patients participated. They

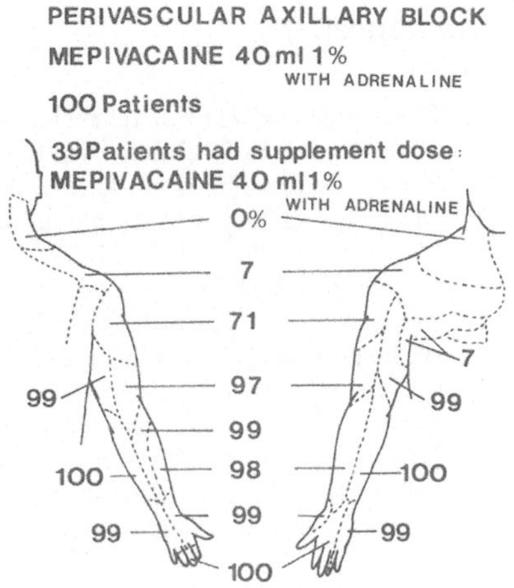

PERIVASCULAR AXILLARY BLOCK
MEPIVACAINE 40 ml 1% WITH ADRENALINE
100 Patients
39 Patients had supplement dose: MEPIVACAINE 40 ml 1% WITH ADRENALINE

Fig. 2. Areas of analgesia in 100 perivascular axillary blocks with 40 ml 1% mepivacaine with adrenaline. Thirty-nine patients had a supplementary dose of 40 ml 1% mepivacaine with adrenaline. Numbers indicate success rate (%) for each cutaneous nerve

were all given the same volume of local anesthetic (40 ml mepivacaine with adrenaline), but with different amounts (mg). Group I received 200 mg, group II 400 mg, and group III 600 mg.

The results of the two investigations showed: (1) increase of injected volume extends the upper area of analgesia and (2) increase of injected amount intensifies the motor blockade. However, neither an increase of volume nor an increase of amount solved the problems involved in the cutaneous area of the radial nerve and the lateral cutaneous nerve of the forearm. Further investigations will have to be made before the optimum dose, for clinical use, is determined.

Incomplete Blocks

Although the frequency of incomplete blocks may be reduced, there is little evidence of total prevention. Dealing with axillary brachial plexus blocks, one has to cope with cases of incomplete blocks. Intravenous supplement or peripheral nerve blocks are generally used in such cases. Reblocks in the axillary region seem less attractive unless a catheter technique is used. The possible benefit of giving a supplementary dose was investigated in our primary study [7]. All patients in the primary study who turned out to have an incomplete sensory blockade were given a supplementary dose of 40 ml 1% mepivacaine with adrenaline. Both the sensory block (Fig. 2) and the motor block were thus intensified during the next 10–15 min, resulting in a success rate of more than 95% in all segmental nerves of the upper extremity, including the radial and the lateral cutaneous nerve of the forearm [7].

The perivascular-axillary-catheter technique may naturally be used to prolong the blockade in surgery lasting a long time, but the possibility of improving an incomplete sensory block is of even greater clinical importance and can be seen as an obvious advance in axillary-block technique.

References

1. Selander D (1977) Catheter technique in axillary plexus block. Acta Anaesthesiol Scand 21:324
2. Vester-Andersen T, Christiansen C, Sørensen M, Eriksen C (to be published) Perivascular axillary block I: an analysis of blockade following 40 ml 1% mepivacaine with adrenaline
3. Hollmén A (1966) Axillary plexus block. Acta Anaesthesiol Scand [Suppl] XXI:53
4. Winnie AP, Collins VJ (1964) The subclavian perivascular technique of brachial plexus anesthesia. Anesthesiology 25:353
5. Vester-Andersen T, Christiansen C, Sørensen M, Kålund-Jørgensen HO, Saugbjerg P, Schultz-Møller K (to be published) Perivascular axillary block II: influence of volume of local anaesthetics on blockade
6. Vester-Andersen T, Christiansen C, Eriksen C (to be published) Perivascular axillary block III: influence of amount of local anaesthetics on blockade
7. Vester-Andersen T, Christiansen C, Sørensen M, Kålund-Jørgensen HO, Saugbjerg P, Schultz-Møller K, Eriksen C (to be published) Perivascular axillary block IV: effect of supplementary dose of local anaesthetics on incomplete blocks

Discussion: Plexus Block Techniques

Zindler:
I would like some practical advice for the beginner. What would you consider the easiest approach with the highest success rate for a brachial plexus block?

Winnie:
The easiest technique, at least in our department, is the interscalene plexus block. Interscalene plexus block is the regional anesthetic method of choice for surgery from the elbow up, including surgery of the upper arm and the shoulder. Unless the other techniques are contraindicated, this is not the ideal technique for, let us say, hand surgery, particularly if the hand surgery is in the ulnar region. Not that it can't be done under interscalene block, but it is more appropriately done with a different technique. So we have trouble weaning our residents away from interscalene block because of this sense of security, although I think that it is the easiest of the three approaches to the plexus. This does not mean that it is also the best in every case and this approach should be used exclusively, just as I don't say a caudal is better than a lumbar epidural anesthetic. Each technique has its place, its advantages, and its disadvantages. One of the advantages of interscalene plexus block is its simplicity.

Bergmann:
Prof. Zindler hat geradezu dazu herausgefordert, das faszinierende Konzept von Herrn Winnie, das er uns dargestellt hat, mit kaudaler, lumbaler und thorakaler Epiduralanaesthesie und axillärem, supraklavikulärem und interskalinärem Plexusblock zu vergleichen.

Richard:
In the standard text books on regional anesthesia, it is stated that a single-needle technique for the lower extremity does not exist. If you think of a perifascial space around the lumbar sacral plexus, shouldn't a single-needle block be possible?

Winnie:
Surely you have read our article entitled "The perivascular technique of lumbar plexus block," in which the same concept is utilized. One finds the space in surrounding this case, the fem-

oral nerve and uses that fascia compartment to force the solution up the sheath to block the entire lumbar plexus. If one turns the patient on his side and places the needle paravertebrally between the musculi quadrates lumborum and the musculus psoas major an injection of 30–40 ml local anesthetic will not only block the lumbar plexus, but also the sacral plexus. So it is possible to extend the intrafascial concept to block the lower extremity.

Lanz:
Dr. Winnie, you convincingly demonstrated the existence of the fascial sheath around the brachial plexus. Dr. Vester-Andersen showed with a dose of 40 ml of local anesthetic a very high rate of blocking the ulnar, the median nerves, indicating that he had the needle tip within this sheath. However, even with the very high volume of 80 ml of a local anesthetic solution he could not block the radial and musculocutaneous nerves. How do you explain this? Are there leaks in the sheath or are there septa? What are the reasons that he had this failure?

Winnie:
I think that one of the differences, other than the fact Dr. Vester-Andersen is using a catheter and I am not, is the level at which the tip of the needle or the catheter is placed. Dr. Vester-Andersen informed us carefully that after penetration of the sheath he advanced the needle opening up the sheath with a fluid load. I believe that a major difference between Dr. Andersen's and our technique mainly exists in that point that the tip of the needle in Dr. Vester-Andersen's technique is lower in the sheath than in our approach. I am saying this because, if you look at a series of cross sections of the sheath and its contents, it is easy to see why the radial nerve can be missed. The radial nerve is in the posterior portion of the sheath and any little tissue, fat, septa, etc., which are found in the sheath might hinder the spread around the sheath to block the radial nerve. However, higher up in the sheath we are not really blocking the radial nerve, we are blocking cords. I think for this reason we should not be blamed for the elusiveness of the radial nerve. We have not looked at the tip of each other's needles after they have been in position. If you position a needle high in the axilla and inject 60 not 80 ml local anesthetic solution, it is reproducibly possible to block the cervical plexus in addition to the brachial plexus.

Zinganell:
How do you identify the perivascular space within the sheath?

You mentioned that you are searching for paresthesias using the interscalene and the supraclavicular approach. But are you searching for paresthesias also at the axillary level?

Winnie:
At the axillary level we don't search for paresthesias. We only utilize the click of the needle entering the fascial compartment. We don't seek paresthesias of peripheral nerves.

Zinganell:
Do you try to enter the axillary artery?

Winnie:
No. We are trying to utilize the click of the sheath as an indication that we are in the compartment. However, Dr. Selander showed us that, even when we are trying to avoid paresthesias, we will obtain them in 40% of the cases. Furthermore, while I am deliberately trying

not to hit the artery, if I hit it, I quickly penetrate the posterior wall and inject my local anesthetic transarterially.

Zinganell:
We are all familiar with the sign of loss of resistance when doing an epidural anesthesia. The sheath around the axillary nerve and vascular compartment is not as firm as the ligamentum flavum. Is the loss of resistance so typical that I can be sure that I have entered the sheath?

Vester-Andersen:
We do not use a loss of resistance technique. We just perforate the sheath in the same manner as Dr. Winnie and many others are doing. But I want to stress that you should make a prestick or prepuncture perforation with a White needle, so that you really have a clear sensation when you perforate the sheath. The first resistance you encounter is the fascia sheath. I would recommend this technique if you want to introduce a catheter. You should have a free path through the skin, the subcutaneous tissues, and then you will have a clear perforation even with a catheter or a stylet. Do not use loss of resistance. If you have perforated you don't feel any resistance during injection and as long as you don't have any change in resistance you can be sure that you stay inside the sheath.

Lanz:
Your anatomic drawings showed the sheath as very long and slender around the brachial plexus, especially in the axillary area. Your X-rays, however, showed a much wider spread, they were not so slender and elongated. Are you losing a lot of local anesthetic out of the sheath?

Winnie:
If you make an injection using radiopaque renographin and you take serial X-rays after injection of 10, 20, 30, and 40 ml, you do indeed see the sheath getting fatter and fatter, just as Dr. Andersen pointed out from his clinical studies. He showed that he was distending the perivascular sheath as he injected the local anesthetic. I would like to emphasize that the hydrodynamics of your injection is a factor only for the first minute or so. If you take X-rays at that stage, you have a very discrete column of dye. If you take X-rays 15–20 min later, you do indeed have a very broad, heavy looking picture of the dye and I am sure the local anesthetic diffuses out of the sheath. So I think that the sheath only plays an important role early in the injection or shortly after the injection in keeping the solution in the area where you want it, getting into the nerves. But then, after that has taken place, I am sure it diffuses through that fascial compartment.

Vester-Andersen:
We have to accept the neurovascular fascial sheath as a rigid tubula structure which is quite firm and looks like your very nice picture in all cases. This is a very different structure and I think there might be some cases, where there is a resistance to this spread of local anesthetic solution even with high volumes. I think it is an anatomical problem.

Winnie:
I didn't mean to imply, nor did my artist, that the vascular sheath is a rigid pipelike structure. Fascia is what is left when everything has been formed. We are utilizing this fascia as a

sheath for the axillary block. The fascia of the surrounding muscles is clearly not a circumferential organization of collagen or anything else. This is a fascia around muscles and there certainly can be, in some cases, dissections away from the axial parts of the structure between any two muscles. All we have said is that the fascia compartment for the most part tends to control the flow pattern of the injected solution. But there clearly is something that we are doing differently, because we can't reproduce with 65 ml of local anesthetic the lowest cervical plexus. I thought from the picture you showed that the catheter was introduced somewhat distally, but obviously it is threaded up.

Ratlitsch:
How long did you have the Venlon needle in situ when doing a continuous axillary block? How often have you done reinjections and have you seen the development of tachyphylaxis in any cases?

Vester-Andersen:
We use this technique as routine even in short operations because we use it to repair incomplete blocks. We do use it for long-term operations, such as microvascular surgery and hand reconstruction. Some of these cases last for 6–10 hours. The continuous axillary blocks are used in our department for postoperative pain relief for a period of 1 or 2 days. We usually use it for wounddressing the day after the operation. I have never seen tachyphylaxis, but we have only done a very few cases and we never were much concerned about it.

Winnie:
We have used a lot of continuous perivascular subclavian blocks, where we left the catheter in for a week, predominantly in patients who have received reimplanted digits and hands. In these cases, we have never seen a development of tachyphylaxis.

Ratlitsch:
If you give the second dose because the effect of the first dose was unsatisfactory, do you replace the needle or do you just inject?

Vester-Andersen:
We just use the catheter as it is. We don't move the catheter. Our basis is that, if the catheter is within the neurovascular sheath, that is sufficient.

Lorenz:
You inject 40 ml of local anesthetic for supplementation of an uncomplete block. Have you made estimations of serum concentrations of your local anesthetics and are you still within the safety margin?

Vester-Andersen:
Before we really allowed ourselves to make a full supplementation of 40 ml, we were much concerned about what would be the risk of intoxication. We measured the plasma concentration after reblocking at 20, 30, and 40 minutes and found that the plasma concentrations were within or below the concentrations which are toxic, independent of whether you inject your supplementary dose at 20, 30, or 40 minutes.

Ratlitsch:
How do you supplement an interscalene block if the surgical procedure is extended?

Winnie:
A simple interscalenus block is more than adequate alone for any procedure, which you do on a shoulder that is closed. As one makes an incision and extends the operation farther and farther from the actual point of the shoulder, then one involves more and more dermatomes. Dr. Ballas in the United States published 300 consecutive open-shoulder operations done under interscalenus block. It was his practice and it has been ours in far fewer cases to utilize a paravertebral block of T_2 and T_3 along with the interscalenus block in much the same way as surgeons long ago used to block T_2–T_3, together with an axillary block, to do radical mastectomy. If you have a patient in whom you can administer high volumes and, as a result, a high mg dose, which alluded to in the axillary paper, you can push this solution medial enough to get your upper thoracic dermatomes as well. But in many cases you don't want to go over 40–50 ml, so this would be a problem and you would have to use a separate paravertebral block. If you inject locally in the axilla, you only block the area distal to the point of injection.

Techniques and Indications of Thoracic Epidural Analgesia

H. J. Wüst

Excellent analgesia during and after upper abdominal surgery can be obtained by a segmental epidural blockade which includes the dermatomes T5 and L3. To achieve this segmental spread with a minimal amount of local anaesthetic for both intra- und postoperative use, the placement of an epidural catheter at the midpoint of the nerve supply to the abdominal wall in the thoracic region is essential [3–5]. Many anaesthetists, however, fear damage to the spinal cord when using the thoracic approach and they prefer therefore to make their injections into the lumbar epidural space below the level of termination of the spinal cord. The experience that over 4,500 epidural anaesthetisations were performed safely in the midthoracic region at the Anaesthesia Department of the University of Düsseldorf lends support to the opinion of Dawkins et al. [4], that this notion has been exaggerated, and anaesthetists could be advised to overcome their reluctance to use a midthoracic approach to the epidural space.

Such a change in attitude is only possible once residents are trained to use an epidural needle at any segmental level of the vertebral column. Before attempting this above the L_{2-3} level, however, the beginner should have successfully performed and managed skilfully at least 100 lumbar epidural anaesthetic injections. Once this degree of proficiency has been attained, the beginner is in a position to undertake further training in the techniques and management of epidural anaesthesia at higher segmental levels. To achieve this aim without danger to the patients, epidural anaesthesia should be a commonly used anaesthetic technique in an institution where, in order to assume the adequate training of residents, the minimum percentage of regional anaesthesia should not be less than 20% to 25% of all anaesthetisations performed.

Management of Epidural Anaesthesia for Surgery

Administrative Considerations

An efficient operating list should be run like clockwork with not more than 5 to 10 minutes elapsing between the end of one case and the start of the next. Regional anaesthesia should not interfere with the time schedule since the administration of regional anaesthetic should not require more than 20 to 30 min and even for the more experienced, it should be possible for each case to be started well in advance. In this way delays are avoided and even the beginner can undertake the necessary preparations carefully and without unnecessary haste. The

Table 1. Contraindications for epidural anaesthesia

Local infection, septicemia		
Coagulopathies, spontaneous or induced	Quick	< 50%
	PTT	> 1 min
	Thrombocytes/ml	< 100,000
Neurological diseases	Poliomyelitis, acute radiculitis	
	Meningitis	

next patient should be sent for in good time and the block should be administered before the preceding case is finished and the patient has left the room. A properly qualified anaesthetic nurse should be available to monitor the termination of the operation while the next case is being started. A rapid turnover is facilitated by the availability of an induction room. In order to simplify the technical aspect of epidural anaesthesia a disposable kit containing needles, catheter and drugs necessary in puncturing the epidural space has been developed according to our needs by Braun Melsungen. This kit has been in use for 2 years.

Preparation of the Patients

A careful review of the history and physical status of the patient should be made to determine whether there are any contraindications to epidural blockade (Table 1). Epidural infections is rare and usually arise from an infection elsewhere in the body. Patients treated with full doses of heparin (20,000–30,000 IU/day), salicylic acid (2–3 g/day) or other agents inducing coagulation must not be given epidural blockade. A subcutaneous minidose of heparin not exceeding 10,000 IU/day does not exclude the use of epidural anaesthesia provided the activated thromboplastine time is not prolonged beyond 60 s (Table 1). Intravenous anticoagulation with 50–100 IU/kg heparin started after insertion of an epidural catheter seems – from our own experience as well as that of other institutions – to be not incompatible with continuous anaesthesia [9, 10, 13, 17, 19]. A close check of the neurological state of these patients during the postoperative period is essential so that the first symptoms of an epidural hematoma are not overlooked.

Premedication

Premedication with 0.5 mg/kg pethidine, 0.5 mg/kg promethazine (Atosil) and 0.5 mg/kg atropine is preferred in this institution. Extensive premedication may be required for the very anxious patient, although wide experience of epidural puncture in this institution as well as personal experience as a patient leads me to support the view that there is very little need for heavy sedation during induction of an epidural blockade. When properly managed induction should be painless except for the slight discomfort of the initial intradermal injection. It cannot be repeated too often that the best premedication is sound emotional support. Heavy sedation is usually avoided provided the anaesthesiologist can win the patient's confidence by skilful and sympathetic handling beforehand. A simple explanation before the operation about the subjective sensation that the patient will experience during induction and afterwards in the recovery room can overcome the fear of a "needle in the back". Special emphasis should be placed on the advantages of early and painfree restoration of function. Patients with underlying pulmonary disease, should be given a special explanation of the respiratory benefits of postoperative epidural analgesia. Effective psychological preparation and good rapport are the most valuable forms of preoperative support in our patients.

Preparation for the Puncture

Before epidural puncture is started, one has to make sure that oxygen can be given by mask. For treatment of complications such as hypotension, convulsions due to inadvertent intravascular injections and total spinal anaesthesia, 1 ampul Akrinor and 1 ampul atropine and diazepam should be prepared. The patient should be connected to the ECG and a safe intravenous infusion should be started; 500 to 1,000 ml Ringer's lactate should be rapidly infused. Blood pressure should be monitored. In this institution the lateral position is preferred for induction of epidural anaesthesia because it is more comfortable for the patient and postural hypotension is not seen. The patient is placed on the operating table in the lateral decubitus with the operative side dependent in order to obtain the benefit of gravity on the spread of analgesia. Often, however, this is not feasible in the traumatized patient because of pain and in this case one has to compromise by using whichever position permits access to the epidural space without discomfort for the patient.

Choice of Puncture Site

Two factors govern the puncture site: The skill of the anaesthesiologist and the segmental nerve supply of the operative site. Puncture should be as close as possible to the centre of the segmental distribution for the operative area, although this aim should be subordinated to the safety of the manoeuvre. As has been stressed before, the beginner should not attempt puncture above the level of the termination of the cord until he is proficient in the execution and management of epidural puncture in the lumbar region, as demonstrated by an acceptably low incidence of dural puncture of less than 2%. The landmark for puncture at the thoracic level is the scapular angle = Th 7/8.

In this institution the following procedure is used before puncture of the epidural space: The patient's back is cleaned mechanically with alcohol containing solutions such as Spitacid, Rapidosept, etc. and sprayed once with a disinfectant solution (Kodan, Braunoderm, etc.). The disinfectant solution should be allowed to work for 5 min. When making the puncture, the rules of strict asepsis should be maintained. The physician is prepared as for surgery. After having prepared the disposable tray by drawing up saline and local anaesthetic through a filter which retains any glass particles from the ampoules, the patient's back is dressed with sterile drapes. The landmarks – the lower angle of the scapula – are shown by a nurse. During epidural puncture, the tip of the Tuohy needle and the epidural canula, which are introduced into the patient, should not be touched. Syringes and canulae should not be put down on the drape in front of the patient and the tip of the catheter should not be allowed to fall on the drape.

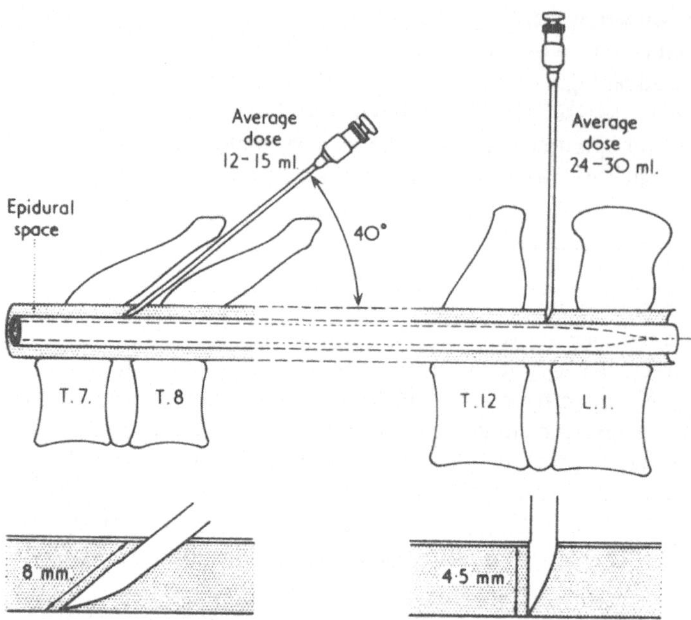

Fig. 1. Schematic drawing of the anatomy of the epidural space at the thoracic and lumbar level. In the thoracic region the vertebral spines and lamina show steep angulation and an overlap making an angle for puncture of 40° necessary. In the upper lumbar region the puncture is made at an angle of 90° in relation to the spinal cord [4]

Median and Paramedian Approach to the Epidural Space

The epidural space can be reached by two approaches, the median and the paramedian approach (Figs. 1, 2).

Median Approach

After having chosen the level of the puncture site, the second and third fingers of the palpating hand – in right handed, the left and in left handed, the right – are used to fix the skin and obtain information as to the cranial and caudal positions of the spinal processes and the lateral extension to the right and left (Fig. 3). Without changing the position of the palpating hand, an intradermal injection of local anaesthetic is made between the second and third finger (Fig. 4). Following this local anaesthetic is infiltrated along a track through which the epidural needle will be passed.

When using the median approach, a Tuohy needle is introduced at an angle of 90° to the skin, the needle being held in the right hand while the left hand fixes the skin. The needle is advanced 2 to 3 cm until bone contact is made. Then the direction of the needle is changed (the angle between the skin the needle is about 30 to 45°) and the needle is advanced further until it is fixed in the ligamentum flavum. Then the stylet of the needle is withdrawn and a freely moving syringe – glass or plastic – containing saline and a little air bubble is connected

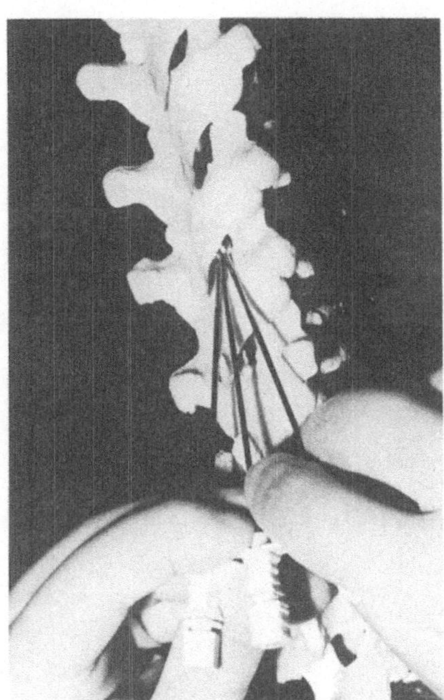

Fig. 2. Direction of the Tuohy needle in the median and paramedian approach to the epidural space

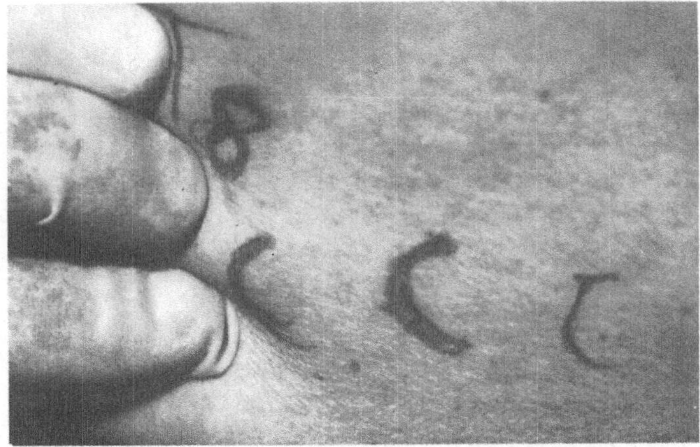

Fig. 3. Fixation of the skin at the puncture site with the left hand in median approach

to the needle. The opening of the Tuohy needle should be turned craniad by rotating the needle.

Paramedian Approach

In the paramedian approach one should obtain similar information relating to the spinal processes as in the median approach. While one finger of the palpating hand is identifying

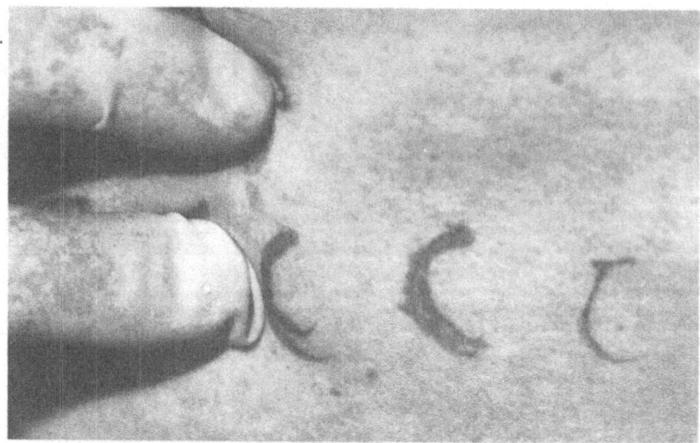

Fig. 4. Fixation of the skin in the paramedian approach

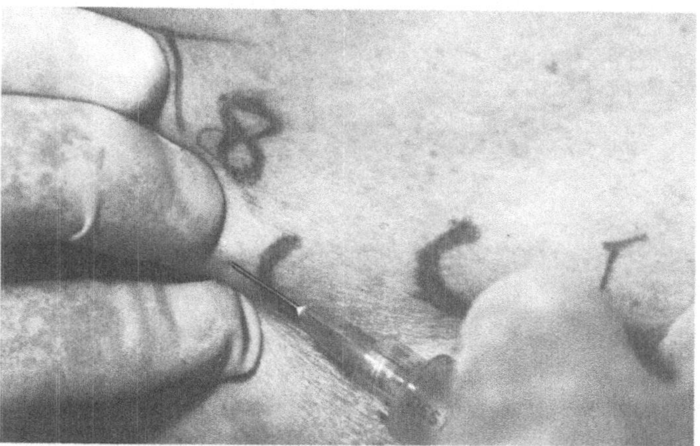

Fig. 5. Intradermic wheel

the interval between the upper and lower spinal processes, the other finger is fixing the skin 1 cm lateral to the spinal processes (Fig. 4). As in Fig. 5 an intracutaneous wheel is made and the suggested track of the puncture is infiltrated down to the lamina. The angle of the needle through which the local infiltration is made is changed until it is fixed in the ligamentum flavum. The needle is then withdrawn and, in our institution it is exchanged for a Tuohy needle, in others for a Crawford needle (Fig. 6). The epidural needle is then advanced from the paramedian or lateral position in a craniomedial direction until it is fixed in the ligamentum flavum.

The midline puncture is often very difficult in the midthoracic region owing to steep angulation and overlap of the vertrebral spines and laminae. The paramedian approach is therefore indicated in this area to avoid the overhang of the spine.

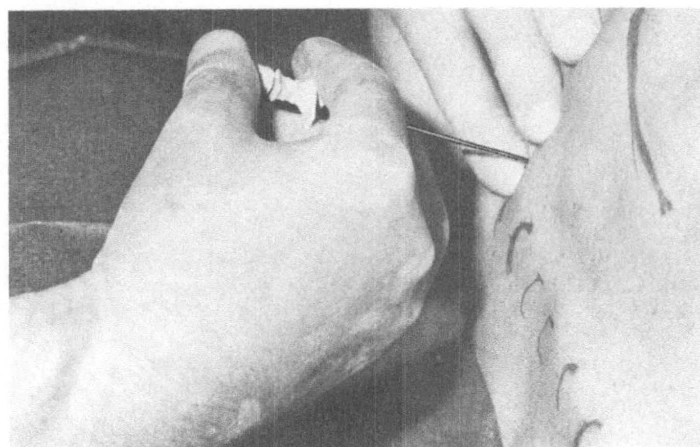

Fig. 6. Puncture of the skin

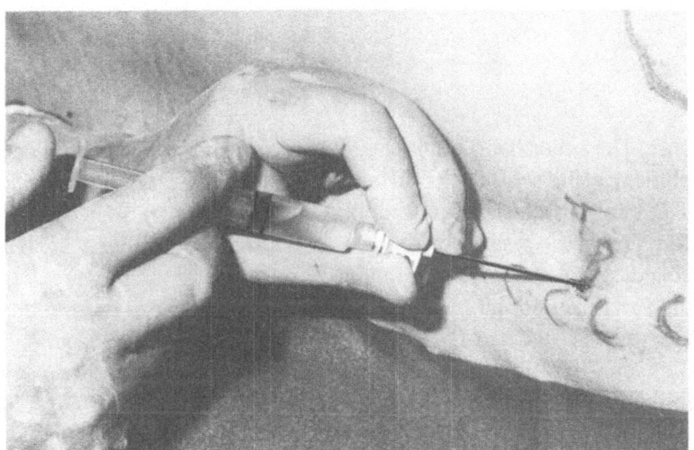

Fig. 7. The setting prior to advancing the needle into the epidural space

Identification of the Epidural Space

In this institution identification of the epidural space is achieved by use of the loss of resistance technique, using a plastic syringe filled with saline and an air bubble (Fig. 7). The needle is advanced further with the left hand (in the right handed) or with the right hand (in the left handed). This hand is supinated with the wrist partially flexed and the back of the carpus braced against the patient's back. When making midthoracic puncture we have found, as Fig. 7 shows, that bracing the ulnar side of the hand against the patient's back is more suitable. The puncture hand must be very steady to apply a gradual, controlled forward movement of the needle as well as an instantaneous braking force as soon as the epidural space is entered. The forward movement should be gradual and continuous, never intermit-

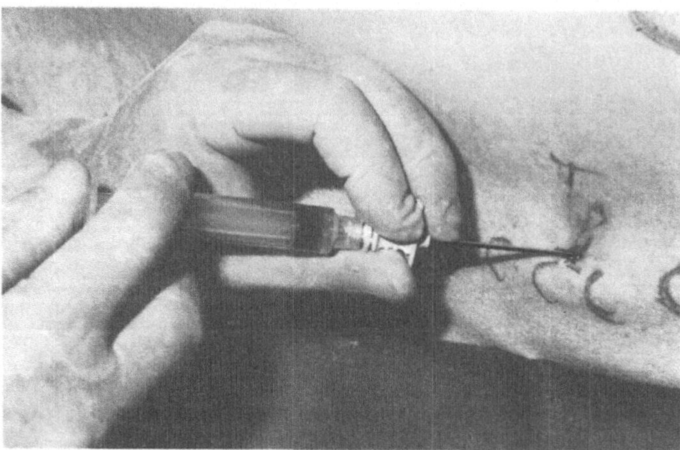

Fig. 8. The epidural space is identified and the saline can be injected very easily

tent. The other hand holds the syringe and the thumb exerts continuous pressure on the plunger while sensing the different resistances encountered during the advance of the needle. This hand is almost entirely concerned with supporting the syringe and interpreting the slight changes of the resistance to injection as the needle advances. When the epidural space is reached, sudden release from this resistance is indicated by free injection of saline (Fig. 8). During further injection of 2 to 3 ml saline, the needle is further advanced 0.5 to 1.0 mm so that the entire tip of the needle is within the epidural space.

Identification of the epidural space by the hanging drop sign of Gutierrez using different indicators for negative pressure in the epidural space such as a Mac Intosh balloon is also used. However, this method is not used in this institution.

Criteria for the Proper Position of the Tuohy Needle

It is unlikely that the dura has been perforated when: (1) no fluid returns, (2) no fluid can be aspirated, (3) if fluid does return, it drops very slowly, (4) the fluid is cold and (5) the glucotest is negative and the pH is lower than 7.5. If these signs are negative, one can be almost certain that the needle is in the epidural space.

Introducing the Epidural Catheter

The epidural catheter is wound around the thumb of the left hand, as shown in Fig. 9, and the free end of the catheter which is not introduced is fixed between the thumb and the second finger. The hub of the Tuohy needle is at the same time held between the thumb and the second finger. The right hand introduces the catheter held at a distance of 10 cm behind the tip of the catheter. In order to maintain strict asepsis, the free end of the tip of the cath-

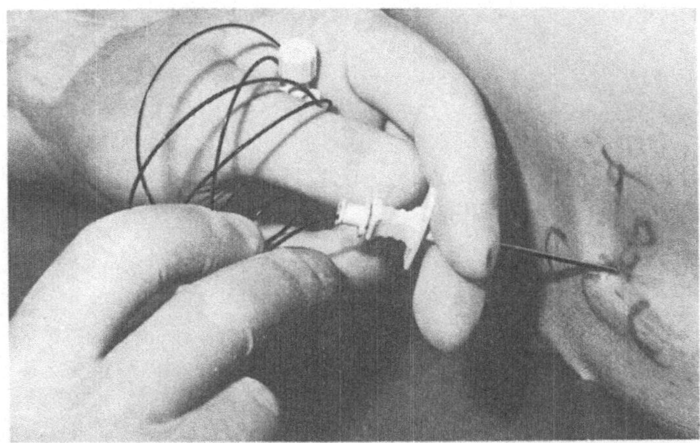

Fig. 9. The epidural catheter is threaded into the epidural space. Notice that the catheter is wound around the thumb and the end of the catheter is fixed between the thumb and the palm to avoid contamination of the catheter by its flailing around

eter should never touch the patient's skin, the physicians clothes or the drape in front of them. If there is any doubt, one should not hesitate to remove the Tuohy needle and the catheter and start again with a new tray. The catheter can be threaded easily because of a more tangential angle of puncture into the epidural space. It is advanced 5 cm so that the third mark on the catheter should have disappeared in the Tuohy needle. The end of the catheter should be observed so blood or liquor cerebrospinalis can easily be seen. The Tuohy needle should never be turned when the catheter is in place, and the catheter should never be withdrawn, because of the danger of shearing the catheter.

The length of catheter which is introduced into the epidural space can in older trays be measured with the aid of the stylet prior to and after removal of the Tuohy needle. Recently this procedure has been simplified by metric gradiations on the catheter. The Tuohy needle is removed slowly over the catheter, the hands being held in the same position as when the catheter was threaded (Fig. 10). The right hand which threaded the catheter, now hinders its withdrawal by holding it at a distance of 1 to 2 cm from the hub of the Tuohy needle while the left hand is removing the Tuohy needle. After removal of the needle the connector and bacterial filter is attached to the catheter. Once again the proper position of the catheter in the epidural space is checked by the aspiration test.

The puncture site is now dressed with sterile compresses from the disposable tray and fixed with fixomull. The drape is not removed from the patient's back before this stage. The catheter is fixed on the patient's back. Before injecting any local anaesthetic solution, it is important to ensure that no blood or cerebrospinal fluid can be aspirated. A negative test, however, does not exclude intravascular or intrathecal placement of the catheter. To exclude such aberrant placement, an injection of 5 ml solution of a local anaesthetic to which adrenaline (1 : 200,000) has been added should be given [8]. Intravascular injection of this solution will cause increased heart rate and blood pressure.

The small test volume of 3 to 5 ml local anaesthetic solution through the epidural catheter, followed by a waiting period of 5 min, should ensure that the injection has not been

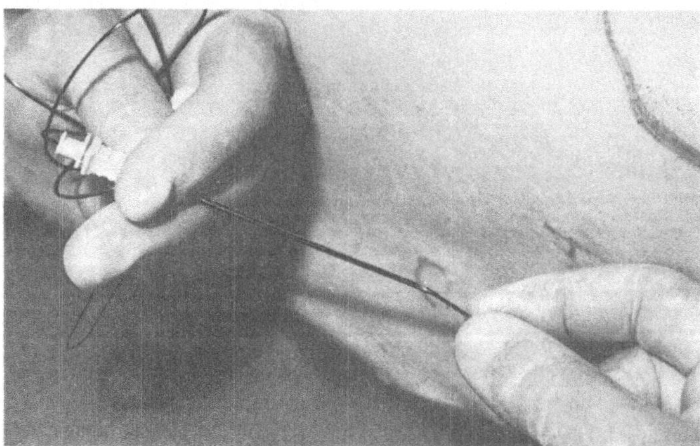

Fig. 10. The Tuohy needle is withdrawn without changing position of the hands

made into the subarachnoid space. However, inadvertent injection into the intrathecal space still occurs. In 6 out of 30,000 epidural blocks performed in this institution, the test dose indicated a negative result. In these patients a very rapid onset of intense motor and sensitive block with cranial spread occurred shortly after the administration of a therapeutic dose. The patients reported difficulty in breathing and the airway had to be quickly secured by intubation and the circulation supported by vasopressors. In none of these patients did cardiovascular or neurological sequelae occur.

Drugs and Dose

The drug of choice used for continuous epidural anaesthesia in this institution is 0.5% and 0.75% bupivacaine used in the postoperative period. Both solutions are used without added adrenaline.

Dose of Bupivacaine

In patients with arteriosclerotic disease and older patients the total dose of local anaesthetics injected for epidural anaesthesia has to be reduced by a third in comparison to healthy younger patients, to avoid an exaggerated spread of the epidural blockade [2]. In 506 patients with and without arteriosclerosis we tested the effect of injecting a total dose of 19 ml 0.5% bupivacaine on the extension of the block related to the puncture site. There were no differences in the extension of analgesia to pin prick in patients with and without arteriosclerosis and between patients who were younger or older when the injection was made in the midthoracic region (Fig. 11). However, when injection was made at L1/2, L2/3 or L3/4 the extension of analgesia was greater in patients who suffered from arteriosclerotic disease than in patients who were free of this disease. Considering the dose needed to block a segment, it was surprising to find that the same dose per segment was necessary at Th8/9 and at L4/5

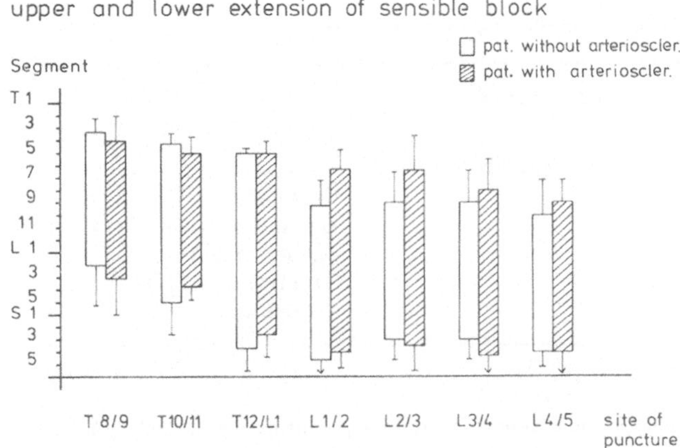

Fig. 11. Upper and lower extension of the sensible block achieved with 19 ml 0.5% bupivacaine. ▫ patients without arteriosclerosis; ▪ patients with arteriosclerosis

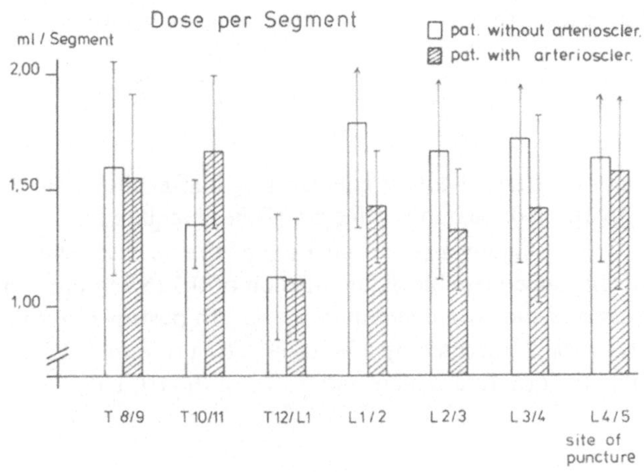

Fig. 12. Dose of 0.5% bupivacaine needed to block a segment in relation to the puncture site when local anaesthetic is injected at the Th8/9 and the L4/5 level. At both puncture sites 1.55 ml per segment is needed regardless of whether the patient suffers from an arteriosclerotic disease or not. When the thoracolumbar approach is used the dose per segment is reduced to 1.2 ml per segment. At the lumbar level smaller volumes are needed in patients with arteriosclerotic disease than in normal patients. ▫ Patients without arteriosclerosis; ▪ patients with arteriosclerosis

(Fig. 12). Again, at these puncture sites no difference was found in patients with and without arteriosclerosis. The dose needed to block a segment was significantly lower when the injection was made via a catheter threaded into the epidural space at the Th12/L1 level. When the same dose was injected at L1/2, L2/3 and L3/4 in patients with and without arteriosclerosis, less local anaesthetic was necessary to block a segment in patients with arteriosclerosis than in patients without arteriosclerosis (Fig. 12). In operations of long duration

Table 2. Combinations with epidural anaesthesia

Volatile anaesthetics	Halothane 0.2 vol% Ethrane 0.4 vol%
Intravenous anaesthetics	Diazepam Etomidate Fentanyl + dehydrobenzperidol Flunitrazepam Gamma-butyric acid Ketamine

Table 3. Indications for combining continuous thoracic epidural anaesthesia with light general anaesthesia

Site of surgery	Type of surgery
Thorax	Lung, mediastinum
Thoracoabdomen	Oesophagus
Upper abdomen	Liver, pancreas, intestine
	Abdominal aorta

half of the initial dose is injected $1\,^1/_2$ h after the initial dose is given. Further injections of 8 to 10 ml 0.5% bupivacaine are given as required.

Immediately after termination of the operation while the patient is still painfree from the intraoperative block, an infusion of 0.125% bupivacaine running at a drip rate of 6 ml/h is started and continued up to the fourth postoperative day. If periods of pain occur the analgesia is corrected by a bolus injection of 8 ml 0.125% or 0.25% bupivacaine. At the same time the drip rate is increased to 12 ml/h [10, 16].

Combination of Light General Anaesthesia with Continuous Thoracic Epidural Anaesthesia

In our institution thoracic epidural anaesthesia is only used in combination with a light general anaesthetic. Volatile and intravenous anaesthetics have been used to induce "social sleep" so that the patient can tolerate intubation and ventilation during the operation (Table 2). From our experience the use of diazepam injected intermittently every $^1/_2$ h at a dose of 2.5 to 5.0 mg or 0.4 vol.% ethrane can be recommended because of the stable cardiovascular function seen with these combinations [11, 12, 13, 14, 18]. Whether the patient should be ventilated or not depends on the situation during surgery. When a Rochar retractor is inserted and the movements of the diaphragm are restrained by the traction of the retractors, controlled ventilation is often indicated to avoid arterial hypoxemia and retention of CO_2.

Indications for Applying Light General and Continuous Thoracic Epidural Anaesthesia

It has been shown that continuous epidural anaesthesia has a beneficial effect, especially in patients with a high risk of complications in cardiovascular function [13] and respiration [1, 15], and of stress response due to surgery [6] and the incidence of deep vein thrombosis [7] during and after surgery. Based on these data we have extended the indications for this combination to include operations in the thorax and in the upper abdomen (Table 3).

Conclusion

Continuous thoracic epidural anaesthesia is, when skilfully managed, a better anaesthetic approach in high risk patients. But it must be stressed once again that the introduction of an epidural catheter at the thoracic level can only be done by a very experienced anaesthesiologist, with these a priori conditions, continuous thoracic epidural anaesthesia can be used for the benefit of patients, especially those with high risk factors.

References

1. Bromage PR (1955) Spirometry in assessment of analgesia after abdominal surgery. Br Med J 2:589
2. Bromage PR (1969) The physiology and pharmacology of epidural blockade. In: Bonica JJ (ed) Regional anesthesia chapt 3. Clin Anesth 2:45
3. Bromage PR (1978) Epidural analgesia. Saunders, Philadelphia
4. Dawkins CJM, Steel GC (1971) Thoracic extradural (epidural) block for upper abdominal surgery. Anaesthesia 26:41
5. Durrans SF (1947) High extradural segmental block. Anaesthesia 2:106
6. Kehlet H, Brandt MR (1980) Effects of neurogenic blockade on the endocrine-metabolic response to surgery. In: Wüst HJ, Zindler M (eds) Neue Aspekte der Regionalanaesthesie 1: Wirkung auf Herz, Kreislauf und Endokrinium. Postoperative Periduralanalgesie, vol 124, Anaesthesie und Wiederbelebung. Springer, Berlin Heidelberg New York, pp 112–118
7. Modig J, Hjelmstedt Å, Sahlstedt B, Maripuu E, Saldeen T (1981) The influence of epidural versus general anaesthesia on the incidence of thromboembolism after total hip replacement. In: Wüst HJ, Zindler M (eds) Neue Aspekte in der Regionalanaesthesie 2, vol 138, Anaesthesiology and intensive care medicine. Springer, Berlin Heidelberg New York, pp 121–127
8. Moore DC, Batru MS (1981) The components of an effective test dose prior to epidural block. Anesthesiology 55:693
9. Rao TLK, El-Etr AA (1981) Anticoagulation following placement of epidural and subarachnoid catheters: an evaluation of neurological sequelae. Anesthesiology 55:618
10. Siepmann HP, Wüst HJ, Liebau W (1980): Postoperative Periduralanaesthesie (Technik und Indikationen) In: Wüst HJ, Zindler M, (eds) Neue Aspekte in der Regionalanaesthesie 1, vol 124, Anaesthesiologie und Intensivmed. Springer, Berlin Heidelberg New York, pp 135–138
11. Wüst HJ, Florack G, Sandmann W, Lennartz H (1976) Kreislaufveränderungen während und nach aorto-femoralen Bypassoperationen (AFB) unter kontinuierlicher Epiduralanaesthesie. Langenbecks Arch Chir 342:594
12. Wüst HJ, Sandmann W, Spirgatis G (1978) Gamma-Hydroxybuttersäure als Adjuvans bei der kontinuierlichen thorakalen und lumbalen Epiduralanaesthesie. In: Frey R (ed) Neue Untersuchungen mit Gamma-Hydroxybuttersäure, vol 110, Anaesthesiology and intensive care medicine. Springer, Berlin Heidelberg New York, pp 123–130

13. Wüst HJ (1983) Der Einfluß des Anaesthesieverfahrens – NLA, Halothan und thorakale Epiduralanaesthesie – und der Operation auf die Herzkreislauffunktion während aorto-femoraler Bypass-Operationen. Med. Habilitationsschrift, Düsseldorf. Springer, Berlin Heidelberg New York
14. Wüst HJ, Florack G, Sandmann W, Richter O, Lemacher W (1980a) A comparison of cardiovascular effects of neurolept halothane or continuous thoracic epidural anaesthesia in patients undergoing an aortofemoral bypass operation. In: Wüst HJ, Zindler M (eds) Neue Aspekte in der Regionalanaesthesie 1, vol 124, Anaesthesiology and intensive care medicine. Springer, Berlin Heidelberg New York, p 12
15. Wüst HJ, Godehard E, Günther D, Sandmann W, Zumfelde L (1980) Modifying effects of anaesthesia on the postoperative pulmonary function in patients undergoing an aortofemoral bypass operation. In: Wüst HJ, Zindler M (eds) Neue Aspekte in der Regionalanaesthesie 1, vol 124, Anaesthesiology und Intensivmedizin. Springer, Berlin Heidelberg New York, pp 175–179
16. Wüst HJ, Liebau W, Richter O, Strasser K (1980c) Tachyphylaxie bei kontinuierlicher thorakaler Epiduralanalgesie mit Bupivacain 0,125% und 0,25%. Anaesthesiol Intensiv Notfallmed 15:159
17. Wüst HJ, Sandmann W, Richter O (1981) Regional anaesthesia pros and cons. In: Rügheimer E, Zindler M (eds) Anesthesiology. Excerpta Medica Int Congress Series, Amsterdam p 538
18. Wüst HJ, Sandmann W, Florack G (1981) Die Kreislaufwirkung von Diazepam, Etomidate und Gamma-hydroxy-Buttersäure während kontinuierlicher Epiduralanaesthesie in: Wüst HJ, Zindler M (eds) Neue Aspekte in der Regionalanaesthesie 2, vol 138, Anaesthesiology and intensive care medicine. Springer, Berlin Heidelberg New York, p 79
19. Wüst HJ (1983) Epiduralanaesthesie und Antikoagulantien, Swiss Med 6a:69

Technique of Lumbar Peridural Anesthesia

A. van Steenberge

Assuming a good technique peridural analgesia and anaesthesia result in a 96% success rate. Side effects are minimised and complications avoided.

Premedication

Children. No premedication is given before the age of 6 months. A dose of 200 μg morphine per kg or 7 μg flunitrazepam per kg body weight is injected intramuscularly 20 min before induction of the peridural anaesthesia just before leaving the ward.

Adults. The night before surgery the usual sedative is given. If surgery is scheduled for early in the morning no premedication is administrated in the ward. Only very anxious patients and those who are late on the programme receive a tranquillizer per os. Elderly and high risk patients (A.S.A. 3) are not given any drug but receive verbal support all the time.

Monitoring

Upon the arrival of the patient in the operating room an intravenous infusion is started. Monitoring of the electrocardiogram of the pulse and blood pressure is set up, either by cuff or by intra-arterial line. The arterial line is used in patients in a poor physical state (A.S.A. 3 or more) or if the surgical procedure requires this precaution. Other forms of monitoring may include a urinary catheter, a gastric tube and a central venous pressure line. The monitoring of the patient under peridural anaesthesia must be as strict as under general anaesthesia. The appropriate equipment and drugs as follows must be ready at any time: (a) an anesthetic apparatus (with the means of positive pressure ventilation), (b) a tested laryngoscope, intubation and suction material, and (c) resuscitative drugs.

Preoperative Sedation

The preoperative sedation in *adults* consists of an intravenous injection of Innovar 0.5 to 1.5 ml fentanyl (0.05 mg/ml) which gives total body analgesia. In long procedures the patient may become restless even with perfect peridural anaesthesia because of immobility, aching joints and the hard surface of the operating table. Droperidol (2.5 mg/ml) provides psychomotor indifference, a potent anti-emetic action and anti-cholinergic effects. Five to ten minutes later we add 0.2 to 0.4 mg flunitrazepam which, besides sedation, induces sleep and amnesia. The patient can be aroused at any time and recovery is immediate at the end of surgery. When upper abdominal surgery, prone positioning or any other ventilatory problem is to be expected, good ventilation is maintained by intubation under light general and good topical anaesthesia. Elderly and high risk patients are given reassurance by constant verbal support alone. Confusion and profound depression could be the price of pharmacological sedation. However, if needed, intubation is carried out under inhalation and topical anaesthesia.

In Children small amounts of flunitrazepam (0.1 mg IV) in addition to the premedication suffice in most instances for the performance of peridural anaesthesia. If not, an assistant can apply a mask for light inhalation anaesthesia. In order to establish good ventilation, planned intubation must be carried out before peridural anaesthesia. Naso-tracheal intubation is a secure method of unhindered ventilation. The administration of 1 to 2 mg/kg Ketalar IM ensures a 10 min period for a quiet peridural procedure.

Technique

Adults. The peridural technique must be performed with the patient in the lateral position with the operating side downwards. The lateral position is comfortable and prevents any excess hypotension. The knees are flexed against the abdomen with the chin against the sternum and head and neck supported by a pillow. The patient's back is in line with the edge of the table or bed. The operator sits in a relaxed position so that no muscular tension is present in his arms and shoulders. His eyes are on a level allowing him to judge the patient's position perfectly. There are no drapes, only a broad disinfected area so that the bony landmarks are visible. Tilting the table 15° with the patient's head down decongests the peridural venous plexuses and decreases the pressure of the cerebrospinal fluid on the dura mater. A nick in a vessel or in the dura mater during the insertion of the needle or the catheter is less likely.

It is important to enter the peridural space on the midline where the space is the widest – up to 9 mm in the lower lumbar area – and free from both vessels and nerve roots. As the conus medullaris terminates at the level of the 2nd lumbar vertebra, the 3rd lumbar interspace is the easiest to locate and the least dangerous to penetrate. A 23-gauge, 2.5 cm needle (the length of the needle is important to prevent piercing the dura mater while infiltrating) is used to infiltrate the skin and the ligaments with plain local anesthetic. A marked needle is introduced with a slight cephalad inclination to a depth of 3 cm, just below the spinous process of the 3rd lumbar vertebra. The marking on the needle facilitates accurate assesment of the depth of penetration. At a depth of 3 cm the dura mater is, in adults, free from puncture; in 92% of our adult patients, the peridural space lies between 3 and 5-cm. Withdrawing the stylet inclined cephalad, a smoothly running 10 ml syringe filled with saline (± 20 °C) and an air bubble is attached to the needle hub. In the loss-of-resistance technique, the advance is slow and constantly controlled, the left hand being braced securely against the patient's back and the thumb of the right hand exerting a constant pressing-releasing movement on the plunger. After entering the peridural space, a few milliliters of saline are injected. For a single-shot injection, the syringe is disconnected, any reflux checked, and, if none, the local anesthetic is slowly injected.

In the continuous peridural technique, the bevel is turned through 360° in four stages and at each stage, a few milliliters of saline are injected. If at any stage resistance to injection is encountered, the needle is cautiously advanced until resistance disappears. One ensures hereby that the bevel of the needle lies entirely beyond the ligamentum flavum. This maneuver facilitates the insertion of the Portex translucent catheter previously tested for permeability. The catheter is marked from 5 cm to 10 cm as well as at 15 cm and 20 cm. It has a blunt, closed end with lateral helically spaced holes at 7 mm, 11 mm, and 15 mm. The marked needle and catheter permit accurate measurement of the cannula in the peridural space. If resistance to the introduction of the catheter is still encountered, a 5-ml syringe filled with 2 to 3 ml air is attached to the needle and injected as a shot after aspiration. If it is still impossible to insert the catheter, the needle should be reinserted, noting the depth from the skin to the peridural space. With relocation of the bevel, the introduction of the catheter is almost always smooth, otherwise another lumbar space must be selected. The catheter is threaded up to 20 cm at the hub of the needle (± 11 cm inside the peridural space); when the needle is removed, the catheter is withdrawn to 4 cm inside the peridural space, while flushing and aspirating with small quantities of saline using a 5-ml syringe to ensure that no blood or cerebrospinal fluid flows back. When the catheter is introduced 4 cm into the peridural space, we inject and aspirate three times and if no blood or cerebrospinal fluid appears, we fix an antibacterial filter, preventing contamination and injection of particles of forein bodies (e.g., glass) The entry site is sealed with nobecutane and, to prevent Kinking, the catheter is taped through a slitted eye patch with a translucent operation site wound dressing (10 cm/14 cm). This membrane checks blood reflux and ensures that shoulder movements will not pull the catheter from the peridural space.

The reason for threading the catheter up to 20 cm and withdrawing it afterwards is to ensure that the part of the cannula left 4 cm within the peridural space lies on the midline. This provides an even bilateral spread of the local anesthetic agent. If on introduction, the cannula hurts a nerve, the needle must be withdrawn at once. Paresthesia indicates a too lateral location of the needle, which would result in an uneven spread of the local anesthetic. Both clear blood and a wet tap necessitate the selection of another peridural space. A pink fluid (blood with saline) requires repeated flushing with increments of saline over a 30-min period. Anesthetization of the lower extremities calls for a 20° Fowler position during the injection and at least 10 min thereafter, so that the large nerve roots (L5–S1) and the spinal cord at its greatest circumference should be blocked. The injection should be given over 2 min (timed by stopwatch) for 20 ml of a warmed (30 °C) local anesthetic agent.

Children

Both peridural and caudal blocks are very easy to perform in newborns, infants, and children. Caudal block requires a higher dosage per spinal segment than peridural block so that the latter appears to be safer as regards toxicity. The preferred space is the second or the third lumbar. For newborn babies and infants, one uses a Butterfly 21 gauge and, for children, a spinal needle gauge 22. A 3-ml Luer-lock glass syringe filled with air is attached to the tubing or the needle. The loss of resistance is very clear and the ligamentum flavum an unmistakable landmark. Age is a better indication of the required dose per segment than body weight (Table 1). The measurement given in Table 1 were provided by Drs. P. Busoni, M. Romiti, and T. Andreucetti and will be published. For the caudal technique, the dosage per segment is about 50% more than for the peridural technique. There is no drop in blood pressure during peridural anesthesia in children.

Table 1. Dose per spinal segment in children

Age (years)	2% Carbocaine (ml)	Dose (mg)
1	0.3	6
2	0.42	10
3	0.55	12
4	0.68	13.5
5	0.71	14
6	0.76	15
7	0.82	16
8	0.88	17
9	0.91	18
10	0.95	19

Peridural Side Effects

Two important characteristics are common in peridural anesthesia and must be considered as part of the technique.

Hypotension. In most patients (A.S.A. 1 and 2) a 20% drop in blood pressure is considered normal. Hypotension can not be prevented by giving an appropriate dose of the local anesthetic agent, since this would restrict the spread to the desired segments. The precise calculation of the dosage remains utopian in spite of the correct location of the catheter and the systematic computation of the exact dosage in relation to the height, weight, lenght of spinal column, and age of the patient. Thus, a rapid perfusion of 500 to 1,000 ml of a warmed Hartmann solution should be given with the patient's legs positioned for a good venous return and oxygen should be administered by mask or nasal catheter. If blood pressure needs to be corrected, 0.5 mg Dihydergotamine given intravenously is the drug of choice. This reduces the venous capacity to near its normal size and there are no effects on the arterial side or on the heart. Blood pressure rises slowly to normal, slightly reducing the heart frequency. This dosage can be repeated and, if pressure recovery is still insufficient, a rapid transfusion of human plasma proteins with a minium of 5% albumin must be used to correct hypovolemia.

Shivering. This must be prevented by warming the patient, the local anesthetic agent (30 °C), and the intravenous solutions (30 °C). If shivering persists, 5 to 10 mg methylphenidate IV will solve the problem.

Conclusion

Having been trained under close supervision, beginners should carefully select their first hundred patients with regard to the ease of performing the peridural block, avoiding any complicated surgical procedures. Once they have gained experience and their good results have convinced those involved, they can begin to broaden their horizons.

Diskussion: Technik der thorakalen und lumbalen Epiduralanaesthesie

Mutan:
Ich bin überrascht, daß Sie bei der thorakalen Epiduralanaesthesie mit 20 ml eine verhältnismäßig hohe Dosis geben. Wir kommen immer mit 7 ml Bupivacain 0,5%ig aus.

Wüst:
Zur Analgesie bei einem Oberbaucheingriff oder einem aortofemoralen Bypass benötigen wir eine Analgesie, die von Th 4–L 2/3 reicht. In den beiden Abbildungen, die ich gezeigt habe, sind die tatsächlich gebrauchten Dosen von Bupivacain 0,5% bei 180 Patienten gezeigt. Bei allen Patienten wurde die Punktion in Höhe des 8./9. Thorakalsegmentes durchgeführt und der Katheter 5 cm in den Epiduralraum eingeführt, so daß die Spitze des Katheters bei Th 7 zu liegen kam. Aus der Dosis, die verabreicht wurde, und der Anzahl der Segmente, die blockiert wurden, errechnet sich eine mittlere Dosis pro Segment von 1,5 ml Bupivacain 0,5%ig.

Lanz:
Sie zeigten, daß Sie gleich große Volumina von Bupivacain 0.5% benötigen, unabhängig davon, ob Sie im lumbalen oder im thorakalen Bereich eingehen. Beim lumbalen Zugang breitet sich das Lokalanaesthetikum bevorzugt auch nach kaudal aus, während beim thorakalen Zugang sich die Analgesie weiter nach oben ausbreitet. Der lumbale Epiduralraum ist aber größer als der thorakale. Es war deshalb zu erwarten, daß Sie bei dem tieferen Zugang im Lumbalbereich größere Volumina an Lokalanaesthetika benötigen müssen als beim thorakalen Zugang.

Wüst:
Diese anatomischen Vorstellungen waren uns auch bekannt, weshalb wir selbst sehr überrascht waren über die Ergebnisse. Bei unseren Untersuchungen über die Dosis-Wirkung-

Beziehung der Lokalanaesthetika in Abhängigkeit von der Einstichhöhe haben wir festgestellt, daß wir zur Blockade eines Segmentes im lumbalen und thorakalen Bereich die gleiche Dosis benötigen. Gehen wir aber im Übergang des thorakalen zum lumbalen Bereich ein, dann benötigen wir plötzlich geringere Volumina, um ein Segment zu blockieren. Wir haben das damit erklärt: Der Epiduralraum ist infolge der Auftreibung des Rückenmarkes in diesem Bereich sehr eng und dadurch wird eine größere Ausbreitung des Lokalanaesthetikums erreicht.

Mutan:
Ich übersehe bisher 200 Patienten. Bei allen Patienten haben wir mit 7 ml eine ausreichende Analgesie erreicht, die es uns gestattete, die Patienten während der Operation unter Sedation spontan atmen zu lassen. Dabei punktieren wir von Th 5 an abwärts. Nach unseren Erfahrungen muß die Anaesthesie mindestens bis zum 4. Thorakalsegment reichen. Wenn Sie unterhalb von Th 8 eingehen, dann ist das zwar in der Mitte des Bauchschnittes, nicht aber in der Mitte der Analgesie, die Sie für einen Oberbaucheingriff benötigen.

Wüst:
Wir führen unsere Punktionen bei Th 8/9 durch und führen den Katheter 5 cm im Epiduralraum vor unter der Vorstellung, daß die Katheterspitze in Höhe des 7. thorakalen Brustwirbels liegt. Bei der Injektion von 20 ml Bupivacain 0,5% erreichen wir eine etwas asymmetrische Ausbreitung, wobei die obere Grenze bei Th 4 ± 2 Segmente und die untere Grenze bei L 3/4 ± 2 Segmente liegt. Diese Ausbreitung der Analgesie benötigen wir insbesondere bei gefäßchirurgischen Operationen, bei denen auch in der Leiste operiert wird. Bei einem reinen Oberbaucheingriff oder bei einem thorakoabdominalen Eingriff punktiere ich bei T 5 bzw. 6. Leider müssen wir unsere Patienten beatmen, denn bei der an unserer Klinik angewandten chirurgischen Technik mit sehr großzügigem Abstopfen des Oberbauches und Zurückhalten des Zwerchfelles durch Haken ist eine Spontanatmung praktisch nicht möglich. Beim Einsetzen der Haken beobachten wir regelmäßig einen Anstieg der Beatmungsdrucke.

Schulte-Steinberg:
Ich kann die Untersuchungen von Herrn Wüst über die Ausbreitung bestätigen: In über 100 Fällen wurde mit 20 ml Bupivacain eine Ausbreitung über eine bestimmte Grenze hinaus nicht erreicht.

Mutan:
Wir führen die kontinuierliche Epiduralanaesthesie mit einer Infusion von Lokalanaesthetika postoperativ fort. Wir haben Bupivacain in 3 verschiedenen Konzentrationen versucht, jedoch waren die Ergebnisse mit der 0,125%igen und der 0,25%igen Lösung sehr unzufriedenstellend, so daß wir seit einiger Zeit Bupivacain 0,5% in der Dosis von 3–5 ml/h infundieren. Mit dieser Technik ließen sich bessere Ergebnisse erzielen als mit den schwächeren Lösungen. Seit ca. einem 1/2 Jahr fügen wir Dolantin der Lokalanaesthetikalösung zu, damit ist unsere Erfolgsrate wesentlich besser.

Crawford:
I am very sorry to hear that both Dr. Wüst and Dr. v. Steenberge in their techniques committed 2 crimes which I would never under any circumstances allow my residents to do. The first is that they inject fluid for loss of resistance and the second is, they fill the canula with

fluid before inserting it. There is the serious possibility of injecting powdered glass into the epidural space from the ampules from which you have taken your fluid for loss of resistance. It reduces the chance of identifying that the canula has entered the cerebral spinal canal. By feeling warmth on your forearm or elbow you do not know if it is cerebral spinal fluid or local anesthetic because the local anesthetic might have come from a warm closet. Loss of resistance should be with air using either syringe or the Mac Intosh balloon. The canula should never be filled. We have over the last 13 years experienced in our department only 3 cases of an imperforated canula in which the holes have not been opened.

v. Steenberge:
First of all, an imperforated canula does occur and the best check is to fill it with some saline. For searching the epidural space I am using saline for the canulas rather than air. But I must say that if you use air, you can inject air to a vessel. Air could escape in very loosy tissues. If your syringe is not hooked up precisely on the needle the air could escape through that. Glass particles could be absorbed into the saline and then be injected into the epidural space. It is quite easy to suck up your saline with the needle hooked to a filter and thus avoid aspirating glass particles into the syringe.

I believe that the saline plays an important role in order to open up the epidural space more easily than with air. This gives you a better access for your catheter. But of course it sounds rational, when using air and there is return, it could be for sure, liquor cerebral spinalis or blood. If you are in the spinal canal with the tip of the needle, the cerebral spinal fluid will flow out and if you are not sure you can even ask your patient to cough and then it spurts out like a fountain.

Star:
I am in doubt about the validity of the filters for retaining bacteria. As far as I know the pores of the filters are usually not small enough to retain bacteria. However, the greatest merit of the filters might be that they can retain a broken glass crystal which otherwise might be injected.

Lorenz:
Welches sind die Kriterien, nach denen Sie das 2. Mal nachinjizieren? Wie stellen Sie bei einem Patienten, der eine Vollnarkose hat, fest, ob die Epiduralanaesthesie noch ausreichend ist?

Wüst:
Die Tiefe der Allgemeinnarkose wird bei der Kombination sehr oberflächlich gehalten, so daß der Patient den Tubus toleriert. Hierzu reichen 0,4 Vol.-% Ethrane bzw. intermittierende Injektionen von 2,5 mg Diazepam aus.

Lorenz:
Sehen Sie einen Vorteil in der Kombination einer Vollnarkose mit einer Epiduralanaesthesie im Vergleich zu einer reinen Allgemeinnarkose mit Hinblick auf Streßfaktoren?

Wüst:
In unserem Krankengut haben wir das Verhalten der Streßhormone während der Operation nicht untersucht. Aufgrund unserer Kreislaufuntersuchungen und im Hinblick auf die Häu-

figkeit von postoperativen Lungenkomplikationen bietet die Kombination erhebliche Vorteile.

Aldrete:
Do you observe tachyphylaxis when you administer the continuous block? This morning it has been said that this phenomenon is not seen with continuous brachiac plexus block. I wonder what are the differences anatomically or physiologically?

v. Steenberge:
We have seen tachyphylaxis in several cases of obstetrical analgesia. In surgical patients we have very rarely seen it.

Wüst:
Im Verlauf der postoperativen Schmerzbehandlung mit der kontinuierlichen Infusionstechnik treten bei allen Patienten immer wieder Schmerzphasen auf. Die Wirksamkeit der zur Korrektur der Analgesie notwendigen Bolusinjektionen nimmt im Verlauf einer 4tägigen Epiduralanaesthesie kontinuierlich ab, d. h., es muß zur Blockade eines Segmentes mehr Lokalanaesthetikum injiziert werden. Die Ursache für dieses Phänomen sehen wir in den physikochemischen Eigenschaften der Lokalanaesthetika. Dr. Raj und Dr. Scott bestreiten allerdings, daß es bei der kontinuierlichen Epiduralanaesthesie mit langwirkenden Lokalanaesthetika wie Bupivacain zur Entwicklung der Tachyphylaxie kommt. Dr. Stanton-Hicks hat jedoch bei gesunden Freiwilligen im Verlauf von 11 h eine Abnahme der Wirksamkeit der zugeführten Lokalanaesthetika beobachtet.

II Komplikationen bei Regionalanaesthesie

Vorsitz: M. d'Arcy Stanton-Hicks, Denver/USA und K. Falke, Düsseldorf

Complications of Regional Anesthesia

M. d'Arcy Stanton-Hicks

Many complications associated with regional anesthesia are described. In order to put them into perspective, it is convenient to classify them into complications due to the pharmalogic agents used and those resulting from the particular technique. Within this classification, one can separate the sequalae into minor and major groups, depending on their seriousness for the patient.

General Complications Occurring With Regional Anesthesia

Toxic Reactions

Local Tissue Toxicity

This is usually the result of too high a concentration of the particular local anesthetic in question or it results from the inadvertent injection of a local anesthetic into the wrong tissue compartment, for example, an epidural dose of local anesthetic into the subarachnoid space or an intraneural injection of local anesthetic [1]. Contamination of local anesthetic solutions with bacteria, chemicals, and foreign material can all be responsible for cellulitis, abscess formation, or even tissue death causing sloughing. Sloughing may also occur when a high concentration of vasoconstrictor is used in conjunction with the local anesthetic. Local infection, as in the case of an epidural abscess is generally not caused by exogenous infection, rather it results by hematogenous spread from an infection site elsewhere in the body (typically pelvic inflammation) and is more likely to occur in the presence of devitalized tissue or in association with a poor immune response.

Systemic Toxic Reaction

Systemic toxic effects of the absorbed local anesthetic occur when the recommended dose of local anesthetic for the given procedure is exceeded or when the local anesthetic is inadvertently injected into a blood vessel or released from a limb suddenly during the administration of an intravenous regional anesthetic. Such toxic effects are manifested in the central nervous and cardiovascular systems. Central-nervous-system effects are biphasic and are manifested first by excitation, twitching, tremors, and ultimately convulsions, a process thought to be the result of a greater sensitivity of the inhibitory systems to the blood local anesthetic concentration [2]. As the concentration increases, facilitatory systems are affected and one sees depression of the cortical and medullary centers with resulting loss of consciousness, vasomotor depression, and depression of the respiratory center, leading finally to apnea if the concentration is high enough.

The toxic cardiovascular effects are similarly biphasic, being dependent on concentration, and occur by two mechanisms [3]. The first is indirect and is a component of central-nervous-system stimulation or depression of the medullary centers by the blood anesthetic concentration, and therefore requires intact autonomic pathways for the effects to be manifested. The second mechanism is direct and comes from the effect of the circulating local anesthetic on vascular smooth muscle and myocardium. Just as local anesthetics interfere with nerve conduction by preventing depolarization, so their effects on vascular tissue are manifested in a similar manner. Local anesthetics stimulate the myocardium at low blood levels with the result that either no change at all or an increase in cardiac output can be expected, but as the blood concentration of local anesthetic rises, negative inotropic effects cause a reduction in stroke volume and cardiac output. Similar biphasic effects on the peripheral vascular system cause an initial stimulation and, therefore, vasoconstriction, followed by vasodilatation as the blood level rises.

Hypersensitive or allergic phenomena associated with local anesthetics are rare complications and are seen mainly in conjunction with the ester local anesthetics. The amide group of drugs seems to be singularly free of this propensity and those instances of reported allergic phenomena are the result not of the local anesthetic, but rather of the preservative (methylparaben) that is included. Most of the so-called allergic reactions are not due to allergy, but are vasovagal or syncopal attacks or the result of the absorbed vasoconstrictor producing tachycardia or palpitations. The massive dose of a vasoconstrictor, usually adrenaline, accompanying an inadvertent intravenous injection of a local anesthetic will produce both alpha and beta adrenergic effects of short duration.

Fetal Uptake of Local Anesthetics

The introduction of local anesthetics into the maternal and thence fetal circulation can occur through any of the common regional anesthetic procedures used during parturition or at term. In the course of epidural anesthesia, unrecognized injection of the therapeutic dose into an epidural vein can be responsible for very high maternal and fetal concentrations of local anesthetic. Similarly, during paracervical nerve block, very high fetal concentrations of local anesthetic can result from its injection into the uterine artery or its rapid absorbtion from the very vascular paracervical tissue.

Fetal toxicity from local anesthetics is manifested by bradycardia, asystole, and central-nervous-system depression of the newborn with consequently low Apgar scores. The concurrent use of a vasoconstrictor such as adrenaline will help to minimize the toxic effects of the absorbed local anesthetic unless it is inadvertently given into a maternal blood vessel, in which case transient tachycardia will be observed in the fetus.

Neurological Complications

Peripheral Nerve Injury

Neural injury may result from a direct toxic effect of the local anesthetic agent or contaminant. The effects may be manifested as neuritis or neurolysis. Intraneural injections of local anesthetics can result in very high internal pressure with subsequent injury to neural components. Although they are not normally neurotoxic when used in the recommended therapeutic concentration, local anesthetics can cause histotoxic changes when these concentrations are exceeded, as might be the case when injections are given repeatedly at the same site over a short period.

A peripheral nerve may be injured directly by the needle, but this complication is more likely to result from the use of regular disponsable needles, which have sharp cutting bevels [4]. Only needles with short, noncutting bevels should be employed for peripheral nerve blocks. During the course of a block, the needle may become damaged after contact with cortical bone forming a hook, which may subsequently damage a nerve.

Central Nervous System

There are many causes of complications involving the central nervous system. Lesions of the meninges, subarachnoid fluid, and neural tissue can occur as a result of the agents used. Chemical, physical, or bacterial contaminants, ischemia or hemorrhage, and trauma from needles. Similar complications may arise from intercurrent neurologic disease and surgical disturbance to the blood supply [5].

While the ED_{50} value of local anesthetics is considerably lower than the dose that causes histotoxic effects, an excessive dose of local anesthetic, which would occur, for example, if an epidural dose were accidentally administered to the subarachnoid space, might produce such a lesion in certain circumstances. Such lesions are arachnoiditis and myelitis, which can cause paresis or paraplegia. Hemorrhage and chemical irritants such as detergents have been responsible for similar sequelae.

Meningitis may be septic or aseptic, the former resulting from introduced infection or from systemic spread, while aseptic meningitis can be due to hemorrhage, pyrogens, chemicals, and even dextrose solutions [6, 7]. Injury to neural tissue such as the leptomeninges may have the same causes as above, in addition to which, needle trauma, abscess, or hemorrhage in the epidural space must be added. Cranial nerves may be injured as a result of the removal of subarachnoid fluid by dural puncture, damage to the blood supply to the abducens nerve, and all of the foregoing causes of spinal neurologic sequelae.

Hemorrhage

Hemorrhage should be a rare sequel to any block procedure performed in patients with no clotting defects. Any bleeding caused by needle passage should be self-limiting and the subsequent hematoma should be small and of little consequence to neural tissue. A special case, however, does exist for hemorrhage within the spinal canal, as it will become loculated and compress the contents of the canal. Furthermore, critical closing pressures in the segmental venous drainage will be rapidly exceeded with consequent stasis and edema exacerbating the neural tissue injury, which will result unless decompression is undertaken.

Miscellaneous Complications

Pneumothorax

This will result if the visceral pleura is torn by a needle during respiration in the course of blocks in the vicinity of the thorax. If the pneumothorax is less than 20%, it may remain symptomless and the air will be absorbed spontaneously. If the puncture hole is larger and air continues to leak, then surgical drainage may be necessary. The incidence of pneumothorax associated with the commonest blocks is as follows: Stellate ganglion block, anterior approach, 0.25%; supraclavicular brachial plexus block, 0.6%–2%; thoracic paravertebral somatic block, 0%–6%; thoracic sympathetic block, 1.4%–7.9%; intercostal block, 0.06%–0.3%. The symptoms of pneumothorax are chest pain aggravated by deep breathing and coughing. A chest radiograph should be taken to confirm the diagnosis.

Headache

This is undoubtedly the most common complication of dural puncture and is presumably due to the leakage of cerebrospinal fluid. The incidence of headache is related to age, sex, race, and type of surgery, being highest in the young female and in pregnant patients. The incidence is variously given as 1.4%–12% and can be reduced with care and by the use of a small gauge needle. Treatment of the headache, which is usually frontal or occipital and is always positional, is bed rest and hydration with large volumes of intravenous fluid and analgesics. If after 24 h the headache persists or if it occurs in an ambulatory patient, an autologous blood patch should be performed [8].

Backache

The symptoms are usually attributed to major anesthesia and occur with the same frequency after general anesthesia. The severity is directly proportional to the duration of the surgical procedure and the backache is probably due to the loss of the lumbar lordosis, which occurs with the supine and lithotomy positions, on the operating table.

Hypotension

This is a common accompaniment of major conduction anesthesia. While it occurs sooner and to a greater degree than is apparently the case with epidural anesthesia, the actual degree of hypotension in either case is directly related to the level of sympathetic blockade which, in the case of spinal anesthesia, tends to be one or two spinal segments higher than the equivalent dermatomal level. In addition, the effects of the absorbed vasoconstrictor and local anesthetic are responsible for systemic circulatory changes that are peculiar to epidural anesthesia. However, whether one considers hypotension to be a complication or an acceptable side effect will obviously depend on the degree and circumstances of the particular surgery and the status of the patient.

Broken Needles and Catheters

Both needles and catheters can separate within the body [9, 10]. While some of the older polyvinyl chloride catheters used for continuous epidural block might stimulate a reaction to their presence if left in situ, the modern teflon and nylon catheters are nonreactive. Unless the separation occurs at the skin, in which case surgical removal is a relatively innocuous procedure, it is usually appropriate to leave the broken portion undisturbed. In fact, the use of nylon and teflon catheters in preference to the previous polyvinyl chloride catheters has reduced the incidence of breakage.

Needle breakage tends to occur close to the hub. Immediate surgical removal is necessary because the shaft will "migrate" in the tissues. The once popular "security bead" regional analgesia needles have a small metal bead attached to the shaft of the needle which is designed to prevent loss of the needle in the tissues. However, the widespread use of disposable needles minimizes the chance of breakage because the metal is not subjected to "fatigue" which otherwise would attend the frequent use of reusable needles.

Complications Associated with Specific Regional Anesthetic Procedures

Brachial Plexus Block

Interscalene Block

This can be considered a block of the trunk. Because of the proximity of the phrenic and recurrent laryngeal nerves, these may be blocked when employing this technique [11]. Pneumothorax has been reported and intra-arterial injection can occur. Because of the confined nature of the space and the volume of anesthetic solution used, it is quite possible to compress the carotid artery and, therefore, this technique is potentially dangerous in patients who have severe arterial compromise due to arteriosclerosis [12].

Supraclavicular Plexus Block

This is the oldest of the plexus anesthetic techniques and its most frequently reported complication is pneumothorax. Arterial injection and neurologic sequalae from needle trauma have been reported to occur with a frequency of up to 6%.

Axillary Plexus Block

This was developed as an alternative to the supraclavicular approach and is essentially a block of the divisions and branches. Pneumothorax is avoided, but arterial penetration frequently occurs and hematomas can occur. The incidence of neurologic sequelae is about the same as with the supraclavicular block.

Infraclavicular Plexus Block

As with the axillary block, hematoma formation is the commonest complication.

Cervical Plexus Block

The most common complication associated with this technique is intervertebral arterial injection. Subarachnoid injection can also occur because of the extraforaminal extension of the dura which occurs in this region.

Stellate Ganglion Block

Accidental intravascular injection (common carotid artery or vertebral artery), block of the recurrent laryngeal nerve, and pneumothorax are the most frequently reported complications of this procedure. However, as is the case for cervical plexus block, it is also possible to enter the dural cuff and, thus, produce a subarachnoid block [13, 14].

Sympathetic Blocks

Thoracic Sympathetic Block

The incidence of pneumothorax is high, although this complication can be reduced by the concurrent use of an image intensifier. Also, because of the proximity of the sympathetic chain to the spinal nerve roots, it is possible to block these roots as well, in which case if a neurolytic solution is used, it could either cause a prolonged somatic block or give rise to reflex sympathetic dystrophy in that spinal segment. Therefore, it is important that only small volumes, accurately placed, are used when performing this type of block. Subarachnoid injection has also been reported.

Splanchnic Nerve Block

This procedure is performed not so much to interrupt the sympathetic fibers in these nerves, but rather to block the visceral afferents mediating pain from the upper abdominal viscera. Pneumothorax and vascular injection are the most common complications associated with this procedure, but reflex sympathetic dystrophy can also occur.

Lumbar Sympathetic Block

Although one of the commonest sympathetic blocks, it is the one regional block procedure having the lowest incidence of complications. Reflex sympathetic dystrophy and vascular injection can occur.

Paracervical Block

The majority of complications attending this block are due to the toxic effects of the local anesthetic on the fetus. Either the local anesthetic is rapidly absorbed from the very vascular pericervical tissues or it is injected directly into the uterine artery [15]. Fetal bradycardia or cardiac arrest can occur. Direct injection into the fetal scalp is also possible, particularly once the head is engaged and the cervix is fully effaced. However, this complication is minimized by use of a guarded needle such as the Kobak needle.

Block of Cranial Nerves

Intrathecal injection, particularly that which can occur during block of the branches of the trigeminal nerve or ganglion, can result in sudden loss of consciousness or respiratory arrest. This form of accident, while only temporary when local anesthetic solutions are used, must be carefully avoided when using neurolytic substances. Injection of anesthetic agents in the sphenopalatine fossa can travel via the inferior orbital fissure where they can cause palsy of the abducens nerve.

Because of the vascularity of the extracranial tissues and the companion vessels associated with the cranial nerves and their branches, inadvertent intra-arterial injection occurs easily and, therefore, extreme care must be exercised if it is to be avoided. Sequelae can range from temporary blindness, loss of consciousness, convulsions, and respiratory arrest to cardiac dysrythmias.

Neurolytic injections into confined spaces such as the inferior orbital foramen during block of the opthalmic division of the trigeminal nerve can cause a disabling neuritis. In actual blocks of the terminal branches of the second and third divisions of the trigeminal nerve the same sequelae mentioned above have been noted. It is now quite apparent that intra-arterial injection of local anesthetic solutions, and likewise embolism such as introduced air, can travel retrograde via these vessels into the internal carotid system, only then to be distributed via its branches to intracranial structures.

Major Conduction Anesthesia

Spinal Anesthesia

The complications can be considered under minor and major headings. Minor sequelae of spinal anesthesia include headache, backache, hypotension, urinary retention, cranial nerve palsy, and neural injury (peripheral nerve). Headacke, backache and hypotension have already been discussed under general complications. Urinary retention is common to both spinal and epidural anesthesia, but its incidence is greater with spinal anesthesia. Cranial nerve palsy most commonly affecting the abducens nerve is now relatively uncommon and its previous incidence was presumably related to techniques of spinal anesthesia involving the removal of large volumes of spinal fluid. Spinal nerve roots and the cauda equina may be injured during traumatic spinal puncture, giving rise to paresthesias and small neurologic deficits, usually, but not always, of short duration [16].

Major sequelae include neural injury, subdural hematoma, anterior spinal artery syndrome, arachnoiditis, and meningitis. Neural injury in this context refers to the transient or permanent loss of neural function in a particular nerve root. Subdural hematoma, while rare, is potentially very serious and can be responsible for paraplegia. Anterior spinal artery syndrome, while also a rare complication, is often associated with arteriosclerosis or the surgical procedure for which the anesthetic has been given. Paraplegia is the invariable result. Arachnoiditis and meningitis have already been discussed.

Epidural Anesthesia

The complications of epidural anesthesia, like those just described for spinal anesthesia, have much in common and can also be divided into minor and major sequelae [17]. Minor complications include: Neural injury (peripheral nerves, cauda equina), dural puncture, headache, backache, urinary retention, massive subarachnoid injection, and broken epidural catheter. Major complications are: meningitis, arachnoiditis, epidural hematoma, epidural abscess, and anterior spinal artery syndrome.

A few observations on the minor complications are in order. Neural injury, backache, and urinary retention probably occur with a similar frequency in epidural as in spinal anesthesia. Headache is not a significant problem in epidural anesthesia and its incidence is similar to that following general anesthesia. Dural puncture, while a cause of headache, is not in itself a serious complication if recognized, but as a conduit for massive injection of the full therapeutic dose, it is a potentially major complication. Cases of paraplegia have been reported following inadvertent injection of large doses of local anesthetic into the subarachnoid space. Meningitis is a serious accompaniment of epidural anesthesia and seems to occur with a similar frequency to that following spinal anesthesia. Arachnoiditis is a rare complication most likely to occur as a result of bleeding or as a toxic reaction to inadvertent subarachnoid injection.

Epidural hematoma is most likely to occur as a result of a blood dyscrasia or during anticoagulation therapy, both situations being contraindications to the use of epidural anesthesia. Unless the bleeding ceases or an immediate laminectomy is performed, paraplegia will ensue. Epidural abscess is similarly serious and generally results from a blood-borne infection, typically from a site in the pelvis. It can, however, be introduced from outside the body, although this is an unusual route. Both epidural abscess and epidural hematoma can be treated if recognized and diagnosed and a decompression laminectomy is immediately undertaken. Pain is generally a constant symptom, even in the presence of epidural analgesia. Motor involvement with flaccid paralysis are constant signs. The onset of signs of epidural hematoma are sudden, whereas the onset of signs during abscess formation may take several days to three weeks to appear. Anterior spinal artery syndrome is a rare complication which is generally associated with arteriosclerosis, although it can also occur as a result of surgical interference of the radicular blood supply.

Summary

The foregoing account of complications that are associated with or that have been the basis of an isolated report, may appear intimidating. However, they must be viewed in relation to the complications and morbidity which are also known to accompany general anesthesia. Most complications are can be prevented and most can be avoided by an appropriate understanding of anatomy, the pharmacology of the drugs used, and through adequate training and expertise of the operator. It is also no accident that centers that have a large regional anesthetic practice also enjoy the lowest incidence of all complications.

References

1. Reisner LS, Hochman BN, Plumer MH (1980) Persistant neurologic deficit and adhesive arachnoiditis following intrathecal 2-chlorprocaine injection. Anesth Analg 59:452–454
2. Munson ES, Gutnick MJ, Wagman IH (1970) Local anesthetic drug-induced seizures in rhesus monkeys. Anesth Analg 49:986
3. Beair MR (1975) Cardiovascular pharmacology of local anesthaetics, Br J Anaesth [Suppl] 47:247
4. Selander D, Dhuner K-G, Lundborg G (1977) Nerve injuries due to injection needles used for regional anaesthesia. Acta Anaesthesiol Scand 2:182
5. Thorsen G (1947) Neurological complications after spinal anaesthesia and results from 2493 follow-up cases. Acta Chir Scand 95:21
6. Rendell CM (1954) Chemical meningitis due to syringes stored in lysol. Anasthesia 9:281
7. Seigne JD (1970) Aseptic meningitis following spinal analgesia. Anaesthesia 25:402
8. DiGiovanni AJ, Dunbar BS (1970) Epidural injections of autologous blood for post lumbar puncture headache. Anesth Analg 49:268
9. Moore DC (1965) Regional block, 4th edn. Thomas, Springfield
10. Frumin MS, Schwartz H (1962) Continuous lumbar peridural anesthesia. Anesthesiology 13:488
11. Ward ME (1974) The interscalene approach to the brachial plexus. Anaesthesia 29:147
12. Siler JN, Lief PL, Davis J (1973) A new complication of interscalene brachial plexus block. Anesthesiology 38:590

13. Moore DC (1954) Stellate ganglion block. Thomas, Springfield
14. Forrest JB (1976) An unusual complication after stellate ganglion block by the paratracheal approach, a case report. Can Anaesth Soc J 23:485
15. Rosefsky JB, Petersiel ME (1968) Perinatal deaths associated with mepivacaine paracervical block anesthesia in labour. N Engl J Med 278:530
16. Noble AB, Murray JG (1971) A review of the complications of spinal anesthesia with experience in Canadian teaching hospitals from 1959–1969. Can Anaesth Soc J 18:5
17. Dawkins CJM (1969) An analysis of the complications of extradural and caudal block. Anaesthesia 24:554

Discussion

Anger:
Why should we use combined epidural and general anesthesia in abdominal and thoracic surgery and what are the advantages?

Stanton-Hicks:
From many studies, published recently, and from the detailed discussion at the two recent symposia in Düsseldorf, it is evident that this combination has a beneficial effect on circulation, stress response due to surgery, and on the incidence of postoperative respiratory and thromboembolic complications than general anesthesia alone. As Dr. Wüst pointed out for upper abdominal and thoracic surgery, one often gives a light general anesthetic to provide "social sleep", so that the patient can tolerate the endotracheal tube. Otherwise, for example, in herniorrhaphy and other peripheral surgical procedures, the combination of epidural and general anesthesia is unnecessary.

Reverse Arterial Blood Flow: A Mechanism for Neurotoxicity from Local Anesthetics

J. A. Aldrete

Introduction

The mechanism for neurotoxicity produced by local anesthetics (LA) has been understood to be produced by the blockade of neural relays, which normally inhibit amygdaloid activity. The generalized depression and muscle rigidity seen before and after convulsions in such cases form part of the suppressive or inhibitory influences on motor pathways [1, 2]. Since LA reach the brain by various routes, most commonly by the circulation, high blood levels can be either the result of overdosage or accidental injection into the lumen of a vein.

In this study, laboratory investigations provide the basis for identification of another mechanism of neurotoxicity through the cephalic circulation that would explain some cases of sudden convulsions, loss of consciousness, apnea, and occasionally death, resulting from injection of small volumes of LA in the head and neck area [3–5].

Methods

The study included four phases.

Phase I

In six rhesus monkeys, 3 mg/kg lidocaine were injected under pressure into the facial artery, while the electroencephalogram (EEG), electrocardiogram (EKG), and direct arterial pressure were being recorded. Through the same vessel, a contrast medium was injected against the flow of arterial blood, followed immediately by roentgenograms of the head, neck, and upper thorax.

Phase II

In three groups of six mongrel dogs each, 3 mg/kg lidocaine were injected into the facial artery (group A) or the facial vein (group B). In group C, only 1 mg/kg of the LA drug was given intra-arterially. Blood samples were then drawn from the internal (IJV) and external jugular (EJV) veins and the internal carotid artery (ICA) 15, 30, 60, and 180 s postinjection. Samples were analyzed with a gas chromatograph for lidocaine concentrations.

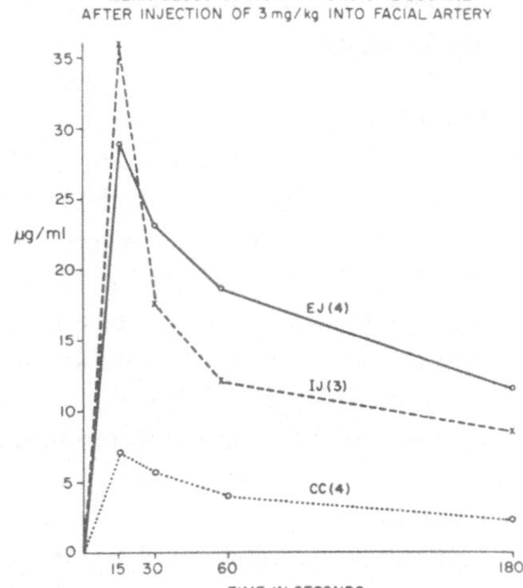

Fig. 1. Blood concentrations of lidocaine 15, 30, 60, and 180 min after the injection of 3 mg/kg into the facial artery of a dog. o——o external jugular vein concentration; x– – –x internal jugular vein concentration; o····o internal carotid artery concentration (with permission from publisher)

Phase III

In baboons, the primates whose cerebral circulation is most similar to that of man, 3 mg/kg lidocaine were injected into the lingual artery centripetally and blood samples were taken from the ICA and jugular veins 6, 30, and 180 s postinjection. In two other groups, injections of 7 mg/kg lidocaine were made into the brachial and femoral arteries also, followed by similar sampling. At the end of the experiment, 2 ml sodium chloride solution containing radioactive microspheres 20 μ in diameter and tagged with strontium (Sr90) were injected into the lingual artery. After sacrifice, the skull contents were obtained and sectioned to identify the distribution of the microspheres by means of a scintillation counter.

Phase IV

In rabbits, lidocaine 10 mg; lidocaine 10 mg plus 5 μg epinephrine, NaCl 0.9% solution alone and with 5 μg epinephrine were injected into the carotid artery, while the EEG, EKG and arterial blood pressure were continuously monitored.

Results

Phase I

Injection of 3 mg/kg lidocaine into the facial artery resulted in electroencephalographic changes 6 s after administration with slight subsequent rises of arterial blood pressure (ABP) and heart rate (HR) 11 s post-injection. Cerebral angiograms could be obtained when contrast medium was injected centripetally under pressure.

Phase II

Blood levels of lidocaine ranging between 5 and 7 μg/ml were found in ICA 15 s postinjection, while IJV and EJV levels exceeded 30 μg/ml at the same time (Fig. 1). When the same amount of lidocaine was injected into the facial vein, ICA levels were less than 3 μg/ml, but peaked at 30 s; in IJV and EJV blood samples, lidocaine peaked at 15 s in doses exceeding 35 μg/ml.

Phase III

Six seconds after injection of 3 mg/kg into ICA, the mean level of lidocaine was 28 μg/kg, whereas in venous samples, the highest levels were noted to be 51 for IJV and 25.7 for EJV 30 s after administration. When 7 mg/kg lidocaine were given into the brachial and femoral arteries, mean values noted at 6 s were 105.5 μg/ml and 20.6 μg/ml. The usual distribution of Sr^{90}-labelled microspheres was as follows: 74.2% into the ipsilateral hemisphere, 10.5% into the contralateral cerebral hemisphere, 6.1% lodged in the cerebellum, and 4.5% in the meninges. The rest (3.7) were not found within the skull contents of the animals and were probably distributed elsewhere in their bodies.

Phase IV

The electroencephalographic changes noted after the injection of 10 mg lidocaine resemble seizure activity appearing from 6 to 10 s after injection and lasting from 30 to 180 s. No changes of ABP or HR were seen in these cases. In contrast, both heart rate and blood pressure rose when epinephrine alone was injected, remaining elevated above central levels for an average period of 12.2 min after the injection of 10 mg lidocaine with epinephrine lasting up to 280 s; the EEG pattern showed seizure activity of the same intensity but lasted for about 320 s. When epinephrine was injected alone, no seizure pattern was observed but the elevations of heart rate and blood pressure were of greater magnitude and longer duration.

Discussion

Elevated bood levels of LA usually result in central nervous system toxicity. The modes of entry of these drugs into the circulation are conventionally: a) direct inadvertent intravenous injection; b) overdosage resulting after absorption from the injection site; and c) when the usual dose is injected into a highly vascular area or applied on mucosas. The studies reported here support early observations and explain several case reports of neurotoxicity occurring shortly after the injection of LA in areas near to arterial vessels. By elimination, when LA is injected into veins, due to subsequent dilution the drug concentration will depend on the amount injected and the rate of administration. Toxic arterial blood levels can result after injection of one-third of the conventional dose. As dilution occurs after overdosage, the blood concentrations will gradually diminish, so, to attain high enough levels to produce neurotoxicity, excessive doses would need to be injected. An alternative would be the administration of conventional doses into a highly vascularized area, where absorption into the circulation will be faster, resulting in high blood concentrations.

One other mechanism of neurotoxicity may be produced by the forceful injection of LA into arteries centripetally. Several clinical cases have been reported where signs of toxicity (somnolence, tremor, analgesia, numbness of the lips, loss of consciousness, respiratory and cardiac arrest) appeared soon after the administration of LA, suggesting intravascular entry [6, 7]. If the LA is injected intravenously, doses approaching one-third to one-half of the recommended maximum safe doses are necessary to produce central nervous system toxicity [8]. Though, in the past, intra-arterial injections have been assumed to be distributed centrifugally [9], depending on the circumstances of injection and site LA may follow a centripetal direction.

From the first set of experiments (Phase I), it was established that a cerebral arteriogram may be produced when contrast medium is injected into a small branch of the external carotid artery, following a distribution pathway through the external, common, and internal carotid arteries. It was also shown that as early as 6 s after the injection of 3 mg/kg lidocaine, electroencephalographic changes were noted with minimal increases of heart rate and systolic and diastolic blood pressure taking place about 15 s postinjections [10].

In Phase II of the study, low blood levels (7.2 μg/ml) of lidocaine were noted in internal carotid blood level 15 s after injection into the facial artery of a dog. When the injection was made into the facial artery, peak ICA blood levels occurred 30 s after injection [11]. When sampling was made 6 s postinjection of 3 mg/kg lidocaine into the lingual artery of a baboon, concentrations above the threshold for neurotoxicity were found in ICA. Similar findings were noted when 7 mg/kg lidocaine were injected either into the brachial or the femoral arteries (Phase III). The observation that most of the radioactively traced microspheres were found in the ipsilateral brain hemisphere indicates the distribution of the blood flow of the individual carotid arteries and confirmed the reversability of the carotid blood flow [12].

The puzzling question of how small volumes of local anesthetic drugs injected aroung the face and neck area may produce central nervous system (CNS) toxicity can finally be answered taking into consideration the volume of blood that may be present at any one time within the brain. For this, extrapolation of a study performed by Penn et al. [13] using computerized axial tomography density measurements indicates that, in the normal adult, there are 3 ml blood for each 100 ml brain tissue, equivalent to about 30 ml blood for a 1,000 g brain. Theoretically, 1 mg lidocaine injected into the ICA could produce blood levels above the toxicity threshold (about 20 μg lidocaine per ml blood) as observed in monkeys [14] and man [15].

Covino [16] suggested the effect that the addition of epinephrine to lidocaine may have on cerebral toxicity and systemic hemodynamics. The studies conducted in Phase IV delineate the effects that lidocaine alone, with epinephrine and epinephrine alone may have on the EEG, heart rate, and arterial blood pressure. The intensity and duration of toxic manifestations depend on the dose given, route and kinetics of administration, protein binding, affinity for nervous tissue and, to a lesser extent, on its metabolism and rate of elimination. Attempts to correlate blood levels of LA to signs and symptoms of neurotoxicity have shown a wide range of results. Foldes et al. [17] made observations in volunteers during the continuous infusion of various local anesthetics: 2-chloroprocaine was the best and lidocaine the least tolerated of the drugs studied. Electrocardiographic alterations were frequently seen at concentrations between 3 and 6 μg/ml lidocaine with signs of toxicity appearing when values between 6 and 12 μg/ml lidocaine were measured in venous blood. With lidocaine, Bromage and Robson [18] noted that venous blood concentrations of 5 to 7 μg/ml produced sedation and obtunded consciousness, whereas 10 μg/ml caused early signs of toxicity. The highest levels observed occurred 20 min after intramuscular injections, 10 min after epidural administration, and 6 min after intratracheal instillation. Larger doses of intravenous procaine [19–21] and lidocaine have been used as analgesic and anesthetic supplements. Doses up to 1,000 mg of the former and 600 mg of the latter per h have been given. However, in most instances barbiturates or benzodiazepine drugs were used continually, thus protecting the patient against neurotoxic manifestations.

Recently, Tucker et al. [22] measured venous plasma levels resulting from epidural, caudal, intercostal nerve, brachial plexus, and sciatic-femoral nerve blocks using 500 mg mepivacaine. The highest blood levels noted resulted after intercostal nerve block (5–10 μg/ml) 9 min after injection. With the addition of epinephrine, peak levels were lower and appeared later, thus confirming its protective effect. The difference in levels found by various authors can probably be explained by the source of sampling. In arterial blood, Munson et al. [14] found 18 μg/ml to be the convulsive threshold in monkeys. These investigators confirmed their findings in unanesthetized monkeys, where arterial blood levels around 20 μg/ml lidocaine were required to produce seizures after they observed mild sedation at about 13 μg/ml [23]. A case report by Bedeyneck [15] noted a concentration of 20 μg/ml in the arterial blood of a patient having a seizure from lidocaine overdose. Again, by sampling arterial and venous blood simultaneously after lidocaine administration, Tucker and Mather [24] noticed higher levels in the former than the latter for periods of up to 1 h.

Various mechanisms for elevated blood levels of local anesthetic drugs have been demonstrated as a result of a distribution process influenced by the site, the route, and the force of injection. These mechanisms have to be considered not only when large volumes are injected, but also when smaller doses are given in the areas of the head and neck. Reversal of the arterial blood flow at the time of injection is one more pathway by which LA reaches high concentrations within the cerebral circulation, even if it is just regionally.

References

1. Usubiaga JE, Wikinski J, Ferrero R et al. (1968) Local anesthetic-induced convulsions in man. An electroencephalographic study. Anesth Analg 45:611
2. DeJong RH (1977) Local anesthetics. Thomas, Springfield, Chap 8
3. Bourne JG (1970) Deaths with dental anaesthetics. Anaesthesia 25:473
4. Tomlin PJ (1974) Death in outpatient dental anesthetic practice. Anaesthesia 29:551
5. Malmin O (1974) The shot that kills: deaths in the dental chair. Exposition, Hicksville, pp 11–17
6. Selden HM (1967) Reactions to local anesthetics. J Mich Dent Assoc 49:41
7. Portman J (1970) Deaths with dental anaesthetics. Lancet 1:627–647
8. Wikinski JA, Usubiaga JE, Morales RL et al. (1970) Mechanism of convulsions elicited by local anesthetic agents. Anesth Analg 49:504
9. Moore DC (1955) Complications of regional anesthesia. Thomas, Springfield, pp 6–22
10. Aldrete JA, Narang R, Sada T et al (1977) Reverse carotid blood flow – a possible explanation for some reactions to local anesthetics. J Am Dent Assoc 94:1142
11. Aldrete JA, Nicholson J, Sada T et al. (1977) Cephalic kinetics of intra-arterially injected lidocaine. Oral Surg 44:167
12. Aldrete JA, Romo-Salas F, Arora S et al. (1978) Reverse arterial blood flow as a pathway for central nervous system toxic response following injection of local anesthetics. Anesth Analg 57:428
13. Penn RD, Walser R, Ackerman L (1977) Cerebral blood volume in man: computer analysis of a computerized brain scan. JAMA 172:1493–1496
14. Munson ES, Gutnick MJ, Wagman IH (1970) Local anesthetic drug-induced seizures in rhesus monkeys. Anesth Analg 49:986
15. Bedeyneck JL Jr, Weinstein KN, Kah RE et al. (1966) Ventricular tachycardia: control by intermittent administration of lidocaine hydrochloride. JAMA 198:553
16. Covino BG (1978) Systemic toxicity of local anesthetic agents (editorial). Anesth Analg 57:387
17. Foldes FF, Molloy R, McNall PG, Koukal LR (1960) Comparison of toxicity of intravenously-given local anesthetic agents in man. JAMA 172:1478
18. Bromage PR, Robson JG (1961) Concentration of lignocaine in the blood after intravenous, intramuscular, epidural and endotracheal administration. Anaesthesia 16:461

19. Wikinski JA et al. (1980) General anesthesia with intravenous procaine. In: Aldrete JA, Stanley TH (eds) Trends in intravenous anesthesia. Year Book Publishers, Chicago, p 198
20. Steinhaus JE, Howland DE (1958) Intravenously administered lidocaine as a supplement to nitrous oxide-thiobarbiturate anesthesia. Anesth Analg 37:40
21. Aldrete JA, Fraser JG (1966) Intravenous lidocaine as a supplement to nitrous oxide anesthesia for radical middle ear surgery. Can Anaesth Soc J 13:397
22. Tucker GT, Moore DC, Bridenbaugh PO, Bridenbaugh LD, Thompson GE (1972) Systemic absorption of mepivacaine in commonly-used regional block procedures. Anesthesiology 37:277
23. Munson ES, Tucker WK, Ausimach B et al. (1975) Etidocaine, bupivacaine, and lidocaine seizure thresholds in monkeys. Anesthesiology 42:471
24. Tucker GT, Mather LE (1975) Pharmacokinetics of local anaesthetic agents. Br J Anaesthesiol 47: 213

Discussion

Zindler:
You give a small amount of local anesthetic to your patient in the dental chair and suddenly, while you inject or shortly after termination of the injection, your patient suffers a cardiac arrest. Do you have any idea, how this retrograde flow of the local anesthetic may cause this disastrous effect on circulation? Does this happen because some of the local anesthetic goes directly to the medullary centers, causing reflex cardiac arrest, or are there other mechanisms known? Is there, finally, a method of local treatment or do you have to start immediate resuscitation?

Aldrete:
I believe that the primary disastrous effect is on the central nervous system leading to convulsions and respiratory arrest. Cardiac arrest will develop due to hypoxemia if resuscitation is not instituted immediately. At least in the USA, where the dentist or the plastic surgeon has neither the equipment nor the capability to ventilate a patient, this happens very frequently. To prevent this disaster, aspiration should be mandatory. There are now a number of devices available in the USA, which aspirate almost simultaneously, while the injection is going on. So, if a vessel is entered accidentally, this is recognized immediately and the point of the needle can be changed.

Stanton Hicks:
It requires an extraordinarily small amount of local anesthetic to produce central nervous effects. If there is a cardiac arrest, presumably there will first be an arrhythmia and it will be just a matter of maintaining normal cardiac and pulmonary resuscitation to restore the normal sinus rhythm. My own experience last week was that, while normally aspirating before injecting in the vicinity of the vertebral artery, I just flushed about one-tenth of a milliliter of local anesthetic because the needle was blocked and that tenth of a milliliter produced a convulsion. It is a very small amount. It's about 1,0 mg lidocaine.

Aldrete:
The blood content of the cerebrum has been estimated to be 3 ml blood/100 g brain tissue. According to that, someone with a brain weight of 1,000 g will have a cerebral blood volume of 30 ml. If you inject 1 mg of a local anesthetic, you will end up with about 30 μg/ml. This blood level is high enough to produce convulsions.

Question:
Has the speed of injection an effect on the reverse flow?

Aldrete:
The speed of injection as well as the size of the needle influences the degree of pressure that we have to apply on the plunger of the syringe. The faster you inject, the greater is the chance of reversing the arterial blood flow. The smaller the needle you are using, the higher the pressure and the greater the chance for this phenomenon to occure. In practice, this can be avoided when the speed of injection is slow and the needles have the greatest possible size and their bevel is may-be a little bit larger. So, hopefully, the lumen of your needle is not completely in the vessel while you aspirate or inject.

Plasma Levels of Bupivacain under Continuous Thoracic Epidural Anesthesia and Analgesia

H. J. Wüst, J. Abel, F. M. M. Thiessen, M. Breulmann, R. Schier, and O. Richter

Continuous thoracic epidural analgesia is more and more widely used in our department to achieve adequate relief from postoperative pain. This rechnique has proved to be of special value following Whipple's and portacaval shunt operations and liver resections. In some patients, however, liver function and thus the metabolism of the local anesthetics might be impaired [5]. The infusion of a total dose of up to 3 g bupivacaine into the epidural space during the course of 4 days may increase the plasma concentration of the drug to toxic levels, causing central nervous symptoms and cardiodepression. To evaluate the safety margin of continuous infusion techniques, especially in patients with impaired liver function, the plasma levels of bupivacaine were determined in 25 patients.

Patients and Methods

The investigation was carried out in 25 patients after having obtained written consent. Nine patients (upper abdominal group) underwent partial or total gastrectomy because of either gastric ulcer or cancer. In ten patients (vascular surgical group), an aortofemoral bypass graft was implanted. Six patients (hyperbilirubinemia group) underwent Whipple's operation because of a cancer of the pancreas causing choleostasis and hyperbilirubinemia of between 15 and 35 mg%. The three groups were comparable with regard to their biometric data and the duration of bupivacaine administration (Table 1).

The liver enzymes GOT, GPT, and bilirubin in serum (total and direct) were in the normal range in the vascular and upper abdominal group, but were elevated in patients who had undergone Whipple's operation.

Anesthetic and Analgesic Technique

In all patients, a preoperative epidural catheter was inserted into the thoracic space Th 8/9 (Table 2). For premedication, the patients received 10 mg diazepam and 100 mg pentobarbital the night before the operation. No premedication was given on the day of operation. After a test dose of 5 ml, the epidural anesthesia was started with 12 to 15 ml 0.5% bupivacain. After 30 min, the extent of sensory block was tested by pin prick. The patients were intubated under hexobarbital and succinylcholine while anesthesia was maintained with 0.4

Table 1. Biometric, laboratory data and duration of bupivacaine administration in three groups of patients

	Abdominal surgery	Vascular surgery	Whipple's operation
	x sd	x sd	x sd
n (m/f)	9 (6/3)	10 (8/2)	6 (4/2)
Age (years)	56.3 + 8	58.4 ± 7.2	52.4 ± 12.9
Height (cm)	168.0 + 3.5	176.4 ± 4.8	175.0 ± 8.4
Weight (kg)	68.6 ± 8.4	77.1 ± 8.1	73.6 ± 17.6
Hgb (g%)	13.6 ± 0.9	15.3 ± 1.4	14.7 ± 3.3
GOT (units)	12.2 ± 2.0	12.2 ± 3.6	33.7 ± 11.4
GPT (units)	12.6 ± 4.3	13.4 ± 7.3	57.5 ± 45.6
Bilirubin (mg%)			
Total	0.4 ± 0.1	0.6 ± 0.3	19.4 ± 14.0
Direct	–	–	14.8 ± 8.7
Duration of bupivacaine infusion (h)	64.1 ± 18.6	66.0 ± 21.4	64.5 ± 22.6

Table 2. Anesthetic protocol

Intraoperative epidural anesthesia

Epidural catheter:	Th 8/9
Premedication:	Evening before 10 mg diazepam + 100 mg pentobarbital Morning –
Induction of the continuous epidural anesthesia:	
	5 ml + 12 ml 0.5% bupivacaine After 30 min pin-prick test (block should indlude Th 5-L 3)
Intubation:	5 mg/kg Hexobarbital 1 mg/kg Succinylcholine + 0.4 vol% ethrane + 50% O_2 : N_2O After 90 min 8–10 ml 0.5% bupivacaine If necessary after 2–3 h additionally 8–10 ml 0.5% bupivacaine

Postoperative epidural anesthesia

Immediately, 0.125% bupivacaine continuous infusion 6 ml/h	
Pain:	Bolus injection 8 ml 0.125% bupivacaine + continuous infusion 0.125% bupivacaine, 12 ml/h
Pain:	Bolus injection 8 ml 0.25% bupivacaine + continuous 0.25% bupivacaine, 6 ml/h
Pain:	Bolus injection 8 ml 0.25% + continuous infusion 0.25% bupivacaine, 12 ml/h

vol.% ethrane and 50% O_2 in N_2O. After 90 min, 8 to 10 ml 0.5% bupivacaine were injected routinely. If necessary, the patients received an additional 8 to 10 ml 0.5% bupivacaine 90–120 min after the last injection. Postoperative analgesia was started with a continuous infusion at the rate of 6 ml/h 0.125% bupivacaine, while tha patient was still painfree. If the patient complained of pain at any time, a bolus injection of 8 ml 0.125% bupivacaine was given. At the same time, the continuous drip rate was increased to 12 ml/h. If further corrections of the analgesia were necessary, the concentration of bupivacaine was increased to 0.25%, at which time the drip rate was decreased to 6 ml/h. If the segmental level of analgesia was found to be unsatisfactory, the patient received a bolus injection of 8 ml 0.25% bupivacaine and the drip rate was increased to 12 ml/h (Table 2).

Arterial blood samples were taken prior to the bupivacaine injection and 10, 20, 30, 60, and 90 min after the first injection and 30, 60, 120, 180, and 240 min after the second injection. In the postoperative period, blood samples were taken every 6 h from the start of the continuous drip until the end of the infusion. After termination of the infusion, blood samples were taken at 1, 2, 3, 4, 6, 12, and 24 h. The plasma levels of bupivacaine were determined using gas chromatography by J. Abel at the Toxicology Institute of the University of Düsseldorf (FRG). Blood gases and the acid-base status were controlled intraoperatively prior to the bupivacaine injection and 30, 60, 120, and 240 min after the start of the operation. Postoperatively, blood gases and the acid-base status were checked daily until the 4th day postoperation.

Since the dose and the rate of the bupivacaine application were adapted to the individual needs for pain relief, the plasma levels had to be analyzed separately for each patient. The results are therefore presented in a descriptive way.

Results

Case 1

The patient (E. Th., age 51 years, 53 kg, female) underwent total gastrectomy. In 73 h of pain relief during and after surgery, a total dose of 815 mg bupivacaine (0.11 mg/kg/h) were injected into the epidural space. The pattern showed an accumulation of bupivacaine in plasma (Fig. 1). To maintain intraoperative analgesia, three bolus injections of 80, 40, and 50 mg bupivacaine (total intraoperative dose, 170 mg) were given at 0, 1.5, and 4 h. The plasma levels of bupivacaine were 0.69 μg/ml plasma at 73 h. The infusion of 0.12% bupivacaine was started immediately after termination of the operation at a rate of 6 ml/h. One hour later, the patient complained of pain and the analgesia was corrected by a bolus injection of 10 ml 0.125% bupivacaine and the drip rate was increased to 12 ml/h. Nine hours later, the patient again complained of pain and analgesia was again corrected by a bolus injection of 8 ml (10 mg) 0.125% bupivacaine, while the drip was still running at 12 ml/h (or 15 mg/h 0.125% bupivacaine). The plasma levels of bupivacaine showed no changes.

After 11 h, the drip rate was decreased from 12 ml/h to 6 ml/h for 3 h. Despite this decrease of the infused dose of bupivacaine, the plasma levels showed a marked increase. Sixteen hours after the start of the infusion, the patient complained of pain and the analgesia was corrected by a further bolus injection of 8 ml 0.125% bupivacaine and the drip rate was increased again to 12 ml/h and maintained at this rate until the end of postoperative epidural analgesia. Without additional bolus injection and an unchanged drip rate, the plasma levels increased slowly and, at the end of the infusion, were found to be 1.93 μg/ml plasma (Fig. 1). The blood gases and the acid-base status were in the normal range (Fig. 1).

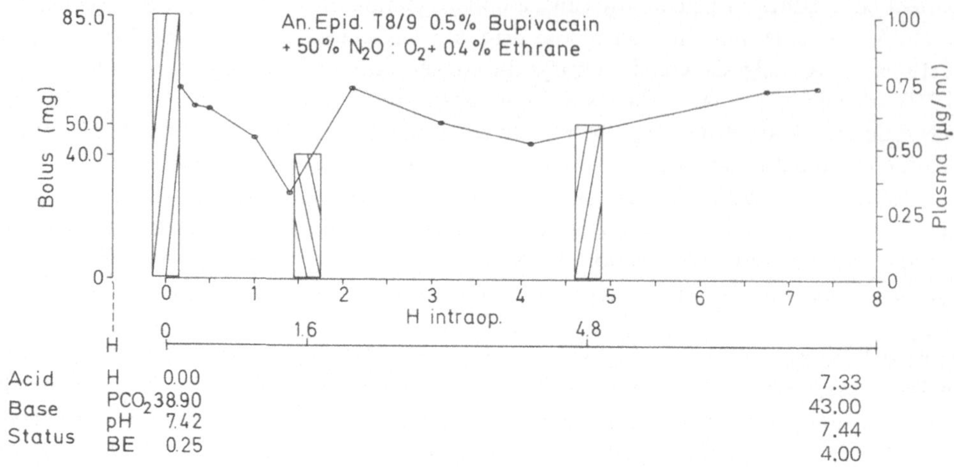

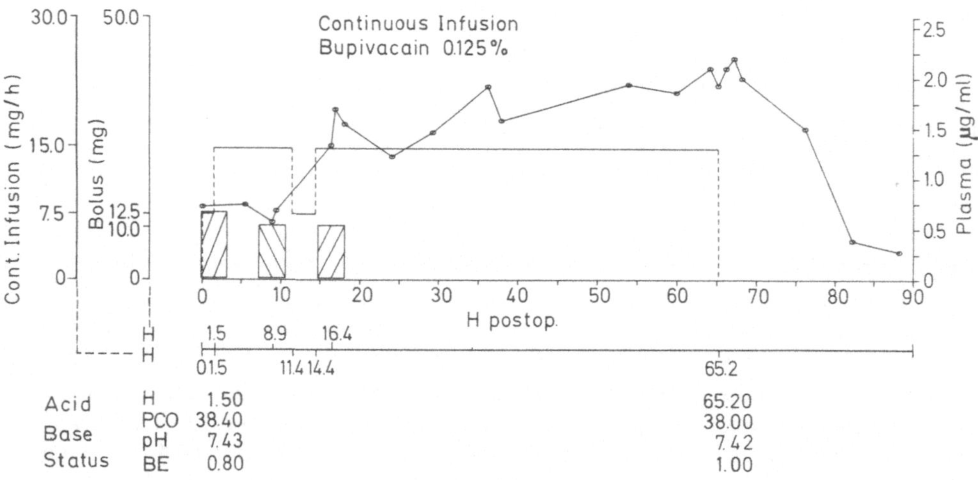

Fig. 1. Case 1 – acid-base status, dosage (bolus injections and the continuous infusion dose is shown in mg/h ——) and the resulting plasma levels during and after operation

Case 2

A completely different pattern was seen in a patient who underwent resection of an aortic aneurysm and in whom an aortofemoral bypass graft was implanted (patient H. M., age 67 years, 75 kg, male; Fig. 2). The intraoperative course of the plasma levels is not shown here. After three bolus injections of 0.5% bupivacaine (total dose, 170 mg), 4 h after the start of the epidural anesthesia the plasma levels were 0.66 µg/ml plasma. For intra- and postoperative pain relief, a total dose of 1,510 mg bupivacaine (0.27 mg/kg/h) was given. In the first

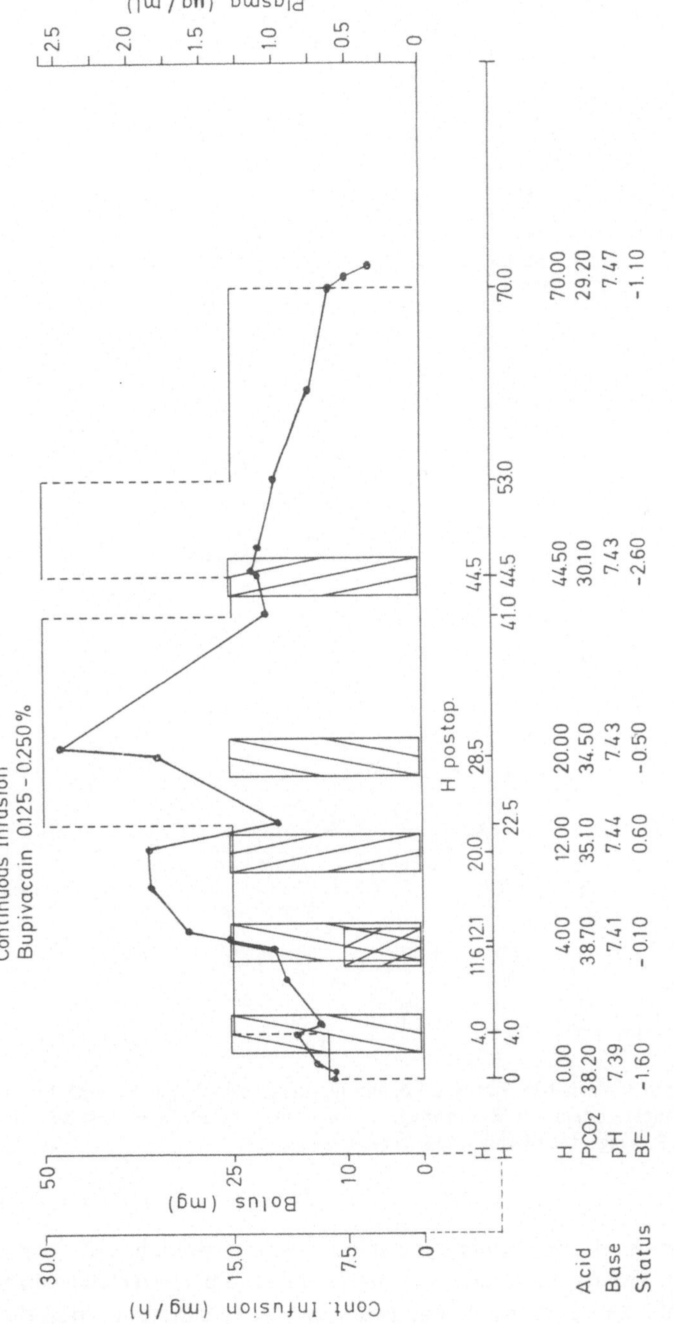

Fig. 2. Case 2 – acid-base status, doses, and resulting blood levels of bupivacaine in the postoperative period. This patient received intraoperatively 170 mg 0.5% bupivacaine in the course of 4 h

28.5 h of the bupivacaine infusion for postoperative pain relief, five corrections of analgesia were necessary. The infusion was started at a drip rate of 6 ml/h (7.5 mg/h) 0.25% bupivacaine. After 4 h, the patient complained of pain and the first bolus injection was given, at which time the drip rate was increased to 15 mg/h. Eleven and twelve hours after the start

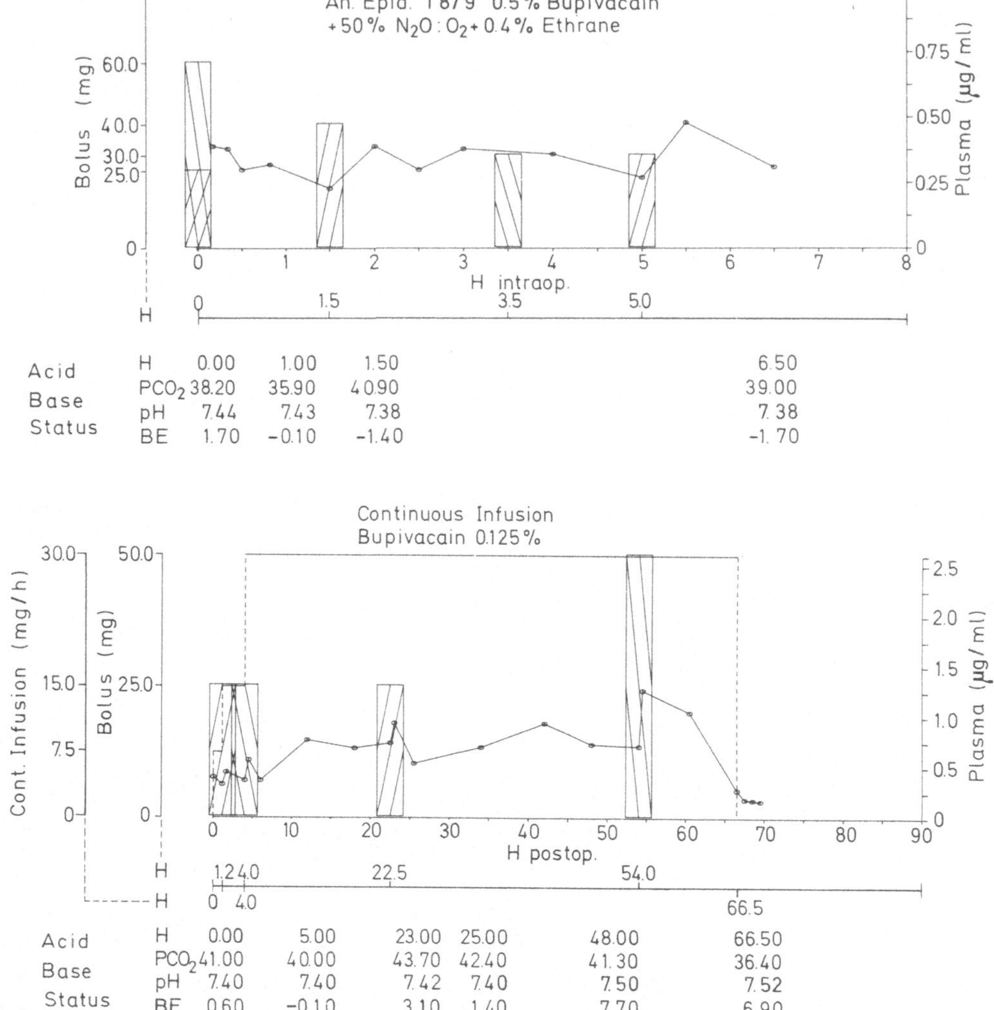

Fig. 3. Case 3 – acid-base status, dose, and plasma levels of a patient with hyperbilirubinemia during and after Whipple's operation. Even though this patient received the highest dose of bupivacaine given in the study (2,334 mg), the plasma levels were very low

of the infusion, two further bolus injections were given, but the drip rate was maintained at 12 ml/h. Twenty hours later, the analgesia had to be corrected again and a bolus injection of 10 ml 0.25% bupivacaine was given. Two and a half hours later, the concentration of the continuous infusion was increased to 0.5% still running at a rate of 12 ml/h. Even with this high dose, the patient complained of pain 6 h later and the block was corrected by an injection of an additional 10 ml 0.5% bupivacaine without changing the drip rate.

Plasma levels increased from 0.66 µg/ml plasma at the beginning to 2.3 µg/ml plasma after 28.5 h. The plasma levels decreased from this point continuously until the 53rd hour.

At that time, the drip rate was reduced to 6 ml/h 0.25% bupivacaine. Plasma levels decreased continuously and were found to be 0.76 μg/ml plasma at the end of the infusion. Even if, on the basis of body weight, the patient received double the dose of local anesthetics given in case 1, the plasma levels were found at the termination of the infusion to be 1.5 times lower than in the first patient. On the 2nd and 3rd postoperative day, the patient showed a respiratory alkalosis (Fig. 2).

Case 3

A similar pattern was seen in a patient with a hyperbilirunemia who underwent Whipple's operation. During the operation and the postoperative epidural analgesia lasting for 66 h, he received a total of 2,334 mg (0.48 mg/kg/h) bupivacaine. Again no accumulation of bupivacaine in plasma was found. At the end of the operation, the patient had received a total of 200 mg 0.5% bupivacaine and the plasma levels were 0.23 μg/ml.

One hour after the start of the infusion 0.125% bupivacaine at a rate of 6 ml/h (7.5 mg/h), the patient complained of pain and in the course of 4 h two corrections were necessary to obtain a satisfactory block. The first time, the patient received 10 ml 0.25% bupivacaine and the continuous infusion was set to 6 ml/h (15 mg/h). Three hours later, an additional correction of the block was necessary. Again 10 ml 0.25% bupivacaine were injected as bolus and the drip rate was increased to 12 ml/h (30 mg/h 0.25% bupivacaine). The plasma levels remained very low in this case. At this rate, plasma levels increased from 0.35 to 0.75 μg/ml. The plasma levels remained very low despite the high drip rate and one additional bolus injection. At the 45th hour, the patient received 10 ml 0.5% bupivacaine to correct the segmental level. At a rate of 6 ml/h (30 mg/h) 0.5% bupivacaine was continuously infused until the end of the epidural blockade. The plasma levels showed a marked decrease until the end of the continuous infusion, inspite of the unchanged rate of infusion. At that point the plasma level had reached a value of 0.23 μg/ml. In the postoperative period the acid-base status showed the tendency toward a metabolic alkalosis (Fig. 3).

As these examples clearly demonstrate – independent of which group the patients belonged to – two different pattern of plasma levels were found: (1) 14 of 25 patients showed a slow but constant increase in plasma levels and, (2) in 11 patients, the plasma levels increased initially until the 1st or 2nd postoperative day, but then decreased or remained stable at a very low level. Even if the total dose and the dose of bupivacaine related to body weight and time did not differ among the three groups, the plasma levels were lower in patients who underwent vascular surgery than in the two other groups (Table 3).

After both upper abdominal surgery and Whipple's operation, the mean values of the bupivacaine levels were higher with a wide variation ranging from 0.23 to 5.3 μg/ml plasma. In four cases they reached toxic levels. In none of our patients, however, were central nervous symptoms or cardiac depression seen.

Elimination of Bupivacaine

The plasma levels of bupivacaine were followed after termination of the infusion for 12 h in four patients with hyperbilirubinemia and in six patients with an arteriosclerotic disease, and for 24 h in six patients who had undergone abdominal surgery (Fig. 4). Starting from a

Table 3. Dosage and plasma levels of bupivacaine in three groups of patients

	n	Total dose of bupivacaine mg x + sd	mg/kg/h x + sd	Plasma level of bupivacaine at the end of infusion µg/ml x + sd
Abdominal surgery	9	1,244.9 ± 699.9	0.26 ± 0.08	2.59 ± 1.66
Vascular surgery	10	1,307.7 ± 758.7	0.24 ± 0.08	1.21 ± 0.4
Whipple's operation	6	1,116.7 ± 713.4	0.25 ± 0.14	1.79 ± 1.8

different level in the three groups of patients, plasma levels showed a marked decrease in the 1st h after upper abdominal surgery and Whipple's operation and only a slight decrease after vascular surgery. The mean values increased by the 2nd h in all three groups, but this increase was more pronounced in patients who had undergone Whipple's operation and was less pronounced in the vascular surgery group. In all patients, a slow but continuous decrease of the blood levels was found during the subsequent period.

Acid-base Status

On average a normal acid-base status was found in our patients. In none of our patients did a significant acidosis or alkalosis develop.

Discussion

The data show that the plasma levels measured in these patients at the end of the infusion were not dose related. The mean plasma levels obtained in the vascular surgery group were lower with less variation than in the other two groups. Both after abdominal surgery and Whipple's operation, the plasma levels were higher, ranging from 0.23 to 5.3 mg/ml plasma. The reason for the differences between the vascular surgery group and the other two groups is not known, but most likely it has to do with the vascularization suggested by Renck [8]. The author found similar plasma levels in two groups of patients with thoracic epidural anesthesia administered for 24 h, in whom three times the quantity of bupivacaine was used in comparison to the thoracic epidural group [8]. The suggestion of Renck [8] is, however, not supported by the results of Appleyard and co-workers [1], who were able to show that the addition of adrenaline to the bupivacaine solution had no significant effect on the uptake of the local anesthetic solution and the resulting plasma levels. The uptake of bupivacaine during administration of continuous epidural anesthetic from the epidural space is, furthermore, influenced, as Renck and co-workers [7] pointed out, by the concentration injected into the epidural space. When infusing 15 to 20 mg/h of a 0.1% bupivacaine solution, a rapid accumulation in plasma occurred over a period of 30 h, but when the same dose per hour was injected in a the tenfold higher concentrated solution (1.0% bupivacaine), the plasma levels were much lower and tended to accumulate less than in the patients who received the weaker solution [7].

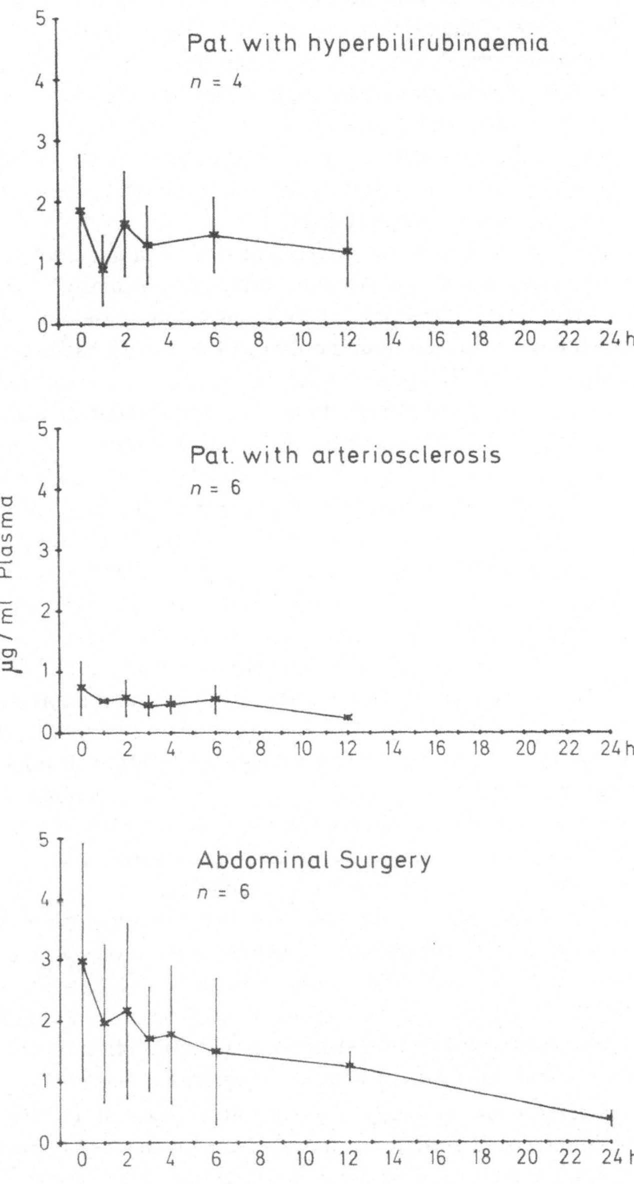

Fig. 4. This figure shows, in some of the patients in the three groups, the decay of the plasma levels after the termination of the continuous infusion. Notice the rapid fall of plasma levels in patients who underwent Whipple's operation and in patients who had abdominal surgery. Free increase until the 2 h may be explained by a redistribution of local anesthetics from a third space, which is followed by a very slow decrease of the plasma levels

Strasser and co-workers [9] showed that the acid-base status in the patient influences the uptake of the local anesthetics. In patients with metabolic acidosis, the plasma levels of etidocaine were found to be significantly higher than in patients with a normal acid-base status [9]. In the present study, however, we were unable to show a correlation between the acid-base status and the plasma levels. The two different patterns of plasma levels that were found in the present study, can thus not be sufficiently explained by the factors influencing uptake of the local anesthetic from the epidural space, such as vascularization [2], blood flow [10], and acid-base status [9].

Renck and co-workers stated in 1975 that accumulation in plasma of long-acting local anesthetics such as bupivacaine or etidocaine regularly occurs in continuous thoracic epidural anesthesia [6]. In the present study, however, increasing plasma levels of bupivacaine with continuous drip were found only in 14 of the 25 patients, irrespective of the group to which they belonged. The plasma levels in four patients were clearly in the toxic range, but without clinical signs of intoxication. This is in agreement with the results of Bromage [3] and Renck et al. [6], who showed that an accumulative absorption from continuous epidurals over a prolonged period is generally better tolerated than a sudden overdosage.

The reasons for the decreasing plasma levels in 11 of our patients is not clear at the present time. In particular, in some of our patients with hyperbilirubinemia and, to some degree, impaired liver function, very low plasma levels were found throughout the continuous epidural analgesia. It is unlikely that, in these patients, an increased metabolism of the local anesthetics in the liver leads to the low plasma levels. Also in hyperbilirubinemia [4] and impaired liver function [5, 10], the plasma levels of amide local anesthetics increased significantly. These controversial results can be partially explained by the fact that the findings of both Chignell [4] and Prescott [5] are based on one single injection of the local anesthetic, while our results are based on a long-term infusion. It might, therefore, very well be possible that the differences are caused, e.g., by a time-dependent enzyme induction of the local anesthetic in the liver or an improvement in liver circulation. These interpretations that the increase in metabolism is due to an improvement of the liver circulation or caused by an enzyme induction are, however, speculative.

Tachyphylaxis clearly occurred in the present study as is did in an earlier published series [11] in all our patients. However, it was not possible to correlate the pattern of the plasma levels with the development of tachyphylaxis. In this context the hemodynamic consequence of pain due to tachyphylaxis has to be stressed [12]. One of the patients in the present series suffered from a myocardial infarction on the 1st postoperative day and died on the 2nd. This patient was in a hypertensive state because of insufficient pain relief during the 1st postoperative day. This case shows once more how important the monitoring and maintenance of sufficient pain relief are for the well-being of patients. To make the continuous technique of epidural analgesia more effective and practicable on the ward, vigorous efforts have therefore to be undertaken to overcome the problem of tachyphylaxis. Local anesthetic solutions with pH values between 7.0 and 7.5 may reduce the rate of tachyphylaxis and thus accumulation.

Conclusion

The present study has shown that there are two patterns of plasma levels in the course of continuous thoracic epidural analgesia: (1) accumulation and (2) after an initial increase, a decrease or a stable plateau until the end of the local anesthetic infusion. At the present time, insufficient explanation of the different patterns and the development of tachyphylaxis can be given. The results show, furthermore, that, from the toxicologic point of view, continuous thoracic epidural anesthesia is a safe technique.

Acknowledgements

We should like to thank Dr. Kazcmarek for his help with the determination of bupivacaine levels in plasma. We would also like express our thanks for the generous financial support of Astra Chemicals, Germany and Sweden.

References

1. Appleyard TN, Witt A, Atkinson RE, Nichols ADG (1974) Bupivacaine carbonate and bupivacaine hydrochloride: a comparison of blood concentrations during epidural blockade for vaginal surgery. Br J Anesth 46:530
2. Bromage PR (1962) Exaggerated spread of epidural analgesia in arteriosclerotic patients. Br Med J II:1634
3. Bromage PR (1967) Physiology and pharmacology of epidural analgesia. Anesthesiology 28:592
4. Chignell CF, Vesell ES, Starkweather DT (1971) The binding of sulfaphenazole to fetal, neonatal and adult plasma albumine. Clin Pharmacol Ther 12:897
5. Prescott LF, Forrest JAH, Adjepen-Yamoak KK, Finlaysen NDC (1975) Drugmetabolism in liver disease. J Clin Pathol [Suppl] 62:82
6. Renck H, Edström H (1975) Thoracic epidural analgesia I. A double-blind study between bupivacaine and etidocaine. Acta Anaesthesiol Scand [Suppl] 57:89
7. Renck H, Edström H, Kinnberger B, Brandt G (1976) Thoracic epidural analgesia II: Prolongation in the early postoperative period by continuous injection of 1,0 % bupivacaine. Acta Anaesthesiol Scand 20:47
8. Renck H (1978) Thoracic epidural analgesia in the management of postoperative pain. Acta Anaesthesiol Scand [Suppl] 70:43
9. Strasser K, Abel J, Breulmann M, Schumacher J, Siepmann HP, Trampisch HJ (1981) Plasmakonzentrationen von Etidocain in den ersten zwei Stunden nach axillärer Blockade bei Gesunden und bei Patienten mit Niereninsuffizienz. Reg Anaesth 4:14
10. Wiklund L, Berlin-Wahlén A (1981) The influence of liver circulation on the pharmacokinetics of local anaesthetics. In: Wüst HJ, Zindler M (eds) Neue Aspekte in der Regionalanaesthesie 2, vol 138, Anaesthesiology and intensive care medicine. Springer, Berlin Heidelberg New York, p 32
11. Wüst HJ, Liebau W, Richter O, Strasser K (1980) Tachyphylaxie bei kontinuierlicher Epiduralanaesthesie mit Bupivacain 0.125% und 0.25% Anaesthesiol Intensivmed Prax 15:159
12. Wüst HJ, Sandmann W, Richter O (1980) Haemodynamische Veränderung durch Schmerzphasen infolge Tachyphylaxie bei postoperativer Epiduralanaesthesie. In: Wüst HJ, Zindler M (eds) Neue Aspekte in der Regionalanaesthesie 1, vol 124, Anaesthesiology and intensive care medicine. Springer, Berlin Heidelberg New York, p 89

Discussion

Stanton-Hicks:

In those patients, in whom the plasma levels began to fall after the 1st or 2nd day, the local anesthetic may have remained as a depot in the epidural space or in the tissues in the paravertebral space.

Wüst:

Unfortunatly we cannot answer this question satisfactorily because we and others have been unable until now to look into the epidural space and find out what is going on. If the local anesthetic stays in the epidural space, I suggest that our block should have been more effective than it has been. Taking the physicochemical properties of the local anesthetics into account, it might be a depot of ionized molecules caused by infusing a high amount of acid solution into the epidural space. These molecules cannot pass into the nerves. But it is also possible that the drug enters the bloodstream more quickly from the acidotic epidural space in one group than in the other and is then metabolized in the liver. A further explanation might be that, in some patients, the drug is metabolized faster in the liver because of an enzyme induction. From our data, the reason for the two different kinetics cannot be found and further research is necessary.

Stanton-Hicks:

These results suggest to me that the drug may not be reaching the liver and the properties that make the drug long acting may be causing it to stay in nontarget tissues, that is, not in nervous tissues, and therefore the drug is not available for blocking. The question is whether the pharmakodynamics are important for preventing further block or acute tolerance from occurring. We don't know. I think the phenomenon that you are seeing is tachyphylaxis whose underlying mechanism is at present not understood.

Observations on Patients Allegedly Allergic to Local Anesthetic Drugs

J. A. Aldrete

Not uncommonly, when patients develop an untoward response during an operative or dental procedure under local anesthesia, it is the local anesthetic agent that appears to be the culprit and, from there on, patients are "labelled" as allergic to that specific drug or, worse yet, to all "caine" drugs [1–3]. This motivated us to investigate several approaches for the purpose of defining the type of untoward reaction suffered by the patient and to attempt to establish whether, in fact, an allergic response had taken place. In our study we tested with various methods and drugs, as well as confirming the patients' acceptability and tolerance of the nonreactive drugs.

Material and Methods

One hundred and nine patients referred to the Anesthesiology Department over a period of 12 years, having antecedents of possible allergy to a local anesthetic drug, were studied as follows:

a) A complete investigation of the incident was made and information was obtained directly from the physician or dentist involved. Specific inquiries were made about the volume and dose of the drug injected, whether it contained vasoconstrictors, preservatives, or any other added compounds, the type of procedure performed and whether any other drugs were applied concomitantly. The type of response was investigated from information given by the patient, the physician or dentist present, and the records available. Evidence of allergy such as erythema, papule, or anaphylaxis, i.e., angioneurotic edema, respiratory embarrassment, cardiac arrest, etc., was sought.

b) Intracutaneous testing was performed with four to six local anesthetics and other solutions as well (Table 4). The volumes and concentrations of the solutions used have been previously described, as have the criteria for quantitatively evaluating the skin responses [4]. Sixteen patients were tested with methylparaben when indicated, while only 72 patients were tested with bupivacaine since it was not available on the market until 1972. This procedure was carried out in the hospital after obtaining the informed consent of the patient, control vital signs were noted, and initially intravenous infusions of crystalloids were given. Once it was found that the reactions noted were of minimal degree and rare, this precaution was not deemed necessary. In every case, however, equipment and drugs used in cardiopulmonary resuscitation were readily available, but were never required.

Table 1. Incidents found by investigation of the events

Type of response	Number of incidents
Rash, edema, and itching	56
Acute anaphylaxis	2
Possible delayed response	3
Signs of mild neurotoxicity	22
Convulsions	11
Convulsions and cardiac arrest	2
Hypotension	9[a]
Vasovagal response	5
Possible drug interaction	2
Surgical or dental trauma	4
Allergy to other drug used	2
Headache	6
Palpitations	11

[a] Hypotension occurred along with other responses

c) In 80 patients, two intramuscular injections of nonreactive anesthetics were given in the same session using 5 ml of the lowest concentration available on the market. These injections were made in the deltoid or anterior thigh regions. Both local and systemic effects were looked for during the following 60-min period.

d) In the first 19 patients, the passive transfer test was performed, in which serum obtained from a possibly allergic individual was injected intradermally into a volunteer previously tested and found to be unresponsive to six local anesthetics. Twenty-four to forty-eight hours later, the same anesthetic drugs were injected at the same injection sites. When positive reactions were noted, the test was repeated after the serum had been heated to 56 °C for 30 min, after which the antibodies are supposed to be lysed and therefore no response should be elecited. This preheated serum was then injected into the volunteers and reactions were noted.

e) Patch tests were conducted in eight patients who received intracutaneous injections in previous studies; the patch was applied on the lateral aspect of the thorax and abdomen and read 48 h later.

f) Observations were also made in 80 volunteer subjects in whom intracutaneous injections with local anesthetic drugs were administered and their responses observed. Those with positive responses returned 24 h later and the injections were repeated 60 min after they had received diphenyl hydramine, 1 mg/kg, intramuscularly.

Results

The results of the investigation, namely the type and degree of incidents, are shown in Table 1. Although in 26 cases complete information on the drugs utilized was unavailable, the

Table 2. Local anaesthetic agents suspected of causing allergy

Drug	Number of cases[a]
Procaine	71 (71)[b]
Tetracaine	12 (12)
Chloroprocaine	5 (5)
Lidocaine	57 (1)
Mepivacaine	7 (2)
Bupivacaine	3 (1)
Cocaine	2 (2)

[a] Several patients were alleged to be allergic to more than one agent
[b] Numbers in parenthesis represent confirmation of allergy

Table 3. Other drug allergies noted in patients supposedly allergic to local anaesthetics

Drug	Number of cases[a]
Penicillin	42
Sulfonamides	19
Other antibiotics	17
Aspirin	26
Codeine	3
Morphine	7
Preservatives	4
Dyes	11

[a] Several patients had allergies to more than one drug

local anesthetic agents suspected of being causative factors in the responses are shown in Table 2. Other drug allergies found when patients were questioned are listed in Table 3; the possibility of drug interaction with sulfa, penicillin, and aspirin may be considered owing to their frequency. The skin responses observed in 109 patients supposedly allergic to local anesthetics are shown in Table 4. The frequency of positive and negative reactions are noted, as well as their intensity.

The results of the two intramuscular injections of the local anesthetic drugs that did not elicit skin response are shown in Table 5. Four patients developed positive reactions. One patient referred to us as having swelling and rash 20 min after the dental injection of 36 mg lidocaine was skin tested and gave a negative response to lidocaine, prilociane, and bupivacaine. The intramuscular administration of lidocaine and prilocaine failed to elicit any untoward reaction. She and her dentist were informed that she could be given both agents. One week later, she tolerated an injection of lidocaine for a dental procedure with no ill effects, however, 2 weeks later, another similar injection produced erythema and several papule, accompanied by itching and edema. Since then, this patient has received prilocaine several times without untoward effects.

Table 4. Results of intracutaneous testing in 109 patients

Drug	No. of patients tested	Positive	Intensity of response			Negative
			+	++	+++	
Procaine	109	71	42	20	9	38
Tetracaine	106	97	57	27	13	9
Chloroprocaine	109	46	28	16	2	63
Lidocaine	109	1	1	–	–	108
Mepivacaine	96	2	2	–	–	94
Prilocaine	109	2	2	–	–	107
Bupivacaine	72	1	1	–	–	71
Methylparaben	16	8	5	3	–	8

Table 5. Incidence and type of response to nonoffending local anesthetics given intramuscularly

Drugs given	No. of patients	Negative	Type of response		
			Pruritus	Positive erythema	Papule
Lidocaine	80	80[a]	–	–	–
Mepivacaine	13	12	1	–	–
Chloroprocaine	8	7	–	1	–
Prilocaine	9	9	–	–	–
Bupivacaine	48	47	1	–	–
Procaine	2	1	–	–	1

[a] One patient with negative response had a reaction to lidocaine later (see text)

Table 6. Skin responses on volunteer subjects given local anesthetic drugs

Drug	Number of reactions
Procaine	12
Tetracaine	21
Chloroprocaine	8
Lidocaine	0
Mepivacaine	0
Prilocaine	0

Observations derived from the passive transfer tests have been previously reported [5] as having confirmed the positive findings of the subcutaneous tests. Epicutaneous testing did not reveal correlation between previous antecedents of drug allergy as shown in Table 6. When the patients returned 24 h later, no cutaneous reactions were seen after the administration of diphenylhydramine.

Discussion

Allergic responses to drugs are a common hazard in medical and dental treatment. In the past when the ester type of local anesthetics were used, they constituted a relatively frequent incidence of drug-elicited reactions [7]. Fortunately, since the advent of local anesthetic drugs of the amide type, these undesirable effects have been more infrequent. Nevertheless, a substantial number of patients who have untoward side effects after receiving local anesthetic drugs are unjustifiably "labelled" as allergic to them. This was evidenced by the apparently high number of patients supposedly allergic to lidocaine and less to other amides (Table 2), in contrast to the very few cases in which this reactivity was confirmed by intracutaneous testing (Table 4) and intramuscular injections (Table 5). Obviously, identification of the manifestations occurring at the time of the supposed "reaction" is useful in ruling out other causes, such as neurotoxicity (intravascular injection) [8], headache, or palpitations (possibly due to the added epinephrine) [9], bradycardia, and hypotension (Vasovagal in origin) [5], and assists in providing a reasonable explanation for the absence of cutaneous response in many of these cases (Table 1). On the other hand, the frequency of positive skin tests to the ester type of local anesthetics was intriguing (Table 4), since many of these patients had in the past received some of these drugs uneventfully. Thus, the frequent false positive reactions noted prompted us to pursue further investigation into this matter. In an earlier report [4], the intracutaneous administration of six local anesthetics to volunteer patients with no drug-allergy history undergoing a surgical procedure failed to show any difference between groups receiving halothane, methoxyflurane, or spinal tetracaine anesthesia. It was evident, however, since only the ester anesthetics elecited reactions, and of these tetracaine most frequently, intrathecal administration did not produce any untoward effects in patients. In this paper, further investigation of such paradoxical responses was conducted in volunteer subjects with no allergic antecendents, who responded in a similar manner to the previously described group [4]. However, when pretreated with an antihistaminic drug 24 h later, no signs of skin response were apparent when the previously reactive local anesthetic drugs were injected. This phenomenon indicates localized histamine release, which may be provoked by the esters without necessarily involving an antigen-antibody reaction (Table 6). This does not preclude the occurrence of an antigen-antibody reaction, but obviously it is extremely rare.

The association of allergy with other drugs in patients supposedly allergic to local anesthetic drugs deserves comment (Table 3). Some cases of penicillin allergy may be related to the use, more frequent in the past, of procaine penicillin, though perhaps some of these moderate cases were more likely due to the former drug than the latter [10]. Sulfonamides and azo-dyes posses and NH_2 radical in the para-position of the benzene ring, similar to the esters, and therefore their linkage in chemical formula suggesting cross-reactivity as a possible mechanism [5].

Lastly, allergy to the preservative methylparaben was initially reported in a patient supposedly allergic to lidocaine [11]. However, the testing solution had been taken from a multiple-dose vial containing the preservative. Skin tests with lidocaine alone failed to produce evidence of allergy, whereas lidocaine with methylparaben or the preservative alone elicited erythema and papules in 8 of the 16 suspected and tested patients. It was felt that the inclusion of these two substances in dental anesthetic solution was not only unnecessary, but may even be the cause of allergic responses and the Federal Drug Administration has recommended its discontinuation following similar reports [12, 13].

From these studies, it is apparent that true allergic reactions to currently used local anesthetic drugs are very rare and, in most instances, moderate, being produced either by local histamine release (easily prevented by an antihistaminic drug, or by cutaneous sensitivity secondary to repeated exposure and, more frequently, produced by esters. Anaphylaxis is fortunately extremely rare and can be investigated by means of the lymphoblast-transformation test [14]. Though skin tests may induce false positive responses, false negatives are infrequent (1 : 109) and therefore it is felt that they are useful, since they allow the clinical anesthesiologist to determine what drugs a patient can safely receive in an emergency. This can be confirmed by the intramuscular injection technique as described [6, 15–17]. By performing these two procedures, patients suspected of being allergic to local anesthetics may still benefit from regional anesthesia techniques once a drug that they can receive without danger has been identified [18, 19].

References

1. Rood JP (1973) A case of lignocaine sensitivity. Br Dent J 135:411–412
2. Goransson K (1976) Hypersensitivity to prilocaine. Dermatologica 152:158–160
3. Selden HM (1967) Reactions to local anesthetics. J Mich Dent Assoc 49:41
4. Aldrete JA, Johnson DA (1970) Evaluation of intracutaneous testing for investigation of allergy to local anesthetic. Anesth Analg 49:173–183
5. Aldrete JA (1973) Reactions to local anesthetic drugs. In: Frazier CA (ed) Allergy and dentistry. Thomas, Springfield
6. Kahn G, Aldrete JA, Ryan SC (1971) Dermic sensitivity to preservatives and local anesthetics, comparison of immediate and delayed hypersensitivity. Ann Allerg 29:480
7. Levine RR (1978) Pharmacology: drug actions and reactions, 2nd ed. Little, Brown, Boston
8. Aldrete JA, Usubiaga LE (1979) New concepts for toxicity for local anesthetic agents. Reg Anesth 4(3):6–11
9. Verrill PJ (1975) Adverse reactions to local anaesthetics and vasoconstrictor drugs. Practitioner 214:380–387
10. Hitschmann OB, Leider M, Baer RL (1950) Dermatitis due to the procaine fraction of procaine penicillin. J Invest Dermatol 15:165–166
11. Aldrete JA, Johnson DA (1969) Allergy to local anesthetics. JAMA 207:356–357
12. Giovannitti JA, Bennett CR (1979) Assessment of allergy to local anesthetics. J Am Dent Assoc 98:701–706
13. Lederman DA, Freedman PD, Kerpel SM, Lumerman H (1980) An unusual skin reaction following local anesthetic injection. Review of the literature and report of four cases. Oral Surg 49:28–33
14. Sabbah A (1978) A study of allergy to local anesthetics using the lymphoblast transformation test. Ann Anesthesiol Fr 17:281–284
15. Aldrete JA, O'Higgins JW (1971) Evaluation of patients with history of allergy to local anesthetic drugs. South Med J 64:1118–1121
16. Sidon MA, Aldrete JA (1971) A patient with multiple allergies: what anesthetic to use. J Am Dent Assoc 82:366–368
17. Arora S, Aldrete JA (1976) Investigation of possible allergy to local anesthetic drugs, correlation of intradermal with intramuscular injections. Anesth Rev 2:13–16
18. Ravindranathan N (1975) Allergic reaction to lignocaine. A case report. Br Dent J 138:101–102
19. Bateman PP (1974) Multiple allergy to local anaesthetics including prilocaine. Med J Aust 2:449–450

Discussion

Schulte-Steinberg:
You see, as far as I understood it, a difference exists between the administration of an ester-type local anesthetic, for example tetracaine, intrathecally or epidurally and a peripheral nerve block. Would you have any objections against giving a patient alleged to be allergic, an intrathecal dose of tetracaine after antihistaminic treatment?

Aldrete:
We have given tetracaine to patients responding positively to the skin test with this drug. We treated them with an antihistaminic and, if they showed no response, then we gave tetracaine intrathecally. But why should one in such a case not choose another drug to which the patient has not responded positively, for example lidocaine or bupivacaine? I prefer to go on the path of safety.

Stanton-Hicks:
We have done skin testing, following which one was always left with the question of whether to use lidocaine in a case with a positive skin test. When lidocaine was subsequently injected, there were no systemic reactions, even when the patient had come from the dentist with a long history of allergy to lidocaine.

Aldrete:
I should mention that, in the USA, methylparaben has in the last 6 months been removed from the dental cartridges. Methylparaben should be removed from all vials because it may produce positive skin-test reactions and make us believe that it was the local anesthetic, the culprit.

Star:
Quite often the dentist combines local anesthetics with adrenaline. It might be also an effect of the adrenaline that the patient experiences palpitations and fainting. Lidocaine is then blamed for this and, for the rest of his life the patient is marked as allergic to lidocaine.

Aldrete:
From the clinical description given by the patient or the doctor/dentist, it is possible to identify what has caused the problem. We should inform the patient and the physician or dentist about what we have done and what we suggest should be used.

Question:
Are there severe allergic reactions after intravenous injections of a placebo?

Aldrete:
Allergic reactions to saline and to distilled water occurred only when the multiple-dose vials contained methylparaben. As far as I know, no allergic reactions to the injection of preservative-free solutions have occurred.

Felius:
Do you have any experience with patients developing malignant hyperthermia after injection of ester-type or amide-type local anesthetics?

Aldrete:
I do not have any personal experience with patients developing malignant hyperthermia during the course of a regional block. But there are reports of patients developing malignant hyperthermia in whom amides, especially lidocaine, were given. It was suggested initially that lidocaine caused the syndrome, but the patients were awake and it is possible that these susceptible patients could also have developed malignant hyperthermia with stress. Wingard tested pigs susceptible to hyperthermia with halothane. In these pigs, he was not able to produce the syndrome with lidocaine either clinically or biochemically. He feels that lidocaine could not produce malignant hyperthermia per se. In our institution we reviewed 32 cases of malignant hyperthermia: 11 patients receiving lidocaine intravenously for the treatment of arrhythmias did not develop the syndrome. More recently, we have done a test determination of the decay of ATP in platelets of patients with a history of malignant hyperthermia. We found that lidocaine was not enlisted in malignant hyperthermia response like halothane or succinylcholine. From this, I feel that you can use ester-type local anesthetics or you may inject amide-type local anesthetics after pretreatment with 8 ml/kg dantrolane 24 h before surgery. But in every case, you should premedicate and sedate the patients heavily, so they do not have stress reactions.

Complications of Epidural Anesthesia in Obstetrics

J. S. Crawford

It would be impossible for me to review even superficially the world literature on this subject within the time allotted for this paper. I intend, therefore, to refer only to our own experience, which is of more than 19,000 epidurals given in an Obstetric Unit. All of these have been continuous lumbar epidurals – none has been a single shot. All injections have been made through a bacterial filter. The test dose has always been 2 ml lignocaine plain (0.5% or 1.0%). Except for brief studies with procaine and etidocaine, the local anaesthetic has invariably been bupivacaine (0.25% or 0.5%, and occasionally 0.375%) and since 1973 it has always been the plain solution.

Maternal Complications

Serious maternal complications have been extremely rare and the two cases that did occur both happened in the early 1970s. One was an epidural abscess, which arose because of haematogenous spread of systemic infection into an epidural haematoma, and the other was a space-occupying lesion in the epidural space due to fibroblastic reaction to a foreign body carried into the space by the epidural needle. Both the patients required a laminectomy and made a full recovery.

The other complications encountered have been of a relatively minor character and have resulted in no residual disability. The most common is total or partial failure to provide analgesia during labour. The incidence of total failure is approximately 4%. The most frequent cause is that the attempt to initiate the epidural was made too late in labour and thus effective analgesia could not be achieved before the mother had delivered. A proportion of the cases of partial relief – which constitute 10%–12% of our series – are due to the same annoying factor. I now believe that it is unwise, except in exceptional circumstances, to attempt to start an epidural on a multigravid with a cervical dilatation of more than 8 cm or a primigravid whose cervix is dilated more than 9 cm. In such situations a spinal block would be a better choice.

Other reasons for total or partial failure include misplacement of the catheter – usually through a paravertebral foramen or too far anteriorly within the epidural space – and a missed segment. Despite experimenting with a number of techniques, we still have no reliable way of eliminating the syndrome of missed segment.

The annual incidence of inadvertent dural puncture has remained consistently at 2% for a decade, reflecting to some extent that we are a training establishment. The routine provision of a post-delivery epidural infusion of Hartmann's solution (1.0–1.5 l in 24–36 h) results in a residual incidence of spinal headache of 25%–30%. For those who develop a headache, an epidural blood patch of up to 20 ml has proved to be remarkably effective. We have now given a blood patch to 169 patients, after either an inadvertent tap or a spinal block, and the success rate has been almost 100% when the approved technique was used. Seven of these patients have had an epidural for a subsequent labour with no evidence of interference with the spread of the local anaesthetic.

On at least seven occasions we have injected the standard top-up dose of bupivacaine intrathecally, without serious consequence – neither severe hypotension nor respiratory embarrassment has resulted. In no instance have we been convinced that the epidural catheter was initially correctly placed and subsequently somehow "wandered" through the dura. Similarly, injections of either the lignocaine test dose or the first dose of bupivacaine into an epidural vein have caused very little distress to the patients involved.

Hypotension due to vaso-motor block has been a relative rarity since we appreciated the absolute requirement to guard against aorto-caval compression and maternal hypovolaemia. If a fall of blood pressure does occur, it is almost invariably corrected rapidly by re-positioning the mother and infusing 1–2 l Hartmann's solution intravenously. We have given ephedrine to only eight labouring patients during the past 13 years and to none of the patients in our most recent series of 300 caesarean sections conducted under epidural block.

We have records of nine cases in which a length of catheter has been broken or sheared off in the epidural space. No action was taken except to reassure the mother and there has been no resultant harm. There has been no instance of prolonged nerve block. However, if the cannula penetrates an intervertebral foramen, and one or two injections of bupivacaine are made through it, there will be sensory and motor loss related to that nerve root which can persist for 24–36 h. Similarly, bladder dysfunction is not related to the autonomic block, but can be a result of the forceps delivery associated with the epidural.

We have records of at least eight mothers who developed a Horner's syndrome – either unilateral or bilateral – during labour under an epidural, without evidence of extensive sensory blockade. I suspect that this occurs much more frequently than we realise. "Marcain shakes" remain an unsolved mystery. They can occur after only one of four or five top-ups, or persist for several hours. I have no idea of their cause or how to treat them successfully. All we do is reassure the mother that they are of no consequence to her or to the baby.

Perinatal Complications

It is now well enough appreciated that an epidural has no adverse effect upon the duration of the first stage of labour. Indeed, by preventing or relieving maternal exhaustion, the epidural helps to avoid the undue prolongation of the first stage. The second stage is undoubtedly likely to be longer than in comparable cases of labour conducted without an epidural, mainly because of the reduction in muscle power and the diminution or suppression of the bearing-down reflex. This should not place the infant in any increased danger. On the contrary, in high-risk cases such as prematurity, intra-uterine growth retardation, breech presentation and multiple pregnancy, this is of significant advantage, as it enables a gentle, well-

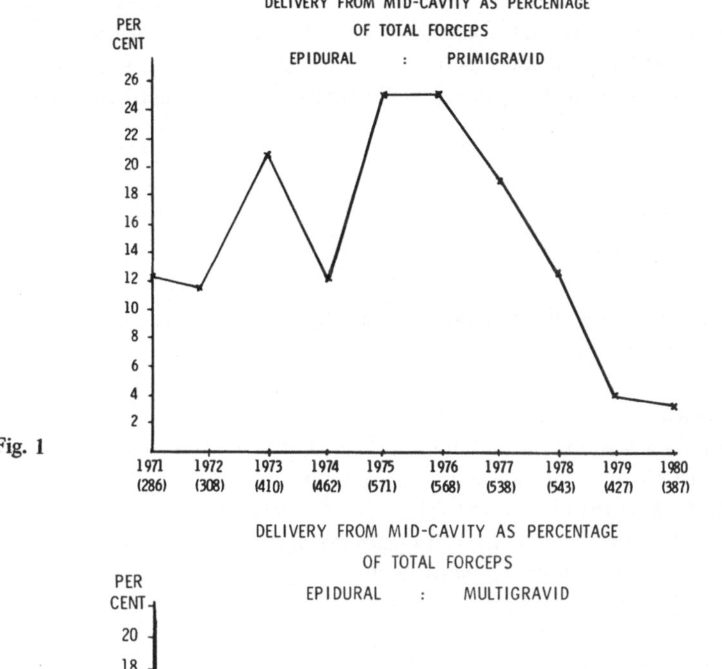

Fig. 1

Fig. 2

controlled delivery to be performed and thus considerably reduces the likelihood of birth trauma.

The major potential complication in this area is that of inexperience or impatience on the part of the obstetrician. Obstetricians have to be discouraged from attempting to expedite the delivery process. Undoubtedly unneccesary birth trauma has been caused by delivery from the mid-cavity in cases in which there was no evidence of fetal distress and the mother was in no way exhausted. Mid-cavity forceps deliveries should be a rarity. Our understanding of this and the results of teaching our obstetric residents the facts can be appreciated from the accompanying figures (Figs. 1 and 2).

The bupivacaine used for our epidurals causes no discernible depression of the neonate. This can be exemplified by the fact that we have given up to 150 ml of the 0.5% solution (300 mg bupivacaine) during a 2–3 h period before delivery by elective section, and yet the clinical condition of the infant at birth and subsequently has been excellent.

If this presentation appears to be more of a list of advantages of obstetric epidural analgesia than of associated complications, the reason is that the complications are so rare and of such little significance as to make it difficult to find any grounds for criticising the application of the technique in a well-staffed and well-organised department.

Discussion

Falke:
Which technique of identifying the epidural space is best to avoid inadvertent lumbar puncture?

Crawford:
I still use a Mac Intosh balloon and I think it is the best way. I allow my residents to use the loss of resistance method with air. Some of them stay with the loss of resistance, some stay with the Mac Intosh balloon. The loss of resistance can be accomplished quite easily with a disposable syringe. You need no glass syringes if you use the proper make of plastic disposable, one which moves forward easily. The position of the patient is the all important thing as van Steenberge said this morning.

(Question:)
One of Dr. Bergmann's slides showed that a cerebral tumor is an absolute contraindication for epidural anesthesia. During a course on epidural analgesia in Kingston, I heard from Dr. Dougthy, however, that a cerebral tumor is an absolute indication to give an epidural for labor. What is your opinion?

Crawford:
In my opinion this is an absolute indication. There is one proviso and I think Gertie Marx made this point some time ago. In her opinion it is more practicable to use a caudal rather than a lumbar epidural if you have a space-occupying intracranial lesion in case you get a wet tap. I still say that this condition, and any chronic neurological disease, is a very strong indication for an epidural in labor.

Bergmann:
I must confess that the contraindications in manifest diseases of the central nervous system I showed this morning only count for spinal and not for epidural anesthesia.

Crawford:
I still do not agree.

Bartel:
Wir führen jährlich bei 2,000–2,500 Geburten eine Single-shot-Epiduralanaesthesie durch. In etwa 10% der Fälle sehen wir oberhalb des Schambeins ein Dreieck, das nicht analgetisch ist. Gibt es dafür eine Erklärung, und wie kann man Abhilfe schaffen?

Crawford:
In some ways it seems to be a missed segment, but we do not see it suprapubicly. Usually it is an oval area in the groin. I have no explanation for it. Sometimes it helps to block the ilio-hypogastric nerve with lignocaine.

Falke:
In my experience unilateral distribution of analgesia is quite common. How do you think one could avoid unilateral distribution and thus increased doses of local anesthetics?

Crawford:
My understanding of the unilateral block is that the cannula has gone around anteriorally and usually you can get bilateral spread by withdrawing the cannula 3 or 4 cm. If that does not work I have to put in another cannula.

Müller:
Wie häufig setzen Sie bei EPH-Gestosen, zur Notfallsektion oder zu sonstigen geburtshilflichen Eingriffen die Epiduralanaesthesie ein? Damit kann der erhöhte Blutdruck gesenkt werden. Bei einer bestehenden Verbrauchskoagulopathie bzw. beim Einsatz von Liquemin droht eine Blutung in den Epiduralraum.

Crawford:
I think this and pre-eclampsia are absolute indications for an epidural in labor and, increasingly, if the patient is going to have a caesarean section. Epidural analgesia will help to reduce the blood pressure, but we do not apply the epidural for that purpose. We give hydralazine, an antihypertensive agent, by pump infusion and an epidural. A coagulation deficit or treatment with heparin is an absolute contraindication.

In-vitro-Untersuchungen zum Einfluß einiger Lokalanaesthetika auf das Zellwachstum – Beitrag zum Mechanismus lokaler Nebenwirkungen

G. Hack und K. Karzel

In letzter Zeit wurde wiederholt über örtliche Gewebsschäden in Verbindung mit Lokal- oder Regionalanaesthesietechniken berichtet. Hierbei ließ sich allerdings ein Kausalzusammenhang mit dem verwendeten Lokalanaesthetikum nicht immer herstellen. Bei klinischen Untersuchungen müssen in diesem Zusammenhang zahlreiche Kovariable berücksichtigt werden, so z. B. die durch einen Vasokonstriktorzusatz induzierte Gewebsnekrose, eine mechanische Irritation des Nerven durch die Kanüle, eine Hämatombildung oder die versehentliche intraneurale Injektion [11, 30, 31]. Der eindeutige Zusammenhang zwischen Hornhautulzera und Langzeitapplikation lokalanaesthesierender Augentropfen [9, 23, 25], beobachtete Anstiege der Kreatininphosphokinaseaktivität nach intramuskulärer Applikation von Lidocain [36] und tierexperimentell nachgewiesene histotoxische Effekte höher konzentrierter Tetracain-, Etidocain- und Bupivacainlösungen [1, 29] sprechen indes für einen direkten gewebsschädigenden Effekt der Lokalanaesthetika. Darüber hinaus könnte auch die für einige Substanzen nachgewiesene antiphlogistische [10, 26] und bakteriostatische [19, 35] (Neben)wirkung auf einer zytostatischen Wirkungskomponente beruhen.

Nach dem bisherigen Kenntnisstand kommen als Voraussetzungen für örtliche Gewebsschäden durch Lokalanaesthetika 2 Faktoren in Frage:

1. die Fixation bzw. Retention der Substanz im Gewebe, somit die Einwirkungsdauer,
2. die relativ hohe Konzentration des Lokalanaesthetikums, welcher die Gewebszellen am Applikationsort ausgesetzt sind.

Zur Klärung möglicher zellschädigender Effekte durch Lokalanaesthetika erscheinen In-vitro-Kulturen tierischer Zellen aus verschiedenen Gründen geeignet:

1. keine modifizierenden oder regulierenden Einflüsse durch übergeordneten Organismus;
2. keine Metabolisierungs- und Eliminationsvorgänge;
3. zeitweise oder permanent in vitro lebens- und vermehrungsfähige Zellen mit hoher Empfindlichkeit gegenüber zytotoxischen Pharmakawirkungen;
4. Suspensionskulturen (Ehrlich-Ascitestumorzellen = EATC): parallele Erfassung zellphysiologischer, biochemischer und morphologischer Parameter; getrennte Ermittlung biochemischer Kenngrößen in Zellen und Kulturmedium möglich;
5. Tumorzellen: intensiver Stoffwechsel, hohe Vermehrungsrate.

Methodik

Die von uns verwendeten EATC [16] wachsen in einem bis auf einen Zusatz von 15% Pferdeserum chemisch definierten Flüssigmedium ([28], leicht modifiziert) im geschlossenen System bei einer Inkubationstemperatur von 37 °C permanent in vitro. Die Inkubationszeit nach Applikation der Lokalanaesthetika betrug einheitlich 24 h. Sowohl vom Ausgangsmaterial als auch nach Abschluß der Inkubation von unbehandelten Kontrollkulturen und den mit 6 verschiedenen Lokalanaesthetikakonzentrationen behandelten Kulturen wurden aliquote Mengen zur parallelen Erfassung von Zellzahl und mittlerem Zellvolumen mit Hilfe des elektronischen Zählgerätes nach Coulter (Coulter Counter^R, Modell ZB, Meßkapillare 200 μm Durchmesser) [7, 17] sowie zellulärem Protein- [24], DNA- [5] und RNA-Gehalt [14] herangezogen. Zur Untersuchung kamen grundsätzlich die Reinsubstanzen, welche in physiologischer Elektrolytlösung gelöst und mit Kulturmedium weiter verdünnt wurden. Die statistische Auswertung der gewonnen Daten erfolgte regressions- und korrelationsanalytisch mit Hilfe der Methode der kleinsten Quadrate unter Berücksichtigung linearer und nichtlinearer Modelle [27]. Zur Bestimmung der mittleren zytostatisch wirksamen Konzentration (ID_{50}) der Prüfstoffe diente das Verfahren von Litchfield u. Wilcoxon [22]. Aus Gründen der besseren Vergleichbarkeit sind auf den Abbildungen für jeden Parameter die prozentualen Abweichungen zu unbehandelten Kontrollkulturen wiedergegeben, deren Werte gleich 100% gesetzt wurden. Nicht signifikante Ergebnisse sind durch unterbrochene Linienführung gekennzeichnet.

Die Untersuchungen erstreckten sich auf folgende Lokalanaesthetika: Procainhydrochlorid (Novocain), Tetracainhydrochlorid (Pontocain), Oxybuprocain (Novesine), Lidocain (Xylocain), Mepivacain (Scandicain), Carticain (Ultracain) und Bupivacain (Carbostesin).

Ergebnisse

Auf Abb. 1 ist der Einfluß der geprüften Lokalanaesthetika in Form von Dosis-Wirkungs-Kurven dargestellt. Für die jeweiligen Anaesthetikumkonzentrationen in mmol/l wurde die beobachtete Hemmung der Zellvermehrung auf unbehandelte Kontrollkulturen bezogen. Wie aus der Darstellung hervorgeht, besitzt Procain eine deutlich geringere wachstumshemmende Aktivität als die beiden anderen esterförmigen Lokalanaesthetika Tetracain und Oxybuprocain. Allerdings zeichnen sich die Dosis-Wirkung-Kurven dieser 3 Verbindungen durch einen vergleichbar steilen Verlauf aus. Im Gegensatz dazu weisen die Lokalanaesthetika vom Säureamidtyp flacher verlaufende Dosis-Wirkungs-Kurven auf. Lidocain und Mepivacain ließen nahezu identische Wirkungsstärken erkennen. Für Carticain ergab sich dagegen eine mäßige und für Bupivacain sogar eine starke Linksverschiebung in den niedrigen Konzentrationsbereich.

Durch den Nachweis eventueller Veränderungen der durchschnittlichen Zellgröße sowie des Protein-, DNA- und RNA-Stoffwechsels sollte ein genauerer Einblick in die möglichen Angriffsorte der Lokalanaesthetika innerhalb des Zellgenerationszyklus erzielt werden. Lidocain verursachte im Konzentrationsbereich zwischen 0,1 und 2,0 mmol/l eine konzentrationsabhängige Hemmung des Zellzuwachses (Abb. 2). Zwischen 2,0 und 4,0 mmol/l zeigte die Zellzahlkurve dagegen einen abgeflachten Verlauf. Unter den übrigen Parametern

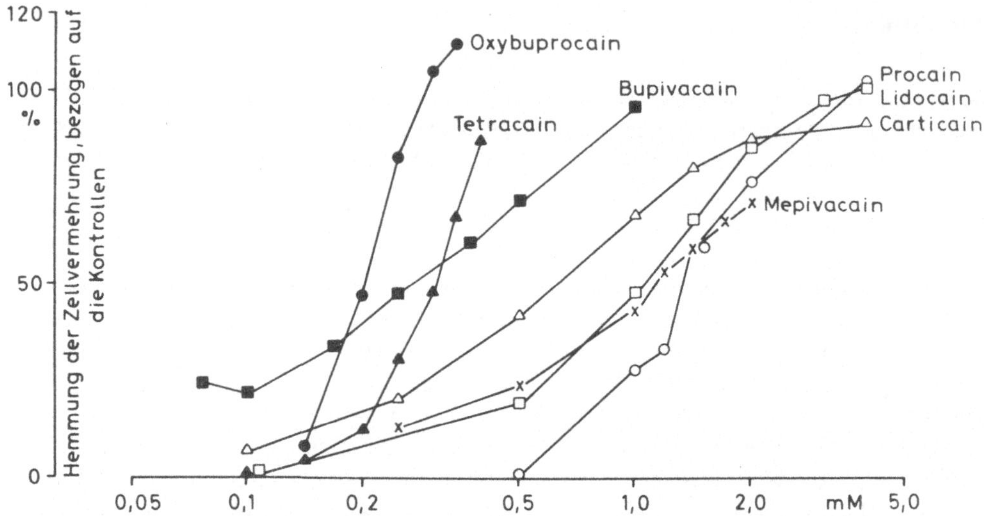

Abb. 1. Einfluß der geprüften Lokalanaesthetika auf die Vermehrung in vitro gezüchteter EATC bei einer Inkubationszeit von 24 h. Die über 100% liegenden Werte entsprechen einem zusätzlichen zytoziden Effekt

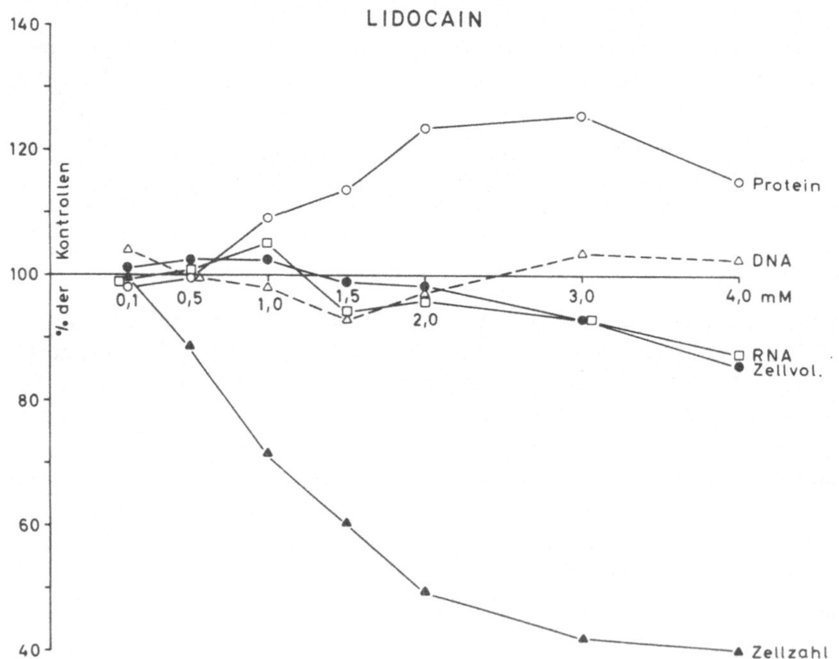

Abb. 2. Prozentuale Veränderungen der Vermehrung, des mittleren Volumens sowie des Protein-, DNA- und RNA-Gehaltes in vitro gezüchteter EATC durch Lidocain (0,1 – 0,4 mmol/l), bezogen auf unbehandelte Kontrollkulturen; Inkubationszeit: 24 h

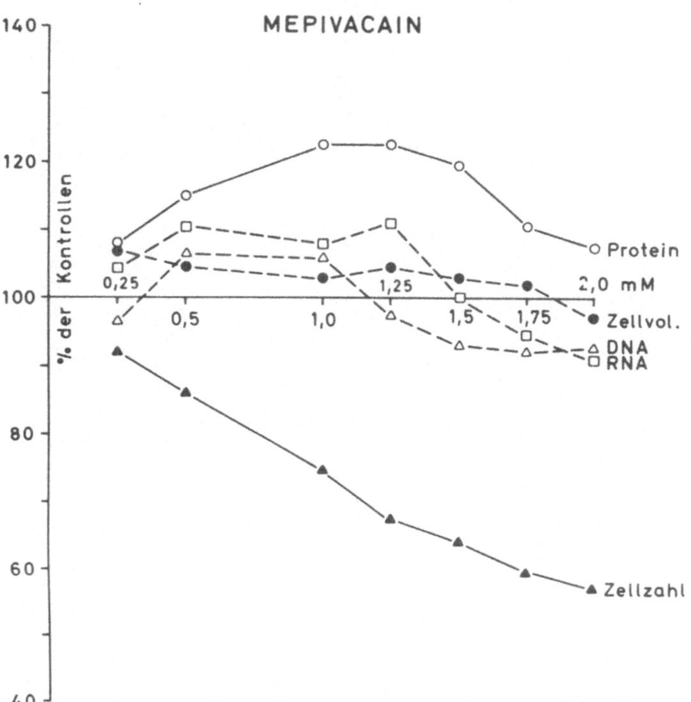

Abb. 3. Prozentuale Veränderungen der Vermehrung, des mittleren Volumens sowie des Protein-, DNA- und RNA-Gehaltes in vitro gezüchteter EATC durch Mepivacain (0,25–2,0 mmol/l), bezogen auf unbehandelte Kontrollkulturen; Inkubationszeit: 24 h

wies der zelluläre Proteingehalt mit einer deutlichen Zunahme bis 3,0 mmol/l die auffälligsten Veränderungen auf. Für den DNA-Gehalt konnte keine statistisch signifikante Abweichung von unbehandelten Zellen nachgewiesen werden. RNA-Gehalt und mittleres Zellvolumen waren erst unter 3,0 und 4,0 mmol/l leicht erniedrigt.

Unter zytostatischen Konzentrationen von Mepivacain mit nahezu linearer Abnahme der Zellzahl ergaben sich nur für den zellulären Proteingehalt signifikante Veränderungen (Abb. 3). Im Vergleich zu den Kontrollen nahm er bis 1,25 mmol/l zu, bei höherer Dosierung jedoch wieder ab, ohne dabei das Kontrollniveau zu erreichen. Die ermittelten Werte für die Nukleinsäuren und das mittlere Zellvolumen divergierten nur um maximal 10% vom Kontrollniveau.

Vergleicht man die durch Lidocain mit den durch Carticain bedingten prozentualen Veränderungen der untersuchten Kenngrößen (Abb. 4), so fallen gewisse Parallelen auf. Auch hier zeigt die Konzentrations-Wirkungs-Kurve für den zytostatischen Effekt im unteren Dosierungsbereich einen steil abfallenden, im höheren dagegen flachen Verlauf. Relevante Zunahmen wies auch hier nur der zelluläre Proteingehalt auf. Mittleres Zellvolumen sowie Nukleinsäurewerte waren unter der höchsten geprüften Carticainkonzentration deutlich vermindert.

Für Bupivacain ließ sich ein zytostatischer Effekt bereits unter der niedrigsten geprüften Konzentration von 0,075 mmol/l nachweisen (Abb. 5). Auch wurden eine Zunahme des zellulären Proteingehaltes im mittleren sowie eine Abnahme des Durchschnittsvolumens der

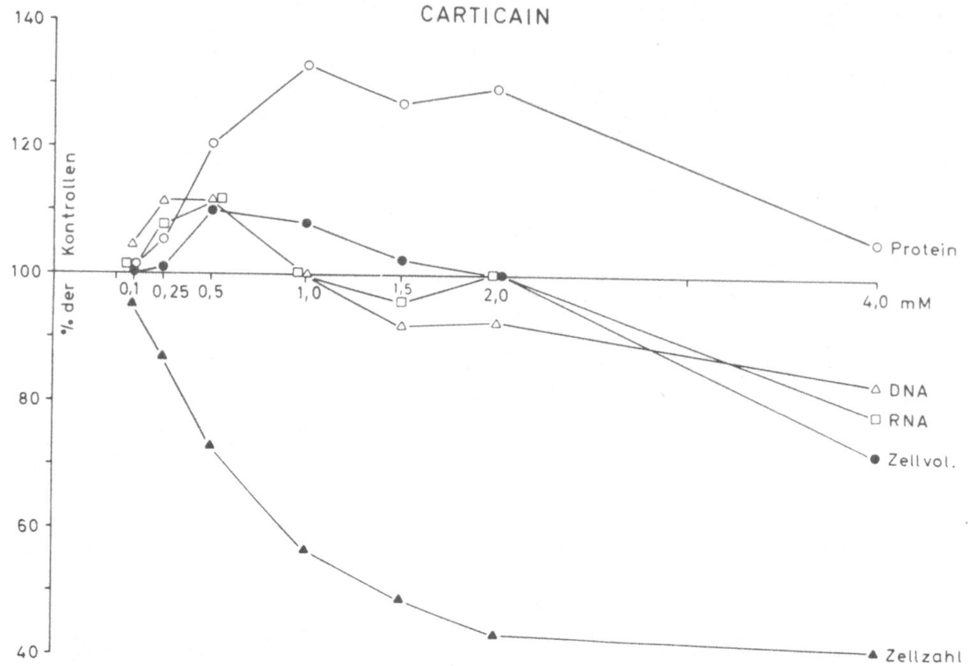

Abb. 4. Prozentuale Veränderungen der Vermehrung, des mittleren Volumens sowie des Protein-, DNA- und RNA-Gehaltes in vitro gezüchteter EATC durch Carticain (0,1–4,0 mmol/l), bezogen auf unbehandelte Kontrollkulturen; Inkubationszeit: 24 h

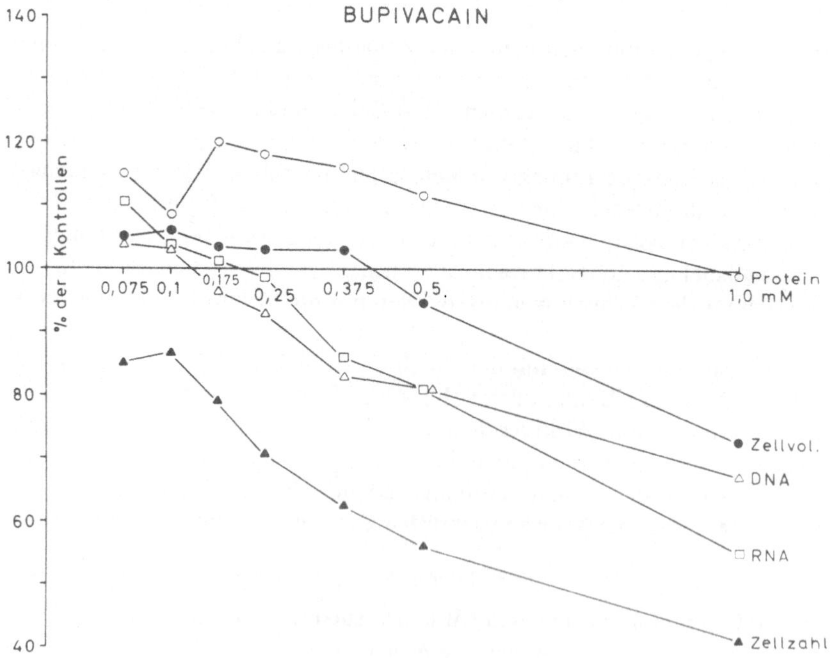

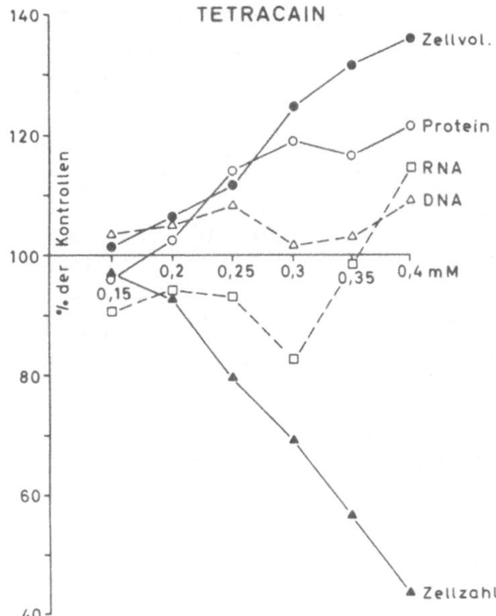

Abb. 6. Prozentuale Veränderungen der Vermehrung, des mittleren Volumens sowie des Protein-, DNA- und RNA-Gehaltes in vitro gezüchteter EATC durch Tetracain (0,15–0,4 mmol/l), bezogen auf unbehandelte Kontrollkulturen; Inkubationszeit: 24 h

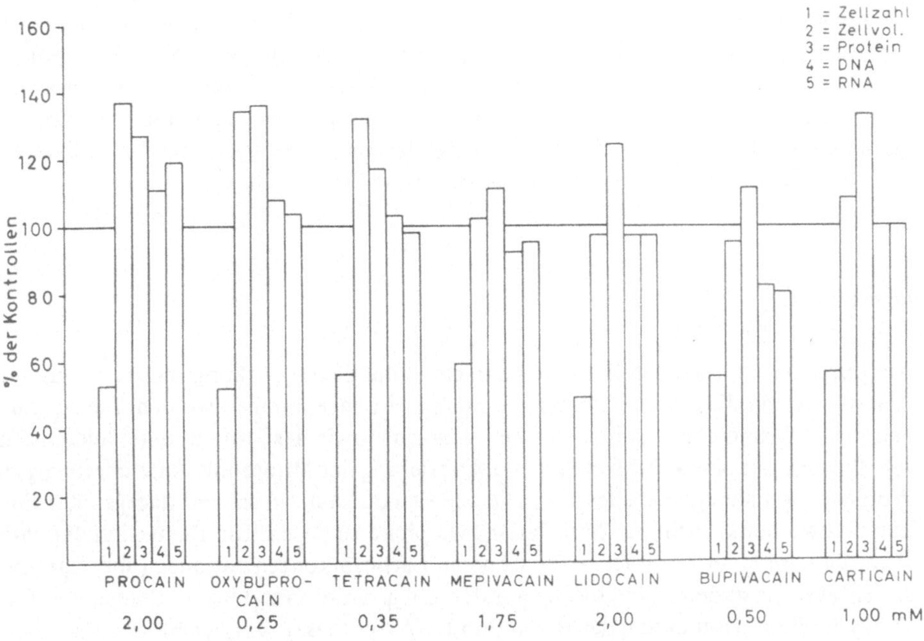

Abb. 7. Vergleichende Darstellung der Veränderungen des mittleren Zellvolumens sowie des zellulären Protein-, DNA- und RNA-Gehaltes durch zytostatisch annähernd äquieffektive Lokalanaesthetikadosen (EATC, Inkubationszeit: 24 h)

◀ **Abb. 5.** Prozentuale Veränderungen der Vermehrung, des mittleren Volumens sowie des Protein-, DNA- und RNA-Gehaltes in vitro gezüchteter EATC durch Bupivacain (0,075–1,0 mmol/l), bezogen auf unbehandelte Kontrollkulturen; Inkubationszeit: 24 h

Tabelle 1. Klinisch übliche Konzentration, C_m- und ID_{50}-Wert für Procain, Tetracain und Lidocain

	Klinisch übliche Konzentration		C_m-Wert[a]	Zytostatische ID_{50}[b]	ID_{50}/C_m
	[%]	[mmol/l]	[mmol/l]	[mmol/l]	
Procain	1,0–2,0	36,7–73,3	8,0	1,35	0,17
Tetracain	0,1–2,0	3,3–66,5	0,6	0,29	0,48
Lidocain	0,5–2,0	18,5–73,9	2,5	1,02	0,41

[a] Untersuchungen am Froschnerven (Sciaticus), pH 7,2–7,3 [33]
[b] Untersuchungen an Ehrlich-Ascites-Tumorzellen, Inkubationszeit 24 h [12]

Zellpopulation im hohen Dosierungsbereich deutlich. Der Trend zur Verringerung des zellulären Nukleinsäuregehaltes zeigte sich bereits unter 0,375 mmol/l.

Unter Tetracain ließen sich für die Nukleinsäuren regressionsanalytisch keine gerichteten Veränderungen nachweisen (Abb. 6). Im Gegensatz zu den Lokalanaesthetika vom Säureamidtyp wiesen diese und andere esterförmige Substanzen eine deutliche Zunahme der mittleren Zellgröße unter den geprüften Konzentrationen auf.

Dies geht aus der zusammenfassenden Übersicht (Abb. 7) hervor, bei welcher äquieffektive Lokalanaesthetikakonzentrationen mit 40–50%iger Reduktion der Zellzahl nebeneinander gestellt sind. Lokalanaesthetika vom Estertyp verursachten Zellvergrößerungen um 32–37% und Zunahmen des Proteingehaltes um 17–36%. Die Nukleinsäurewerte zeigten nur bei Procain deutliche Zunahmen. Bei den Substanzen vom Amidtyp bildet demgegenüber der zelluläre Proteingehalt allein den Gipfel des jeweiligen Wirkungsprofils. Der zelluläre DNA- und RNA-Gehalt ist einzig bei Bupivacain um rund 20% deutlich erniedrigt.

Diskussion

Aufgrund der vorliegenden Befunde kann ein einheitlicher Wirkungsmechanismus der Lokalanaesthetika für die Zellwachstumshemmung nicht angenommen werden. Für Procain ergeben sich aufgrund der Zunahme des Zellvolumens sowie des Protein- und Nukleinsäuregehaltes Hinweise auf eine kolchizinähnliche Arretierung der Mitose mit Anreicherung großer Prophase- und Metaphasezellen. Für alle anderen Substanzen scheint dagegen der Einwirkungsschwerpunkt mehr im Bereich der Interphase zu liegen. Die Reduktion der Nukleinsäuresynthese unter Bupivacain und höheren Carticainkonzentrationen (über 2,0 mmol/l) spricht für eine gezielte Einwirkung auf den Zellgenerationszyklus im Bereich des G1- und S-Stadiums (Hemmung der RNA- und DNA-Synthese). Vergleicht man die beim Menschen üblichen klinischen Konzentrationen und die minimale anaesthetisch wirksame Konzentration, den sog. C_m-Wert, einiger Lokalanaesthetika [33] mit den von Hack [12] für das vorliegende Zellmodell ermittelten zytostatischen ID_{50}-Werten (Tabelle 1), so wird ersichtlich, daß die Lokalanaesthetika die Zellvermehrung bereits unterhalb des klinisch relevanten Konzentrationsbereiches hemmen. Zu ähnlichen Befunden kamen Sturrock u. Nunn [32], die für Procain, Lidocain und Bupivacain bei In-vitro-Studien an Fibroblastenkulturen ED_{50}-Werte ermittelten, die sich als 10fach niedriger erwiesen als klinisch übliche Dosierungen.

Grundsätzlich gilt jedoch, daß sich In-vitro-Befunde nur mit Einschränkungen auf klinische Bedingungen bzw. Verhältnisse im intakten Organismus übertragen lassen. Neben der großen Schwankungsbreite für den C_m-Wert, die durch den chemischen Aufbau des jeweiligen Lokalanaesthetikums [4, 8, 34], den pH-Wert im Gewebe, die Dissoziationskonstante sowie die Elektrolytverhältnisse am Wirkort [6, 20] und einen variablen Markgehalt der Nervenfaser [15] bedingt ist, sind unterschiedliche Verteilungskoeffizienten und Proteinbindungskapazitäten zu berücksichtigen. Zudem dürfte bei der einmaligen örtlichen Injektion von Lokalanaesthetika die Einwirkungszeit in der Regel zu kurz sein, um Gewebsschäden auszulösen, zumal die meisten betroffenen Gewebe eine weniger hohe Zellumsatzrate aufweisen als EATC oder z. B. embryonale Gewebe. Anders liegen allerdings die Verhältnisse bei der chronischen Anwendung von Tetracain oder Oxybuprocain als Oberflächenanaesthetika oder von Bupivacain als Langzeitlokalanaesthetikum im Rahmen einer postoperativ weitergeführten Analgesie über den Periduralkatheter. Die eingangs erwähnten Kreatininphosphokinaseerhöhungen nach intramuskulärer Lidocaininjektion [36] sowie histologisch verifizierte Muskelzellalterationen nach Gabe von Bupivacain [2, 3, 21] geben einen deutlichen Hinweis darauf, daß auch in adulten Geweben mit geringer Proliferationstätigkeit lokale Schädigungen durch Lokalanaesthetika prinzipiell möglich sind.

Nicht nur im Hinblick auf eventuelle Toxizitätserscheinungen im systemischen Bereich, sondern auch in Anbetracht einer möglichen lokalen Gewebsschädigung sollten Lokalanaesthetika somit nur in der geringstmöglichen Konzentration und nicht über einen unkontrolliert langen Zeitraum zur Anwendung kommen.

Zusammenfassung

Ziel der vorliegenden Untersuchungen war, einen Beitrag zum Mechanismus örtlicher Nebenwirkungen von Lokalanaesthetika (Procain, Tetracain, Oxybuprocain, Lidocain, Mepivacain, Carticain und Bupivacain) zu leisten. Am Modell von permanent in vitro in Suspensionsform wachsenden EATC sollte anhand von Bestimmungen der Zellzahl, des mittleren Zellvolumens sowie des zellulären Protein-, DNA- und RNA-Gehaltes geprüft werden, ob und gegebenenfalls in welchen Konzentrationsbereichen Lokalanaesthetika Einflüsse auf die Zellvermehrung und den Vermehrungsstoffwechsel ausüben. Für alle Substanzen konnte eine Hemmung des Zellwachstums im klinischen Konzentrationsbereich nachgewiesen werden, wobei von den esterförmigen Lokalanaesthetika Oxybuprocain und Tetracain, von den amidförmigen Bupivacain die stärksten Effekte aufwiesen. Für die Zellwachstumshemmung der geprüften Substanzen kann kein einheitlicher Wirkungsmechanismus angenommen werden. Während sich für Procain gewisse Hinweise für einen kolchizinähnlichen Effekt im Bereich der Metaphase finden, scheint für alle anderen Lokalanaesthetika der Einwirkungsschwerpunkt mehr in der Interphase zu liegen. Bei Bupivacain dürfte die zytostatische Wirkung auf einer gezielten Hemmung der Nukleinsäuresynthese beruhen, während bei anderen Substanzen vom Säureamidtyp eine Verlängerung der gesamten Generationszeit diskutiert werden muß.

Literatur

1. Adams HJ, Mastri AR, Eichholzer AW, Kilpatrick G (1974) Morphologic effects of intrathecal etidocaine and tetracaine on the rabbit spinal cord. Anesth Analg (Cleve) 53:904
2. Benoit PW, Belt WD (1970) Destruction and regeneration of skeletal muscle after treatment with a local anaesthetic, bupivacaine (Marcaine[R]). J Anat 107:547
3. Benoit PW, Belt WD (1972) Some effects of local anesthetic agents on skeletal muscle. Exp Neurol 34:264
4. Büchi J, Perlia X (1971) Structure-activity relations and physiochemical properties of local anesthetics. In: Lechat P (ed) Local anesthetics. Pergamon, Oxford (International encyclopedia of pharmacology and therapeutics, Section 8, vol 1) p 70
5. Ceriotti G (1952) A microchemical determination of desoxyribonucleic acid. J Biol Chem 198:297
6. Condouris GA, Lagomarsino WE (1966) Adreanalectomy in rats and its influence on local anesthesia of peripheral nerves. J Pharmacol Exp Ther 152:417
7. Coulter WH (1956) High speed automatic blood cell counter and cell size analyzer. Proc Soc Natl Electr Conf Chicago 12:1034
8. Covino BG, Vasallo HG (1976) Local anesthetics. Mechanisms of action and clinical use. Grune & Stratton, New York
9. Cullen BF (1979) Cellular effects, teratogenicity and toxicity of anesthetics (Abstr.). ASA Annual Meeting 1979 Refresher Course Lectures: 217
10. Eifinger FF (1963) Infiltrationsanästhesie und Pulpitis-Therapie. Dtsch Zahnarztl Z 18:1129
11. Fink BR (1973) Acute and chronic toxicity of local anaesthetics. Can Anaesth Soc J 20:5
12. Hack G (1978) Zur Frage des cytostatischen Effektes einiger Lokal- und Inhalationsanästhetika – Untersuchungen an Suspensionskulturen von Ehrlich-Ascitestumorzellen. Habilitationsschrift, Universität Bonn
13. Hack G, Karzel K (1981) Suspensionskulturen von Ehrlich-Ascitestumorzellen als Arbeitsmodell zum Nachweis zelltoxischer Anästhetikawirkungen. Anaesthesist 30:88
14. I-San Lin R, Schjeide OA (1969) Microestimation of RNA by the cupric ion-catalyzed orcinol reaction. Anal Biochem 27:473
15. De Jong RH (1970) Physiology and pharmacology of local anesthesia. Thomas, Springfield
16. Karzel K (1965) Über einen in vitro in Suspension wachsenden permanenten Stamm von Ehrlich-Ascitestumorzellen. Med Pharmacol Exp 12:137
17. Karzel K, Hack G (1972) Zellvolumen und Volumenverteilung bei einem permanent in vitro in Suspensionsform wachsenden Stamm von Ehrlich-Ascitestumorzellen. Arzneimittelforsch 22:1793
18. Karzel K, Breull W, Hack G (1970) Zur quantitativen Bewertung von Pharmaka-Einflüssen auf Lebens- und Stoffwechselvorgänge von Zellkulturen in Suspensionsform. Arzneimittelforsch 20:1843
19. Knothe H, Hoppe WF (1965) Experimentelle Untersuchungen über die antibakterielle Wirkung verschiedener Oberflächenanästhetika. Dtsch Zahnarztl Z 20:840
20. Levy RH (1974) Local anesthetic structure, activity and mechanism of action. In: Eger II EI (ed) Anesthetic uptake and action. Williams & Wilkins, Baltimore, p 323
21. Libelius R, Sonesson B, Stamenovic BA, Thesleff S (1970) Denervation-like changes in skeletal muscle after treatment with a local anaesthetic (Marcaine[R]). J Anat 106:297
22. Litchfield JT Jr, Wilcoxon F (1949) A simplified method of evaluating dose-effect experiments. J Pharmacol Exp Ther 96:99
23. Nowak A, Zschausch K (1971) Medikamentöse Hornhautschäden. Dtsch Arztebl 68:2331
24. Oyama VJ, Eagle H (1956) Measurement of cell growth in tissue culture with a phenol reagent (Folin-Ciocalteu). Proc Soc Exp Biol 91:305
25. Pau H (1971) Hornhautschädigungen durch Anästhetika. Bekanntgabe der Arzneimittelkommission der Deutschen Ärzteschaft. Dtsch Ärztebl 68:2637
26. Rost A (1967) Tierexperimentelle Untersuchungen über die entzündungshemmende Wirkung von Hostacain und Oxyprocain forte. Dtsch Zahnarztl Z 22:367
27. Sachs L (1972) Statistische Auswertungsmethoden, 3. Aufl. Springer, Berlin Heidelberg New York
28. Schindler R, Day M, Fischer GA (1959) Culture of neoplastic mast cells and their synthesis of 5-hydroxy-tryptamine and histamine in vitro. Cancer Res 19:47

29. Schubert HJ, Nolte H, Rudolph R (1977) Histotoxische Veränderungen durch Bupivacain und Etidocain nach perineuraler und subduraler Injektion. In: Meyer J, Nolte H (Hrsg) Die Pharmakologie, Toxikologie und klinische Anwendung langwirkender Lokalanästhetika. Thieme, Stuttgart, S 17
30. Selander D, Dhuner KG, Lundborg G (1977) Peripheral nerve injury due to injection needles used for regional anesthesia. An experimental study of the acute effects of needle point trauma. Acta Anaesthesiol Scand 21:182
31. Stöhr M, Mayer K (1976) Nervenwurzelläsionen durch Neuraltherapie. Dtsch Med Wochenschr 101:1218
32. Sturrock JE, Nunn JF (1979) Cytotoxic effects of procaine, lignocaine and bupivacaine. Br J Anaesth 51:273
33. Truant AP, Takman B (1959) Differential physico-chemical and neuropharmacologic properties of local anesthetic agents. Anesth Analg (Cleve) 38:478
34. Tucker GT (1975) Plasma binding and disposition of local anesthetics. In: Dal Santo G (ed) Biotransformation of local anesthetics, adjuvants, and adjunct agents. I. A. C. Little Brown, Boston, p 33
35. Winther JE, Praphailong L (1969) Antimicrobial effect of anesthetic sprays. Acta Odontol Scand 27:205
36. Zener JC, Harrison DC (1974) Serum enzyme values following intramuscular administration of lidocaine. Arch Intern Med 34:48

Reaction on the Skin and in the Epidural Space after Continuous Epidural Anesthesia

H. J. Wüst, W. Wechsler, and W. Hort

For many years, continuous epidural anesthesia has been the method of choice for the provision of analgesia during and after operations in our department. Two cases of anterior spinal artery syndrome [3] have occurred during the course of aortofemoral-bypass surgery. The etiology of the developing paraplegia, such as epidural hematoma caused by intraoperative heparization or local neurotoxic damage due to local anesthetics, has been discussed.

Recently, during the course of 1 month, superficial necrosis of the epidermis (5 to 8 cm in diameter) around the epidural puncture site occurred in five patients. The local tissue tolerance to local anesthetic solutions depends to a high degree on the pH value, the tonicity, and the electrolyte content of the solution [4]. It was therefore decided to study the pH, electrolyte content, osmolality, and in vitro propensity to cause hemolysis in local anesthetic solutions normally used for epidural anesthesia. Furthermore, the epidural spaces in seven postmortem specimens from patients who had had epidural analgesia for 4 days, were examined with regard to local tissue reactions.

Method

Commercially available solutions of 0.5% bupivacaine, 1% etidocaine, 2% and 3% chlorprocaine, 1% lidocaine, and 1% mepivacaine in two preparations were randomly allocated for determination of pH, PCO_2, sodium, calcium, and osmolality. One or two milliliters of these local anesthetic solutions were mixed with 10 ml freshly prepared bank blood, after 5 to 10 min the blood samples were centrifuged, and the free hemoglobin in the serum was determined spectro-photometrically. The pH was determined using a pH-meter (Beckman), the sodium and calcium by flame photometry, and the osmolality using an osmometer (Knaur). In the second series, five samples from three different batches of 1% mepivacaine (preparations 1 and 2) were analyzed.

Postmortem specimens from seven patients, of whom five had intraoperatively received heparin, were prepared by W. Hort (Director of the Pathological Institute of the University Düsseldorf, FRG) and histologically examined by W. Wechsler (Director of the Neuropathological Institute at the University of Düsseldorf).

Table 1. Physicochemical properties of local anesthetics used for regional anesthesia (first series)

Drug	Batch #	n	pH 25 °C x ± sd	PCO_2 mmHg x ± sd	Na^+ mmol/l x ± sd	Ca^{++} mmol/l x ± sd	Osmolality mmol/l x ± sd	Drug added ml	n	Free hemoglobin/S mg%
Bupivacaine prep. 1 0.5% 5-ml glass ampule	821700	5	6.03 ± 0.07	–	135 ± 1	–	279 ± 2	1.0	5	–
Bupivacaine CO_2 0.5%	2230	3	6.14 ± 0.07	653 ± 2	131 ± 0	–	286 ± 1	1.0	3	–
Bupivacaine prep. 2 0.5% 5-ml glass ampule	25220	3	5.97 ± 0.01	–	130 ± 5	–	277 ± 2	1.0	3	–
Bupivacaine prep. 2 0.5% 20-ml ampule	BFK17-7	2	5.92 ± 0.03	–	132 ± 0	–	279 ± 2	1.0	3	–
	BFE12-10	2	5.89 ± 0.01	–	135 ± 1	–	275 ± 2	1.0	2	–
Etidocaine 1%	BD1131	2	6.00 ± 0.01	–	117 ± 0	–	276 ± 0	1.0	3	–
	BDE122	2	6.00 ± 0.01	–	117 ± 0	–	276 ± 0	1.0	2	–
Chlorprocain 2%	B751	2	3.80 ± 0.01	–	108 ± 0	–	298 ± 2	1.0	2	–
Chlorprocain 3%	B021	2	3.80 ± 0.01	–	78 ± 1	–	282 ± 0	1.0	2	–
Lidocaine 1% 5-ml glass ampule	4737	2	6.53 ± 0.02	–	121 ± 1	–	292 ± 1	1.0	2	–
Lidocaine 1% Pharmacy University of Düsseldorf	44245	1	4.50	–	111	–	285	1.0	1	–
	44569	1	4.50	–	44	–	142	1.0	1	–
	45277	1	4.50	–	119	–	290	1.0	1	–
Mepivacaine prep 1 1%	88363/C	3	6.39 ± 0.01	–	–	5.33 ± 0.09	97 ± 0	2.0	1	70.4
								1.0	1	0.5
								1.0	1	1.5
Mepivacaine prep. 2 1%	BFD14-2	2	6.02 ± 0.02	–	133 ± 0	–	318 ± 1	2.0	1	–
	BFH28-2	1	6.01 ± 0.01	–	134 ± 0	–	322 ± 1	1.0	1	–

Table 2. Physicochemical properties of two preparations of mepivacaine (second series)

Drug	Batch #	n	pH 25 °C x + sd	Na^+ mmol/l x + sd	Ca^{++} mmol/l x + sd	Osmolality mmol/l x + sd	Drug added ml	n	Free hemoglobin mg%
Mepivacaine prep. 1 1%	B21730	5	6.33 ± 0.0	2.3 ± 0.2	5.2 ± 0.1	86.0 ± 1	2.0	5	–
							1.0	5	–
							0.5	5	–
	B1131	5	6.35 ± 0.0	2.3 ± 0.5	5.2 ± 0.1	88.0 ± 2	2.0	5	–
							1.0	5	–
							0.5	5	–
	B1850	5	6.37 ± 0.0	2.1 ± 0.8	5.2 ± 0.2	87.0 ± 1	2.0	5	–
							1.0	5	–
							0.5	5	–
Mepivacaine prep. 2 1%	BGD51-1	5	6.01 ± 0.01	130.3 ± 1.0	–	318.8 ± 2	2.0	5	–
							1.0	5	–
							0.5	5	–
	BGC49-1	5	6.01 ± 0.00	130.7 ± 0.8	–	320.8 ± 2	2.0	5	–
							1.0	5	–
							0.5	5	–
	BFK42-2	5	6.05 ± 0.00	130.3 ± 1.2	–	313.6 ± 4	2.0	5	–
							1.0	5	–
							0.5	5	–

Results

Only slight variations with regard to pH, sodium, and osmolality were found (Table 1) among the different preparations of bupivacaine. In the 1% solution of etidocaine the sodium content was somewhat lower than in the bupivacaine solution. The osmolality of the solutions was within the normal range. This was also the case in the two solutions of chlorprocaine, where a very low pH (3.8) and sodium content (108 mmol and 78 mmol/l) were found (Table 1). In the two preparations of lidocaine studied, it was found that, in the solution of one batch prepared in our pharmacy, the sodium content and osmolality were very low. Owing to a very low sodium content, the sample from batch 44,569 was hypo-osmolar in comparison with blood (Table 1).

There were striking differences in sodium content and osmolality between the two preparations of mepivacaine 1%. Preparation 1 contained 5.3 mmol/l calcium instead of sodium. The solution was hypo-osmolar in comparison with blood. Preparation 2, on the other hand, contained sodium and was iso-osmolar. Free hemoglobin in serum was only seen in one test with mepivacaine (Solution 1) when 2 ml solution were mixed with 10 ml blood. In this experiment, the free hemoglobin content increased from 0 to 70 mg%. The differences in sodium and calcium content and in osmolality were confirmed by the examination of five samples from three different batches of each drug preparation of mepivacaine (Table 2). In this series no hemolysis was induced by 1% mepivacaine preparation 1 (Table 2).

Neither inspection of the epidural space, the dura mater, and the spinal cord nor the histologic examination showed signs of epidural bleeding (Fig. 1) or reactive changes of the tissues in the epidural space (Fig. 2).

Discussion

The present investigation has shown that most local anesthetic preparations used for epidural, infiltration, or intravenous anesthesia are normotonic in comparison with blood. Only preparation 1 of mepivacaine and one solution of 1% lidocaine prepared in the pharmacy of the University of Düsseldorf were clearly hypo-osmolar in comparison with blood.

The injection of hypo-osmolar solution into tissue leads to an interstitial edema, which might be followed by a necrosis. Both Lundborg in 1975 [2] and Selander and co-workers in 1979 [4] showed that injection of hypo-osmolar solutions near to neural tissues causes damage to the nerves. The hypo-osmolar solution of 1% lidocaine that was prepared in our pharmacy for clinical use in our reusable epidural trays caused superficial lysis of the epidermis in five patients. Shortly after this accident, disposable epidural trays were introduced at this institute, which contain lidocaine, for skin infiltration. Neither before nor since have we seen such skin reactions. It is therefore suggested that the superficial lysis of the epidermis was caused by the hypotonic lidocaine solution used at that time.

Mixing hypotonic solutions like aqua destillata causes hemolysis in vitro. This test is used in the daily laboratory routine to determine the osmotic resistance of erythrocytes, whose normal range is between 0.44% and 0.32% NaCl [1]. It is therefore suggested that the osmotic fragility of erythrocytes in the units of bank blood tested varied in the same range, so that the hemolytic response to a hypotonic agent changed from one blood unit to another as these were taken from different individuals.

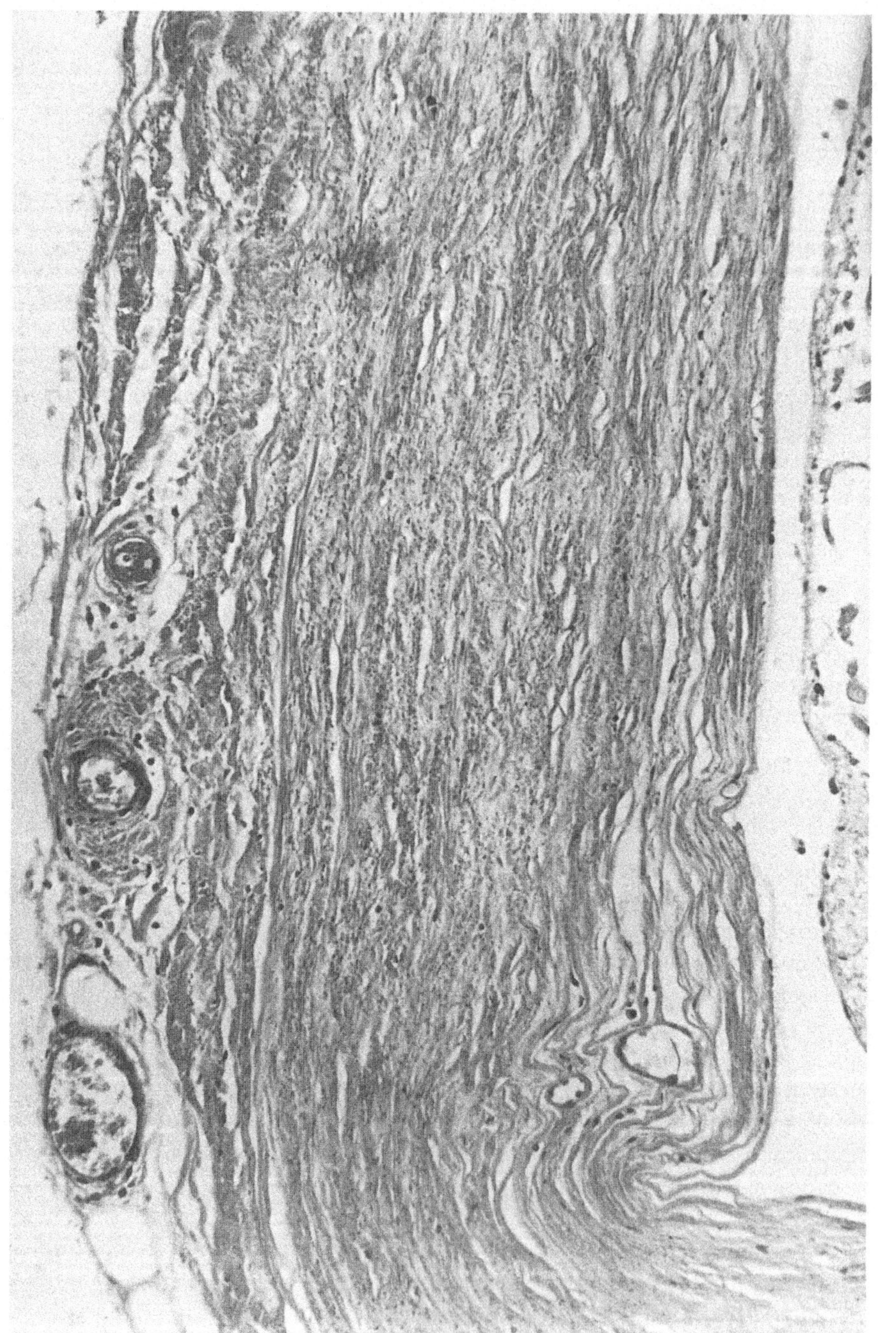

Fig. 1. Cross section of the dura at T 8 upper part shows the epidural side of the dura mater. x 32. There are no signs of reactive proliferation or inflammation

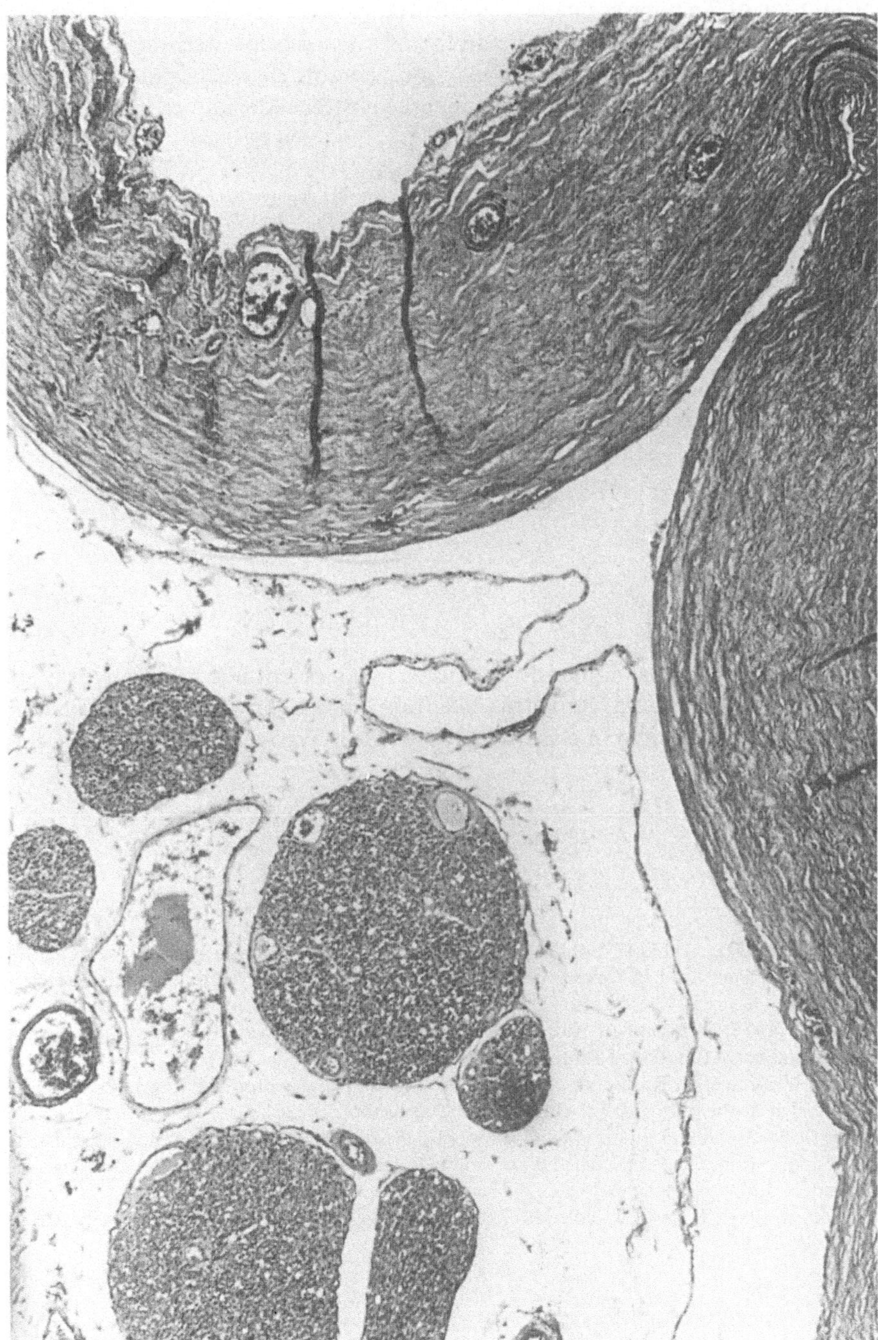

Fig. 2. Cross section of the dura at T 8. x 32. No signs of reactive proliferation or inflammation are found

The infusion of 2 g bupivacaine in a concentration of 0.125% to 0.5% into the epidural space over a period of 4 days in seven patients, five of whom received heparin intra-operatively, produced no signs of an epidural hematoma or local neurotoxic reactions in the epidural space. This is in agreement with the results published by Selander and co-workers in 1979 [4].

Conclusion

The experiments have shown that there are commercially available hypotonic preparations of local anesthetics. The injection of a hypo-osmolar solution might cause tissue necrosis. Until there is clear experimental evidence that solutions that are hypo-osmolar in comparison with blood can be injected without damaging the patient, such preparations should be used with great caution. The findings in the epidural space support our clinical impression that continuous catheter epidural anesthesia is a safe clinical method.

Addendum

Recently, in a prospective randomized study using hypo- or isotonic preparations of mepivacaine for IV regional anesthesia, Dr. Petruschke from Minden showed that significant hemolysis (50 mg/ml free hemoglobin in plasma) occurred when hypo-osmolar solutions were injected [5].

References

1. Blume KG, Busch D, Arnold H, Löhr GW (1971) Klinische Untersuchungen zur hereditären, nicht sphärozytären hämolytischen Anämie bei Pyruvatkinasemangel der Erythrozyten. Klin Wochenschr 49:228
2. Lundborg G (1975) Structure and function of the intraneural microvessels as related to trauma, edema formation and nerve function. J Bone Joint Surg 57 A:938
3. Sandmann W, Kremer K, Rötzscher M, Knieriem HJ (1975) Ungewöhnliche Komplikationen nach Ersatz der terminalen Aorta abdominalis. Aktuel Probl Chir Orthop 10:361
4. Selander D, Brattsand R, Lundborg G, Nordborg C, Olsson Y (1979) Local anesthetics: importance of mode of application, concentration and adrenaline for the appearance of nerve lesions. Acta Anaesthesiol Scand 23:127
5. Petruschke H, Gergs P, Meyer J, Nolte H (1982) Zur Frage der Hämolyse bei i.v.-Regionalanaesthesie. Anaesthesist 31:517

Discussion

Müller:
Ihre Ausführungen über Heparin und rückenmarknahe Leitungsanaesthesien haben mich etwas irritiert. Ich möchte das kurz anhand eines Fallberichts erläutern. Unsere neurochirurgi-

sche Abteilung bekam vor ca. 5 Wochen eine 72jährige Patientin, bei der in einem auswärtigen Krankenhaus eine linksseitige Endoprothese in Spinalanaesthesie durchgeführt worden war, eine Woche nach der Operation wegen einer Paraplegie überwiesen. Bei präoperativ normalem Gerinnungsstatus war die Lumbalpunktion mit einer 25-G-Nadel nach Auskunft des Kollegen völlig unproblematisch. Die Operation dauerte $1-1^1/_2$ h. Intraoperativ wurden 2 Konserven, postoperativ weitere 3 Konserven am 2. postoperativen Tag gegeben. Die Patientin hatte am Operationstag laut Kurve 3mal 5,000 IE Liquemin erhalten. Die Paraplegie wurde erst am 2. postoperativen Tage bemerkt, da die Patientin nach der Operation somnolent und nicht kooperativ war. Vor der Operation konnte sie am Stock gehen.

Bei der von den Neurochirurgen präoperativ durchgeführten Lumbalpunktion konnte kein Liquor gewonnen werden. Die Myolographie zeigte einen Stopp bei Th11. Bei der Laminektomie über 3 Etagen fand man ein ausgedehntes Hämatom, das sich nicht vollständig herausspülen ließ. Da die Laminektomie nicht über die ganze Ausbreitung des Hämatoms erweitert wurde, kann man ein Angiom oder einen Tumor als mögliche Blutungsquelle nicht ausschließen. Die Patientin hat den Eingriff überstanden, ohne daß sich die Paraplegie gebessert hat.

Aufgrund des geschilderten Falls muß man fragen, wann Liquemin präoperativ abgesetzt werden muß, wie und ob es labortechnisch kontrolliert werden muß, wann man intra- oder postoperativ bei liegendem Epiduralkatheter oder während oder nach einer Spinalanaesthesie wieder mit Heparin beginnen darf. Ist nicht zu fordern, daß man zumindest innerhalb der ersten 24 h den neurologischen Status des Patienten kontrollieren muß?

Wüst:
At our last meeting in 1979 in Düsseldorf, the problem of heparin and regional anesthesia was discussed in a panel. It was stated then that all types of regional blocks should be omitted in the presence of a minidose of heparin. They are allowed, however, when the PPT is no longer than 60 s and the Quick test is not lower than 50%. But you are on the safe side if you stop minidose heparin at least 12 h before regional anesthesia is started. But, in the face of the questionable prophylactic effect of minidose heparin on the incidence of deep vein thrombosis and thromboembolism, in 34% to 50% of your patients heparin has no effect and will therefore not prevent thromboembolism, the question must be asked why should heparin be given at all?

Regional anesthesia per se is much more effective because of the increased arterial and venous flow and because of a much smaller deterioration of coagulation and the fibrinolytic system.

Intraoperative heparinization, for example, in vascular surgery, may be started 1 to $1^1/_2$ h after the epidural cannula has been inserted. But there is, as we have always pointed out, a slight risk of an epidural hematoma and, therefore, close control of the postoperative neurologic status is required.

Stanton-Hicks:
As Dr. Wüst pointed out, I think, that if your surgeons are using minidose heparin subcutaneously for postoperative thromboembolic prophylaxis, then any thought of major conduction anesthesia is contraindicated.

The experience of many centers that are using heparin after an epidural catheter has been placed has shown that it can be used, provided that the catheter or the patient is not allowed to be moved before heparin has either been reversed or allowed by time to reverse.

We still don't have an accurate laboratory means of determining heparin levels. Until we have such a method, I think the use of low-dose heparin should be avoided in patients in whom a regional block is planned. It is probably redundant to use minidose heparin in patients in whom you are going to apply a continuous epidural technique, because the technique itself will provide a prophylaxis against thromboembolic phenomena.

Aldrete:
Perhaps we should not forget that there are alternatives to minidose heparin to prevent thromboembolism. In a recently published multicenter study performed in Europe, the effects of dextran and of minidose heparin on the incidence of thromboembolism were compared. There were no differences found concerning the incidence of thromboembolic events between the two treatments, except the incidents of bleeding were greater in cases treated with heparin. So I think we should not lose the prospect that we can use regional anesthesia and, at the same time, lower the risk of thromboembolism by dextran.

Stanton-Hicks:
I think one must compromise with one's own surgeons as to whether or not they should use heparin. The only point I wish to make is that I see no contraindication to the use of heparin once the epidural catheter has been placed in a patient. Then it is generally safe.

Crawford:
This point is specifically important in the obstetric field, where you quite frequently get patients who developed a thrombophlebitis while they were on the pill before they became pregnant or in a previous pregnancy. Two things I find very odd. The suggestion by some people that it is all right to give an epidural block to a patient on minidose heparin. That seems to me to be a total inconsequence or contradiction. The idea of giving minidose heparin is to interfere with the coagulation of the patient's blood and, if one interferes with coagulation, an epidural block must be forbidden unless there are absolute outstanding indications to use it. The second point is that, if we have got a mother who has been on Warferin and then had heparin during her pregnancy and she comes to require a cesarian section or might go into labor with an epidural block, I am satisfied to start the epidural block once the heparin has been stopped and the hematologists have told me that the coagulation is normal. As I already said, I think 10% of patients do bleed when you put a cannula into the epidural space and I ought to allow a couple of hours for that bleeding vessel to be sealed off before I start to recommend heparin. But I don't mind when patients are going to walk about once the epidural is finished, the labor is over, and the cesarian section is finished. The mother can get up while she is still on her anticoagulant because she is going to remain on anticoagulant therapy for at least 6 weeks postnatally.

Stanton-Hicks:
I just fear that, in such cases, one does run the risk that the movement of a catheter could erode a vessel and cause an epidural hematoma while the patient is on heparin. The catheter is placed before the patient is heparinized and is left inside for 1 to 3 days, depending on how long the patient needs postoperative analgesia after aortofemoral-bypass operation. The patient is completely heparinized during surgery and, provided that there has been no heparin given within half an hour before the end of surgery, there should be sufficient time for the degradation of the heparin dose so that the patient can now be moved off the operating table.

Neural Complications of Axillary Plexus Block

D. Selander

Neural complications following axillary plexus blocks have a reported incidence of less than 2%, while the corresponding figure for supraclavicular plexus blocks varies between 2.2 and 7.5%. This difference may depend on trauma to the nerves during the search for paresthesias, [1, 3] which is obligatory in supraclavicular blocks but not in axillary blocks. To test this idea, we studied the incidence of neural complications after axillary blocks performed with or without searching for paresthesias [8] (Table 1). In one group of 290 patients, paresthesias were used to locate the axillary plexus, in the other group of 243 patients, the pulsations of the axillary artery were used to ensure correct placement of the injection needle within the neurovascular sheath. Signs of postblock nerve lesion were found in eight patients (2.8%) in the paresthesia group and in two patients (0.8%) in the nonparesthesia, or artery group, in both of which there were reports of accidental paresthesias during the block procedure. This difference supports the impression that searching for paresthesia may injure nerves and thus increase the risk of postblock nerve lesions.

Symptoms of nerve lesions appeared within 1–21 days after the operation and varied from light paresthesias of a few weeks' duration to severe ache, sensory impairment, and paresis lasting more than a year. The most severe cases were found in the paresthesia group. The symptoms originated in the median nerve in seven cases, the ulnar nerve in five, and the radial nerve in one case. The frequency of inury to the various nerves corresponded well to their position within the axillary neurovascular sheath: the median and ulnar nerves, which run above the axillary artery, are most likely to be hit by the needle, whereas the radial nerve, which runs behind the axillary artery, is least likely to be injured. (Fig. 3).

The peripheral nerve consists of a number of fascicles held together by the epineurium (Fig. 1). Each fascicle is surrounded by a multilayered sheath, the perineurium, inside which the nerve fibers are embedded in the endoneurium [2]. The various structures are well

Table 1. Incidence of nerve lesions after axillary blocks performed with or without searching for paresthesias. Number of patients with symptoms of postanesthetic nerve lesion

	Patients	Nerve lesion (patients)	%
Paresthesia group	290	8	2.8
Artery group	243	2	0.8
Total	533	10	1.9

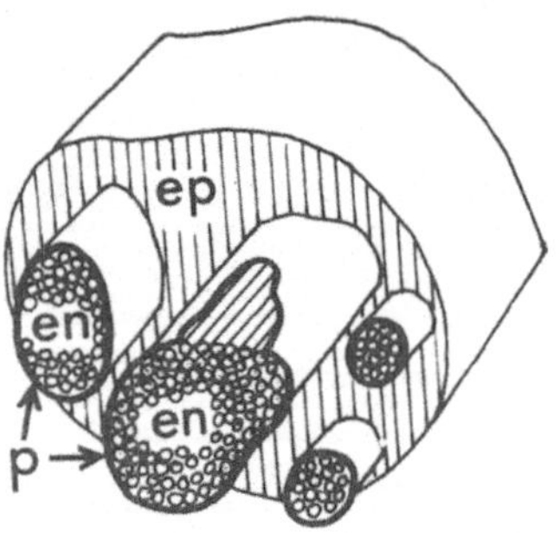

Fig. 1. Schematic drawing of a peripheral nerve. ep = epineurium; p = perineurium; en = endoneurium. Note that all tissues are well vascularized

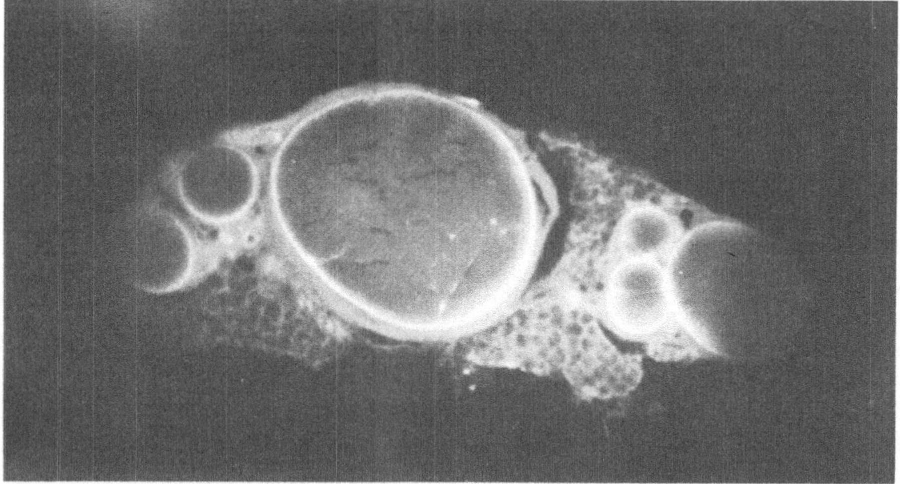

Fig. 2. Fluorescence micrograph of cross-sectioned sciatic nerve from the rabbit. The perineurial barrier prevents the topically applied red-fluorescent Evans Blue Albumin (EBA, here white) from entering the endoneurial space

vascularized by anastomosing microvessels [4]. The endothelium of the endoneurial blood vessels and the inner layer of the perineurium form diffusion barriers with a selective permeability (Fig. 2). Together, these barriers form a blood-nerve barrier (BNB), [5, 11], which maintains a specific endoneurial milieu for optimal nerve-fiber function. It is obvious that any of these structures can be injured during an axillary block procedure.

Besides mechanical trauma, the nerves may be subjected to toxic and ischemic traumata. Mechanical trauma can be induced by the needle, intraneural injection, and compression. The injection needle can penetrate and damage nerves and blood vessels. In animal experiments, we found that the use of a short-beveled (45°) needle significantly decreased the risk of fascicular damage compared with a standard, long-beveled (14°) needle (Fig. 4), [6]. We also found that the orientation of the bevel was of importance for the size of the fascicular lesion. Figure 4 shows the endoneurial injury caused by a standard needle that penetrated the fascicle with its bevel plane parallel with the nerve fibers, whereas Fig. 5 shows the injury caused by the same needle after penetrating with its bevel transverse to the nerve. Clinically, we found that puncture of axillary blood vessels was significantly more common with long-

Fascicle injury after intraneural injection.

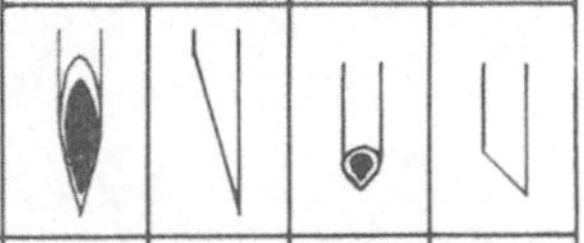

	Long bevel		Short bevel	
n	15	15	15	15
Fascicle injury	9	5	0	3

Fig. 3. Incidence of fascicular injury after intraneural injections with long- and short-beveled needles (rabbit sciatic nerve in situ)

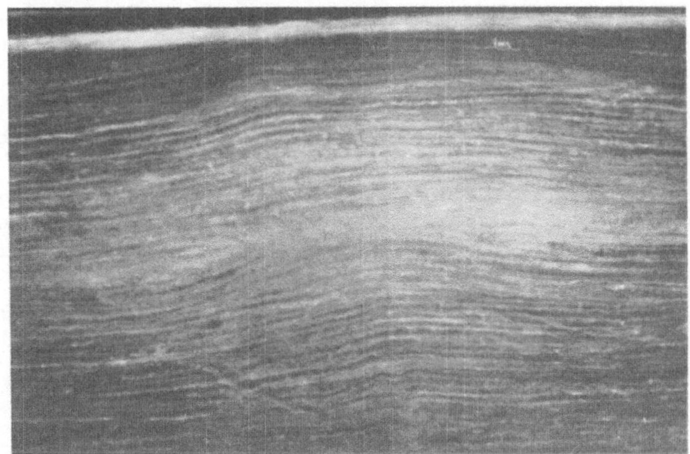

Fig. 4. Endoneural lesion caused by long-beveled injection needle which pierced nerve with bevel plane parallel with nerve fibers

beveled needles than with short-beveled needles. A late effect of bleeding and local trauma is the development of scar tissue in or around the nerve. This may disturb neural microcirculation and axonal transport and thereby cause deterioration of nerve function.

Toxic trauma can be caused by the injected local anesthetic. Factors of importance are concentration, pH, osmotic tonus, and additives. After injection of 0.05 ml normal saline and 0.5% plain bupivacaine in the rabbit sciatic nerve, we found an equal degree of axonal degeneration [9] (Table 2). The degeneration increased with increasing bupivacaine concentration, but in our experiments, the most significant changes were seen with 0.5% bupivacaine with adrenaline (5 μg/ml). This indicates that adrenaline enhances the toxicity of the local anesthetic, probably by inducing a local ischemia of the nerve [10].

Ischemic trauma can be caused by vasoconstrictive drugs as mentioned or by internal or external compression. Internal compression was experimentally found after intraneural

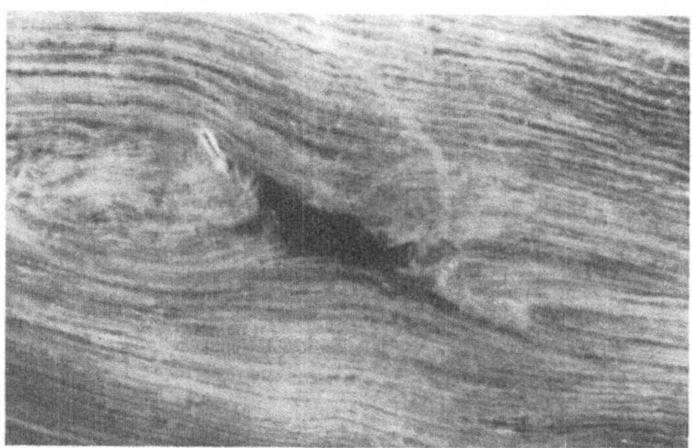

Fig. 5. Endoneurial lesion caused by the same needle as in Fig. 4, but with bevel plane transverse to nerve fibres

Table 2. Axonal degeneration 10–14 days after intrafascicular injection of saline or bupivacaine in rabbit sciatic nerves

Agent	Conc. mg/ml	Axonal degeneration		
		0 → +	++	+++
Physiol. saline		11	4	1
Bupivacaine	5	10	6	–
Bupivacaine	10	4	7	5
Bupivacaine with adrenaline 5 μg/ml	5	–	11	5

Degrees of axonal degeneration: 0 → +: None or insignificant, ++: Significant but < 50% of axons, +++: ⩾ 50% of axons

(intrafascicular) (Fig. 6) injections, where the endoneurial pressure could be elevated to levels high above the capillary perfusion pressure for 10–15 min, which resulted in ischemia of the corresponding nerve segment [7]. External compression can be caused by incorrect positioning of the arm, by plaster casts, or by a tourniquet used to achieve a blood-free field. In the rabbit, nerve conduction distal to the inflated tourniquet ceased after 65 min of ischemia, but was fully regained after more than 6 h of ischemia (Fig. 7). However, the combination of compression and ischemia, such as found under the tourniquet, led to permanent loss of nerve conduction in less than 4 h. The loss of nerve conduction coincided with the appearance of endoneurial edema [4].

Most nerve lesions following axillary plexus block appear to be primarily the result of a direct trauma to the nerves caused by needles or intraneural injections. However, it seems clear that both toxic and ischemic factors are important for the extent of the lesion. Thus, the risk of neural complications due to axillary blocks may be decreased by careful handling of the nerves, which means:

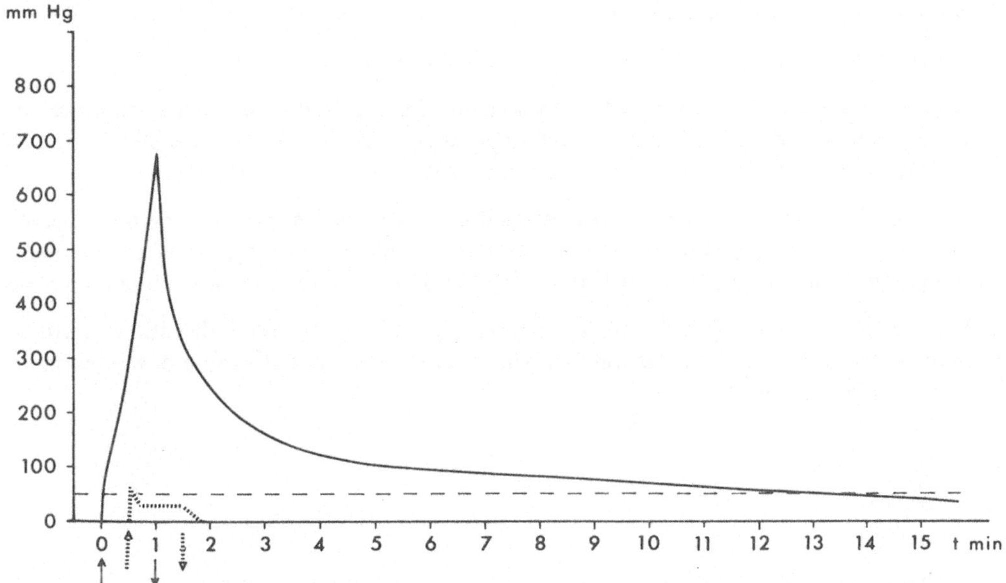

Fig. 6. Pressure recordings during intraneural injections in rabbit sciatic nerve of 0.1 ml tracer solution. (—— endoneurial injection; – – – epineurial injection.) Interrupted horizontal line indicates estimated capillary perfusion pressure

ischemic period	tibial nerve (subjected to ischemia)		sciatic nerve (subjected to ischemia and compression)	
	original	recovery	original	recovery
2h				
4h				
6h				
8h				

Fig. 7. Recovery of impulse transmission in rabbit nerves 1 h after 2–8 h of ischemia or ischemia plus compression. Lack of recovery coincides with the appearance of endoneurial edema [4]

1. Avoid rough, repeated paresthesias;

2. Use short-beveled, fine-caliber needles or a catheter technique

3. Chose local anesthetic solutions withoutadrenaline. Long-acting drugs, such as bupivacaine and etidocaine, and the use of catheter techniques makes adrenaline unnecessary unless, blood absorption for some reason, must be minimized

4. Avoid prolonged ischemia since this may itself cause a nerve lesion or worsen other nerve lesions. It is recommended that the time of ischemia should not be longer than 2 h and the tourniquet pressure not higher than 100 mm Hg (13.3 kPa) above the systolic blood pressure

5. Every case presenting symptoms or signs of postoperative nerve lesion should be carefully examined and subjected to a close follow-up in order to determine the cause of the lesion and to provide adequate treatment.

References

1. Bonica JJ (1954) The management of pain, 2nd edn. Lea and Febiger, Philadelphia, pp 227–228
2. Key A, Retzius G (1876) Studien in der Anatomie des Nervensystemes und des Bindegewebes. Samson and Wallin, Stockholm
3. Moore DC (1955) Complications of regional block. Thomas, Springfield, pp 112–118
4. Lundborg G (1970) Ischemic nerve injury. Scand J. plastic reconstr. Surg [Suppl] 6:3
5. Lundborg G (1975) Structure and function of the intraneural microvessels as related to trauma, edema formation and nerve function. J Bone Joint Surg 57A:938
6. Selander D, Dhunér KG, Lundborg G (1977) Peripheral nerve injury due to injection needles used for regional anaesthesia. Acta Anaesthesiol Scand 21:182
7. Selander D, Sjöstrand J (1978) Longitudinal spread of intraneurally injected local anesthetics. Acta Anaesthesiol Scand 22:622
8. Selander D, Edshage S, Wolf T (1979a) Paresthesiae or no parestesiae? Acta Anaesthesiol Scand 23:27
9. Selander D, Brattsand R, Lundborg G, Nordborg C, Olsson Y (1979b) Local anesthetics: Importance of mode of application, concentration and adrenaline for the appearance of nerve lesions. Acta Anaesthesiol Scand 23:127
10. Selander D, Karlsson L, Månsson LG, Svanvik J (1980) Adrenaline, neural ischemia and local anesthetic nerve toxicity. 7th World congress of anaesthesiologists, Hamburg, paper no 777
11. Waksman B (1961) Experimental study of diphteric polyneuritis in the rabbit and guinea pig. III. The blood-nerve barrier in the rabbit. J Neuropathol Exp Neurol 20:35

Discussion

Stanton-Hicks:
You did not mention the use of a nerve stimulator for seeking the nerves. Would you advocate that or do you feel, from your studies, that it is sufficient to use a short-beveled needle?

Selander:
First of all, it is sufficient to use a short-beveled needle. Secondly, I think that the use of a nerve stimulator is all right as long as you use it carefully and follow up your patients afterward to see that there are really no complications. I do not know whether anyone has found any. I do not think it has been described. Until now I have not tried it myself, I must confess.

van Steenberge:
What was the outcome of paresthesias in the plexus block given in the ulnar region? Is it good or did you do definite damage to the nerve by your plexus block?

Selander:
I think there are some examples of that. You can get definite persistent damage of nerves. In many cases, there are other factors contributing to and complicating the situation, like a shoulder-finger-hand syndrome or maltreatment. In such a case, the anesthesiologist has possibly not recognized that there was a preexisting nerve lesion, or it was hidden by the operation or by the plastic cast or by anything else that makes that you miss it in the beginning. It may lead to a situation where there is no recovery.

van Steenberge:
Is there any therapy for that?

Selander:
No, if it does not recover, it does not. You can try a sympathetic block. Most patients will recover, but it may take time, sometimes up to a year. If it lasts longer or if it gets worse, it is usually recommended to do a neurolysis and see what the situation is like.

Zindler:
Are there other preexisting diseases, for example diabetes, which are more liable to permanent lesion? We had one patient who had some permanent lesions after a plexus block. Finally, it turned out to be a diabetic neuropathy with a more peripheral lesion. Could this be a relative contraindication for a plexus block?

Selander:
Yes, it is a relative contraindication. We have the impression that some systemic diseases, for example diabetes, SLE, and some other diseases, make the nerve more susceptible to injuries than in normal patients. So, even if you often think that regional anesthesia would be the best for your patient, who may have other complications as well, you should be careful and, I think, extremely careful with adrenaline in a diabetic.

Stanton-Hicks:
The axillary block is often employed for frequent shunt revisions in the diabetic patient, who may well have a neuropathy, because of the much lower morbidity of regional anesthesia compared with that associated with general anesthesia.

Ergebnisse einer Umfrage nach katheterbedingten Komplikationen bei Epiduralanaesthesien

J. Ungemach, A. Lorentz und H. Lutz

Die kontinuierliche Epiduralanaesthesie wurde in der heute praktizierten Form erstmals 1949 von Curbello [2] beschrieben. Ein Bericht Bonicas [1] über 3637 Epiduralanaesthesien zeigt aber, daß diese Technik der Regionalanaesthesie nicht frei von Komplikationen ist.

Da die Untersuchungen Bonicas bereits 25 Jahre zurückliegen und an einem relativ kleinen Krankengut vorgenommen wurden, erschien es uns notwendig, die Ergebnisse für die heutige Praxis zu überprüfen. Deshalb unternahmen wir den Versuch, anhand einer Umfrage zu klären:

1. welche schwerwiegenden Komplikationen durch das Einführen eines Katheters im Epiduralraum auftreten können,
2. wie häufig sie beobachtet werden.

Methode

Im Jahre 1980 verschickten wir einen Fragebogen an 622 deutsche Anaesthesieabteilungen und 406 geburtshilflich-gynäkologische Kliniken (Tab. 1). Neben den aufgeführten Komplikationen wurde nach der Gesamtzahl der in den Jahren 1970–1980 durchgeführten Narkosen, der Häufigkeit der verschiedenen Techniken, insbesondere der Katheterepiduralanaesthesie gefragt. Wenn Epiduralanaesthesien unter Verwendung von Kathetern durchgeführt worden waren, sollten ergänzende Angaben über die Art der Operation, über die Indikation für den Epiduralkatheter, über die Höhe der Punktionsstelle und über das verwendete Kathetermaterial gemacht werden.

Die Antworten wurden auf Lochkarten übertragen und statistisch ausgewertet (Tab. 2)

Ergebnisse

Von den 1028 angeschriebenen Abteilung antworteten 473 (278 Anaesthesieabteilungen und 195 Frauenkliniken). An 201 anaesthesiologischen und 84 geburtshilflich-gynäkologischen Abteilungen wurden kontinuierliche Katheterepiduralanaesthesien durchgeführt. 73 Antwor-

Tabelle 1. Fragebogen über kathederbedingte Komplikationen bei Epiduralanaesthesie

Bitte zurück an:
Institut f. Anästhesiologie
und Reanimation am Klinikum
der Stadt Mannheim
Postfach 23
6800 Mannheim 1

Katheterbedingte Komplikationen bei Epiduralanästhesie

Folgende schwerwiegende Komplikationen sollen erfaßt werden:

Nervenwurzelirritation, Hautabszeß, peridurales Hämatom, periduraler Abszeß, Abscheren d. Katheters bei dessen Einführen, Abriß d. Katheters beim Entfernen, Sekundäre Duraperforation

Indikation:** a) postop. Schmerzbekämpfung
b) geburtshilfliche Anästhesie
c) langdauernde Operationen mit entspr. Indikation (Urol., Traumatol., Allgemeinchir.)
d) medik. Sympathikolyse bei Gefäßerkrankungen
e) andere

	Zahl d. Anästh.	Zahl d. Kath.PDA	Art d. Komplikation*	Art d. Op	Höhe d.Punktionsstelle	verwendeter Katheter	Indikation** zur Kath.PDA	Bemerkungen
1970								
1971								
1972								
1973								

Tabelle 2. Statistische Auswertung der Fragebogenaktion

		Anaesthesie	Frauenklinik
Abteilungen	Σ 473	278	195
Statistisch verwertete Angaben	212	164	48
Keine KEDA durchgeführt	188	77	111
Statistisch nicht verwertbare Angaben	73	37	36

Tabelle 3. Statistische Auswertung der Fragebogenaktion

Zahl der erfaßten Anaesthesien			2521782
Zahl der KPD			135663
In Anaesthesie			95747
In Frauenklinik			39916
Varianzbreite:	Anaesthesie:	Anaesthesiezahl/Jahr und Abteilung:	626 – 24385
		KEDA-Zahl/Jahr und Abteilung:	1 – 1356
	Frauenklinik:	KEDA-Zahl/Jahr und Abteilung:	1 – 1134

ten (37 Anaesthesie- und 36 gyn.-geburt. Abteilungen) waren nicht verwertbar, da die Angaben ungenau waren. Die Angaben weiterer 188 Abteilungen (77 Anaesthesie- und 111 Frauenabteilungen), die nur "single-Shot"-Epiduralanaesthesien durchgeführt hatten, wurden ebenfalls bei der Auswertung der Fragebogen nicht berücksichtigt (Tab. 3)

Tabelle 4. Prozentualer Anteil der KEDA an der Anaesthesiezahl/Jahr (Angaben der Anaesthesie-Abteilungen)

	[%]	[n]
1971	2,87	3
1972	2,38	6
1973	3,1	8
1974	4,64	13
1975	4,62	20
1976	3,29	37
1977	3,66	59
1978	4,23	85
1979	4,02	103
1980	4,23	47

Häufigkeit der Verwendung von Epiduralkathetern

An den verschiedenen Anaesthesieabteilungen wurden in den Jahren 1970–1980 2521781 Narkosen durchgeführt. Die Anzahl der Narkosen in geburtshilflich-gynäkologischen Abteilungen ist nicht berücksichtigt.

In diesem Zeitraum wurde 135663 (95747 an Anaesthesieabteilungen, 39916 an Frauenkliniken) mal, d. h. bei etwa 5,3% der insgesamt durchgeführten Narkosen, ein Epiduralkatheter verwendet. Die Gesamtzahl der Anaesthesien und der Anwendung der kontinuierlichen Epiduralanaesthesie in den einzelnen Abteilungen zeigte keine Normalverteilung, sondern eine Kurve mit nach links verschobenem Gipfel. Daraus folgt, daß der Anteil großer Anaesthesieabteilungen mit einer entsprechenden Gesamtzahl an durchgeführten Narkosen, die einen Epiduralkatheter verwendet haben, gering ist, während der Anteil von kleinen Abteilungen, an denen die kontinuierliche Epiduralanaesthesie seltener durchgeführt wird, in der vorliegenden Untersuchung groß ist. So beantworteten überwiegend kleine Abteilungen, in denen 2 bis 4000 Narkosen/Jahr durchgeführt werden, den Fragebogen.

Die Zahl der berichteten kontinuierlichen Epiduralanaesthesien nimmt zwar, wie aus Tab. 4 hervorgeht, zu; der prozentuale Anteil der Katheterepiduralanaesthesien bleibt aber, in Relation zu der Gesamtzahl der Narkosen, etwa gleich. Der Anteil der Katheterepiduralanaesthesien betrug in den Jahren 1971–1973 2–3%. Er stieg in dem Zeitraum 1974–1975 auf 4,6% an und pendelte sich in den folgenden 5 Jahren bei 4% ein.

Indikationen für einen Epiduralkatheter

Als häufigste Indikation zur Verwendung eines Epiduralkatheters wurde eine lange Dauer der Operation, die postoperative Schmerzbehandlung und die Geburt angegeben. In der Mehrzahl der Fälle ergaben sich mehrere Gründe, weshalb ein Katheter verwendet wurde (Tab. 5). Am häufigsten wurde ein Epiduralkatheter für eine Geburt (21,1%) oder wegen der Dauer der Operation (17,5%) gelegt. Die postoperative Schmerzbehandlung war nur sehr selten (0,8%) eine Indikation für die kontinuierliche Epiduralanalgesie. Etwas häufiger (1,8%) wurden Lokalanaesthetika zur Sympathikolyse über einen Epiduralkatheter injiziert.

Tabelle 5. Indikationen zur KEDA (Anaesthesie)

	[%]
Lange Operationsdauer	75,4
Geburtshilfliche Anaesthesie	60,4
Postoperative Analgesie	42,2
Sympathikolyse	12,4
Rippenserienfraktur	1,5
Malignomschmerzen	1,0

Tabelle 6. Katheterbedingte Komplikationen 1

		Anaesthesie	Frauenklinik
Kopfschmerzen	31	10	21
Arachnoiditis	3	3	–
Hautrötung der Einstichstelle	14	14	–
Hämatom an der Einstichstelle	3	1	2
Rückenschmerzen	3	3	–

Tabelle 7. Katheterbedingte Komplikationen 2

	[n]	[$^0/_{00}$]
KEDA-Zahl 135 663	Σ 134	0,98
Abscheren des Katheters bei Legen der KEDA	27	0,21
Abriß des Katheters beim Entfernen	13	0,1
Duraperforation des Katheters bei Legen der KEDA	26	0,19
Spätere, sekundäre Duraperforation des Katheters	7	0,05
Intravasale Lage des Katheters	11	0,08
Knotenbildung	3	0,02
Wurzelirritation	37	0,27
Subkutaner Abszess	2	0,01
Epidurales Hämatom	2	0,01
Andere	5	0,04

Komplikationen

Tabelle 6 führt die Komplikationen auf, die bei der Auswertung nicht berücksichtigt wurden, da die mitgeteilten Antworten zu ungenau und unsicher erschienen. Viele der Komplikationen waren nicht eindeutig auf die Anwendung eines Katheters zurückzuführen.

Verwertbar waren 134 Komplikationen, die auf einen Epiduralkatheter zurückgeführt werden können. Bei einer Gesamtzahl von 135 000 Katheterepiduralanaesthesien trat bei 1 von 1000 Anaesthesien eine katheterbedingte Komplikation auf (Tab. 7).

Katheterabriß

Beim Einführen in den Epiduralraum wurde 27mal der Katheter abgeschnitten. 13mal wurde ein Abriß beim späteren Entfernen des Katheters beobachtet.

Duraperforation

Die Dura wurde beim Legen des Katheters 26mal perforiert. Sekundäre Perforationen bei der 2. oder 3. Injektion wurden 7mal, entsprechend bei 0,05 von 1000 Anaesthesien beobachtet.

Intravasale Lage des Katheters

11mal wurde eine intravasale Lage des Epiduralkatheters berichtet.

Wurzelirritation durch den Epiduralkatheter

Die Irritation einer oder mehrerer Nervenwurzeln war mit 37 berichteten Fällen die häufigste Einzelkomplikation der Katheterepiduralanaesthesie. Ihre Häufigkeit liegt bei 0,27 ‰.

Epidurale Infektionen und Hämatome

Zur Bildung eines Knotens im Epiduralraum kam es in 3 Fällen. Ein subkutaner Abszeß sowie ein epidurales Hämatom wurde je zweimal beobachtet. In einem Fall entwickelte sich ein epiduraler Abszeß.

5 weitere Komplikationen, die sich nicht eindeutig in die gefragten Kategorien einordnen ließen, wurden berichtet. Mit Hilfe des Rankorrelationskoeffizienten nach Spearman wurde geklärt, ob die Häufigkeit von Komplikationen von der jährlichen Narkose- und Katheterepiduralfrequenz abhängt. Überraschend für uns zeigte sich, daß zwischen der Anaesthesie- und Katheterepiduralfrequenz und der Komplikationsrate kein Zusammenhang nachweisbar war. Dies gilt auch für jede Einzelkomplikation.

Diskussion

Die Ergebnisse einer Umfrage an deutschen Anaesthesieabteilungen und geburtshilflich-gynäkologischen Kliniken, die 2,5 Mio Anaesthesien und 135000 Epiduralanaesthesien erfaßte, haben gezeigt, daß mit *einer* katheterbedingten Komplikation bei 1000 Epiduralanaesthesien zu rechnen ist.

Über bleibende neurologische Schäden berichtete Bonica [1] in 0,08% bei über 3600 Epiduralanaesthesien. Hellmann [4] kommt in einer Untersuchung bei 26000 Epiduralanaesthesien, die in seiner Klinik durchgeführt wurden, zu dem Schluß, daß schwere Komplikationen sehr selten sind. Er berichtet von 2 Paraplegien und von totalen Spinalanaesthesien in 0,04% der Fälle. Über katheterspezifischen Komplikationen berichtete Dawkins [3] anhand einer Zusammenstellung von 350 Untersuchungen bei 32000 kontinuierlichen Epiduralanaesthesien. Sekundäre Perforationen der Dura wurden 18mal und Knotenbildung sowie Abbruch eines Katheters je 1mal beobachtet. Passagere Störungen der Nervenfunktion traten in 0,1% und bleibende Ausfälle in 0,02% der Fälle auf.

In der vorliegenden Umfrage wurden 134 Katheter-bedingte Komplikationen bei 135000 Epiduralanaesthesien berichtet. Aufgrund der Übereinstimmung in der Art der jetzt beobachteten Komplikationen mit den Untersuchungsergebnissen von Dawkins [3], ist davon auszugehen, daß die berichteten Komplikationen katheterspezifisch sind. Bei einem Vergleich der Frequenz der Einzelkomplikationen in beiden Studien fällt auf, daß die Häufigkeit von technisch bedingten Komplikationen, wie Katheterabriß, Wurzelirritation etc. seit Dawkins [3] Untersuchung zugenommen hat. So berichtet Dawkins [3] je 1 Fall von Knotenbildung und Abriß des Epiduralkatheters bei 32000 Epiduralanaesthesien. In der vorliegenden Studie wurden bei 135000 Epiduralanaesthesien 40 abgerissene Katheter beobachtet.

Die Tatsache, daß ein Katheterabriß in der Regel auf eine unsachgemäße Handhabung zurückzuführen ist, oder auf Materialfehler, weist auf eine mangelnde Praxis bei der Durchführung der Epiduralanaesthesie. Deshalb überrascht es nicht, daß kein Zusammenhang zwischen der Häufigkeit von Komplikationen und der Anaesthesiefrequenz besteht.

Zusammenfassung

Eine Umfrage an deutschen Anaesthesieabteilungen und geburtshilflich-gynäkologischen Kliniken, erfaßte 2,5 Mio Anaesthesien und 135000 kontinuierliche Epiduralanaesthesien. 134 katheterbedingte Komplikationen wurden berichtet. Auffällig hoch ist, mit 30%, der Anteil an Komplikationen, der auf eine mangelhafte Technik hinweist.

Schwerwiegende Komplikationen, wie Hämatom und epiduraler Abszeß, kommen vor, wurden aber extrem selten berichtet.

Literatur

1. Bonica JJ (1957) Peridural Block: analysis of 3637 cases and a review. Anesthesiology 18:723
2. Curbello MM (1949) Continous peridural segmental anesthesia by means of a urethral catheter. Curr Res Anesth 28:12
3. Dawkins CJ (1969) An Analysis of the complications of extradural and caudal block. Anesthesia 24:554
4. Hellmann K (1965) Epidural anaesthesia in obstetrics: a second look at 26, 127 cases. Can Anaesth Soc J 12:398

Discussion

Stanton-Hicks:
Is not an incidence of an epidural haematoma of 0,01% similar to the percentage of haematomas which occurs in an obstetric population?

Crawford:
In 10% of cases, you get blood, when you are putting in the needle or the canula, but that is not a haematoma causing symptom. I am sure that the incidence of a haematoma is in a very low order of magnitude like Dr. Ungemach reported. But with respect I think that is a magnificent study and you have in my opinion had the same trouble which everybody has when trying to do big surveys. You are not getting honest reports. The reason is that I do not believe that you had in 135,000 epidurals a wet tape rate of only 0,01%.

Ungemach:
Die Zahlen sind von berichteten Katheterepiduralanaesthesien und enthalten möglicherweise eine hohe Dunkelziffer.

Zindler:
Sie haben bei den Patienten, die Sie nicht ausgewertet haben, einen Fall einer Arachnoiditis aufgeführt. War es tatsächlich eine, und hat ein Zusammenhang mit der Epiduralanaesthesie bestanden? Wissen Sie etwas Näheres darüber?

Ungemach:
Wir haben diesen Fall nicht mit ausgewertet, da es eine Antwort unter vielen war und wir nicht speziell danach gefragt hatten. Es ist nur dieses eine Mal angegeben worden. Wir wissen nichts über die näheren Umstände und Symptome.

Müller:
In diesem Zusammenhang möchte ich auf die sehr schöne Literaturzusammenstellung über Komplikationen von Herrn Neumark hinweisen. Danach waren bei 750,000 Epiduralanaesthesien 8 epidurale Hämatome berichtet worden. Spontane Hämatome wurden von 1850 bis 1964 über 50 in der Weltliteratur berichtet. Spontane Abszesse waren mit 250 veröffentlichten Fällen weit häufiger als Hämatome.

Bakterienfilter bei Periduralanaesthesien

R. H. Borst, N. Ekmekci, H. Fleischer, S. Schielke, R. Stehle und A. Turanoglu

In unserer Abteilung ist die Katheterperiduralanaesthesie (KPDA) eine gebräuchliche Methode zur Behandlung von postoperativen oder posttraumatischen Schmerzzuständen. In einer früheren Mitteilung – beim Zentraleuropäischen Kongreß 1977 in Genf – berichteten wir über unsere Anfangsergebnisse bei der bakteriologischen Untersuchung nach Langzeitperiduralanaesthesie [3].

Wir fanden bei den damaligen Untersuchungen, wobei die Gesamtzahl der Patienten mit 23 relativ gering war, bei einer durchschnittlichen Liegedauer des Periduralanaesthesiekatheters (PDA-Katheter) von 6, 8 Tagen eine mit 48% erschütternd hohe Kontamination der Katheterspitze (Abb. 1). Aus der Spülflüssigkeit konnte der Bakteriologe bei 22% der Fälle Bakterien züchten, und die Haut im Bereich der Einstichstelle erbrachte bei 30% einen positiven Abstrich [3].

Wir haben danach von der Durchführung einer KPDA ohne Filter Abstand genommen und in der Folgezeit nur noch diese Anaesthesieform unter Verwendung eines Bakterienfilters – des Millipors – durchgeführt. Inzwischen überblicken wir 100 Patienten nach einer KPDA mit einer durchschnittlichen Liegezeit von 5,5 Tagen. Nach Einführung des Bakterienfilters, den wir alle 2 Tage wechseln, ging die Kontaminationsrate – wie man der Abb. 1 entnehmen kann – auf 20% zurück, die Spülflüssigkeit war nur noch bei 14% der Fälle infiziert.

Bakteriologische Untersuchungen

Ich kann hier nur kurz auf die Technik der bakteriologischen Untersuchungen[1] eingehen. Die zur bakteriologischen Untersuchung anstehenden Materialien, wie Katheterspitze, aspirierte Flüssigkeit nach Durchspülung des noch liegenden PDA-Katheters mit steriler Kochsalzlösung und Watteträger mit Abstrich an der Einstichstelle, wurden zur Bakterienvermehrung in Traubenzucker-bouillon und in Thioglykolatmedium (Fa. DIFCO-Detroit) gebracht. Die Ansätze wurden danach bis 5 Tage bei 37 °C bebrütet. Trat ein mikrobielles Wachstum auf, so wurde auf feste Nährböden überimpft (Blutagar, Endoagar und Sabouraud-Nährböden). Die weitere Bebrütung erfolgte sowohl ärob als auch anärob.

---

[1] Die Untersuchungen wurden durch Herrn Prof. Dr. R. Haas, 8960 Kempten, Augartenweg 20, durchgeführt, wofür wir ihm an dieser Stelle danken möchten

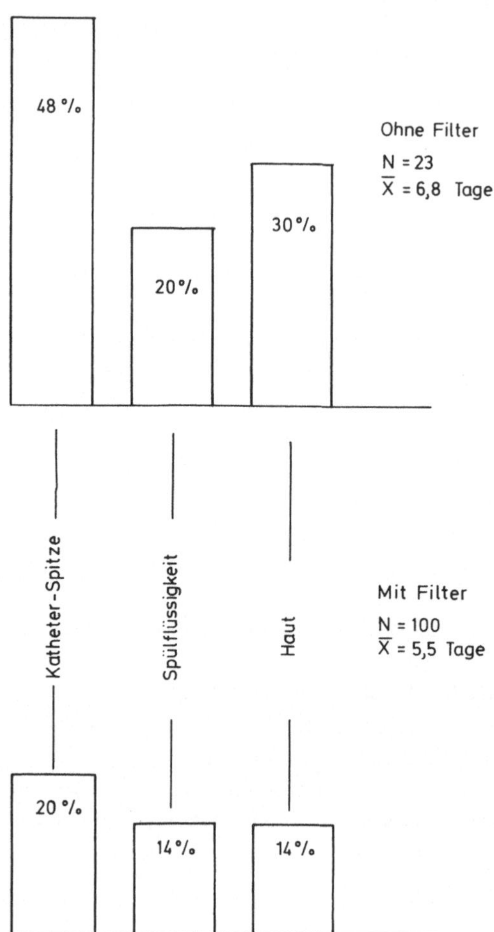

Abb. 1. Kontaminationsraten bei Langzeit-KPDA. *Oben:* Injektionen des Lokalanaesthetikums, in % ohne Bakterienfilter, n = 23, $\bar{x}$ = 6, 8 Tage, *unten:* unter Verwendung eines Bakterienfilters, n = 100, $\bar{x}$ = 5,5 Tage. Rückgang der Kontamination der untersuchten Materialien Katheterspitze, Spülflüssigkeit aus dem Katheterlumen sowie der Haut an der Einstichstelle

Wir wollen mit dieser kurzen Schilderung nur darauf hinweisen, daß mit diesen Methoden der Bakteriologie eine starke Anreicherung von Bakterien gesichert war, so daß auch eine ganz geringe Kontamination mit nur wenigen Bakterien, z. B. an der Katheterspitze, schließlich zu einem Erregernachweis führte. Dies mag zu Diskrepanzen in den Prozentzahlen zu der in der Literatur angegebenen Kontaminationsrate bei KPDA führen [2, 4, 6, 8].

In Tabelle 1 sind die nachgewiesenen Keime aufgelistet. Der Staphylococcus aureus führt den – man möchte sagen beängstigenden – Reigen der pathogenen Keime an (9/6/8). Es folgen Enterokokken (4/2/2) und die Kolibakterien (3/1/0). Weitere Keime, wie nicht hämolytische Streptokokken, Klebsiellen, Citrobacter freundii, wurden in Einzelfällen gefunden. Bei den fakultativ pathogenen Keimen findet sich der Staphylococcus albus je 3mal an der Katheterspitze, in der Spülflüssigkeit und an der Haut.

Wenn man diese Auflistung von Keimen sieht, ist man als Kliniker mit Recht beunruhigt über die möglichen Auswirkungen der bakteriellen Kontamination, z. B. entzündliche Pro-

Tabelle 1. Übersicht über die an den Untersuchungsmaterialien nachgewiesenen pathogenen, fakultativ pathogenen und sonstigen Keimen

Keimart		Katheterspitze	Spülflüssigkeit	Haut
Pathogen	Staphylococcus aureus	9	6	8
	Enterokokken	4	2	2
	E. coli	3	1	–
	Nichthämolytische Streptokokken	2	–	–
	Klebsiellen	1	–	–
	Citrobacter freundii	–	1	–
	Candida albicans	1	–	–
Fakultativ pathogen	Staphylococcus albus	3	3	3
	Alkaligenes (Achromobacter)	–	1	–
Sonstige	Aerobe Sporenbildner	1	–	1

zesse im PDA-Raum wie Abszesse [1, 7] und Übergreifen der Entzündung auf den intrathekalen Raum. Glücklicherweise haben wir – und das sei hier eingeflochten – in keinem Fall klinische Hinweise auf derartige Komplikationsmöglichkeiten finden können.

Liegedauer des PDA-Katheters/Kontamination

Abbildung 2 zeigt die Kontaminationsquoten in Abhängigkeit von der Liegezeit des PDA-Katheters. Bis zu 2 Tage lagen allerdings nur 2 Katheter, die in beiden Fällen in den 3 Untersuchungsmaterialien keine Infektion zeigten. Nach 3–4tägiger Liegedauer – ähnlich wie auch nach 5–7 Tagen – waren um die 20% der Katheterspitzen kontaminiert. Erstaunlicherweise ging die Kontaminationsrate bei längerer Liegezeit – über 7 Tage – auf 14% zurück.

In der Spülflüssigkeit dagegen fand sich in dem zuletzt genannten Zeitraum die mit 29% höchste Kontaminationsrate. Möglicherweise kommen mit längerer Liegezeit körpereigene Abwehrmechanismen in Gang, die in den PDA-Raum eingedrungene Keime abtöten.

Aufschlüsselung der Kontaminationsquote nach Art der Operation

In Tabelle 2 sind die Kontaminationsquoten nach der Art der Operationen aufgeschlüsselt. Erstaunlich ist, daß nach aseptischen Operationen mit 29% positive Befunde an der Katheterspitze vorlagen im Gegensatz zu Darmoperationen mit rund 15%. Hierbei muß erwähnt werden, daß Patienten nach Darmoperationen häufig Antibiotika zur „Kurzzeitprophylaxe" erhielten. Septische Operationen hatten mit 36% den höchsten, Patienten ohne Operationen mit 12,5% den niedrigsten Anteil.

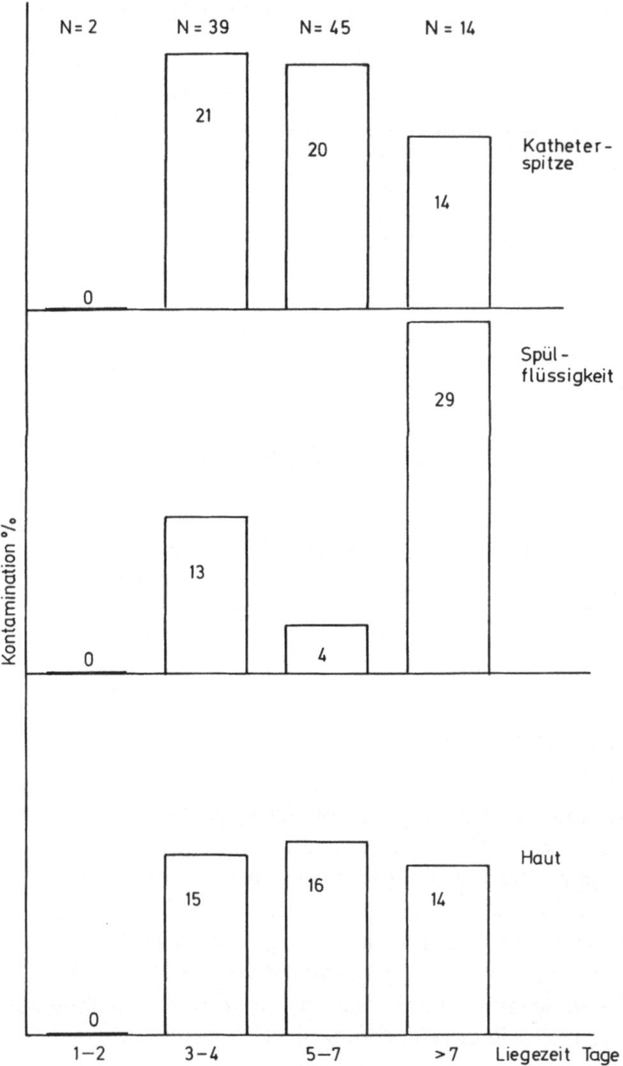

Abb. 2. Kontamination in Abhängigkeit von der Liegezeit

Tabelle 2. Kontaminationsraten (%) in Beziehung zum chirurgischen Eingriff

	Aseptische Operationen (n = 14)	Darm-Operationen (n = 68)	Septische Operationen (n = 11)	Keine Operation n = 8
Katheterspitze	29	15	36	12,5
Spülflüssigkeit	29	16	9	12,5
Haut	14	15	9	25

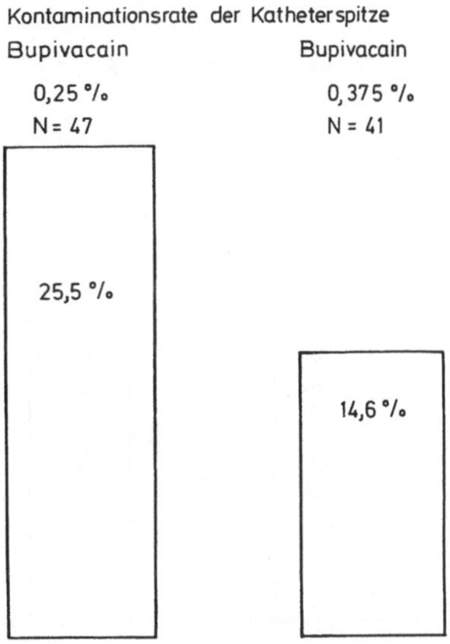

Abb. 3. Kontaminationsraten der Katheterspitze (%)

Konzentration Bupivacain/Kontaminationsrate

Abbildung 3 stellt für die Katheterspitze die Ergebnisse bei Verwendung von 0,25%iger bzw. 0,375%iger Bupivacainlösung mit Adrenalinzusatz dar. Bei Verwendung von 0,25%igem Bupivacain war die Kontaminationsrate mit 25,5% deutlich höher als bei Verwendung von 0,375%igem Bupivacain mit 14,6% kontaminierten Katheterspitzen.

Antibiotika/Kontaminationsquoten

Schließlich war für uns noch die Frage interessant, inwieweit die Verabreichung von Antibiotika sich in der Keimbesiedelung niederschlägt (die Antibiotika wurden allerdings nicht wegen der Tatsache der KPDA sondern aus anderen Gründen verabreicht). Aus Abb. 4 ist ersichtlich, daß in der Patientengruppe ohne Antibiotika bei 26,5% der Fälle ein positiver bakteriologischer Befund an der Katheterspitze vorlag, dagegen nur bei 14% – was einer deutlichen Abnahme entspricht – in dem Patientenkollektiv mit Antibiotika. Die Antibiotikagabe hatte keinen Einfluß auf die Besiedelung des Katheterlumens, wie an den nahezu identischen Prozentzahlen der Spülflüssigkeit zu erkennen ist. Bei der Haut dagegen reduzierte sich die Kontamination von 22% auf 8% bei Antibiotikagabe.

Einfluß des Alters auf die Kontamination

Eine Beziehung zum Alter der Patienten haben wir nicht nachweisen können. So lag z. B. die Kontaminationsquote an der Katheterspitze bei Patienten bis 50 Jahren bei 17%, bei über 50jährigen Patienten bei 21%.

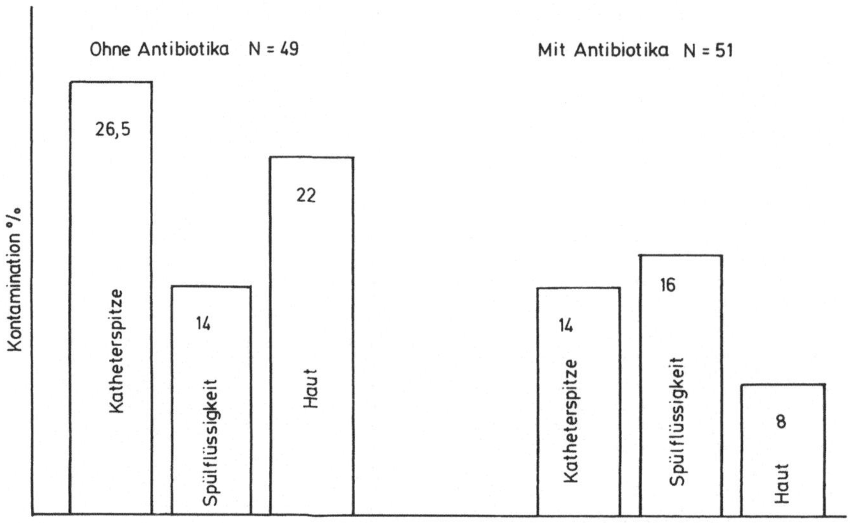

Abb. 4. Einfluß der Antibiotikaapplikation auf die Kontaminationsquote der Untersuchungsmaterialien

Als Resümee unserer Untersuchungen möchten wir folgern, daß man bei allen Maßnahmen im Zusammenhang mit einer KPDA äußerst strenge hygienische Kautelen einhalten sollte. Die Sicherheit aus hygienischer Sicht wird für den Patienten mit der Verwendung von Bakterienfilter erhöht. Man sollte daher Langzeit-KPDA ohne Filter nicht durchführen.

Literatur

1. D'Arcy Stanton-Hicks M (1976) Questions and answers. Anesth Analg (Cleve) 55:133
2. Barreto RS (1962) Bacteriological culture of indwelling epidural catheters. – Anesthesiology 23:643
3. Borst RH (1977) Bakteriologische Untersuchungen bei Langzeit-Katheter-Peridural-Anästhesie. Vortrag Zentraleuropäischer Kongreß 1977, Genf
4. Dannemiller FJ (1976) Questions and answers. Anesth Analg (Cleve) 55:132
5. Edwards WB, Higson RA (1943) Present status of continuous caudal anesthesia for obstetrics. Bull NY Acad Med 19:507
6. James FM, George RH, Naiem H, White GJ (1976) Bacteriologic aspects of epidural analgesia. – Anesth Analg (Cleve) 55:187
7. Saady A (1976) Epidural abscess complicating thoracic epidural analgesia. Anesthesiology 44:244
8. Strasser K, Hirsch I, Tomaschoff E (1974) Bakteriologische Nachuntersuchung von Epidural-Kathetern. Anaesthesist 23:351

Diskussion

Zindler:
Man ist immer wieder über die hohe Kontaminationsrate überrascht. Wieviele Ihrer Patienten haben einen Abszeß bekommen?

Borst:
Wir haben glücklicherweise in keinem Fall unserer "single shot" oder kontinuierlichen Katheterepiduralanaesthesien einen Abszeß gesehen.

Zindler:
Sie haben eine Hautkontamination bei Epiduralanaesthesien ohne Filter bei 30% der Fälle und mit Filter bei nur 14%. Welchen Effekt hat der Filter? Bei solchen Untersuchungen ist immer die Frage, ob man nicht im Verlauf der Studie merkt, wie gefährlich die Sache ist und entsprechend die Vorsichtsmaßnahmen verstärkt. Ich glaube, Ihre Zahlen, die ganz plausibel erscheinen, werden bei den nächsten 100 Epiduralanaesthesien ganz anders sein, und ich glaube, man darf nicht zu weitreichende Schlüsse daraus ziehen.

Borst:
Ich stimme Ihnen zu, daß diese Untersuchungen sehr schwierig sind. Sowohl beim Herausziehen des Katheters kann eine Infektion der Katheterspitze aus dem Stichkanal erfolgen als auch bei positivem Befund an der Katheterspitze kann der Stichkanal und sekundär die Haut infiziert werden. Ich würde mich freuen, wenn diese Untersuchung mit einer Kontaminationsrate von 20% nicht repräsentativ ist. Herr Ungemach hat eine ähnlich hohe Kontaminationsrate bei seinen Untersuchungen gefunden. Nach 1–2 Tagen konnte er ohne Bakterienfilter bei 52% Bakterien nachweisen, wobei es sich vorwiegend um Staphylokokkus aureus handelte.

Falke:
Bei welchen Patienten führen Sie länger als 7 Tage eine Epiduralanaesthesie durch?

Borst:
Bei diesen Patienten handelt es sich in der Regel um Schwerverletzte mit einer Zertrümmerung des Beckens oder der unteren Extremität. Auch bei einer Pankreatitis kann es sein, daß der Heilverlauf protrahiert ist, und wir würden deshalb eine längerdauernde Epiduralanaesthesie machen. In der vorliegenden Studie haben wir uns generell nach den Bedürfnissen des einzelnen Patienten gerichtet. Es wurde nicht vorherbestimmt, für wie lange bei dem einzelnen Patienten die Epiduralanaesthesie durchgeführt wurde, sondern wir haben den Epiduralkatheter für 3 oder sogar 10 Tage belassen, je nachdem, ob es uns für den Patienten günstig erschien.

Stanton-Hicks:
You showed the real nature of these complications. They are in the majority of the cases bloodborn. The bacteria reaches the catheter by blood, occasionally they are entering the epidural space from the puncture sit. With long term indwelling catheters the epidural abscess is usually occuring from an infection elsewhere in the body. The fact, however, that we do not get infections in patients who have epidural catheters for 4–8 weeks to relieve chronic pain, must be due to the bactericidal nature of the local anaesthetic solution. Obviously the bactericidal effect is related to the concentration of the local anaesthetic. As you showed it is stronger with the 0,375% solution than with a 0,25%. It does look therefore as if there is a great deal of protection just from the continuous local anaesthetic solution.

Rasterelektronenmikroskopische Befunde an Epiduralkathetern

H. J. Wüst und K. A. Rosenbauer

Bei Untersuchungen an Biomaterialien [1, 3, 7] hat es sich gezeigt, daß sowohl das Material von Venenverweilkathetern als auch deren Oberflächenbeschaffenheit [2, 4, 5, 7] einen großen Einfluß auf die Entstehung von Abscheidungsthromben haben.

Da auch in der Anaesthesiologie Kunststoffkatheter benutzt werden, wie etwa Katheter aus Polyamid, die im Regelfall 3–4 Tage im Epiduralraum eines Patienten belassen werden, schien es naheliegend, zunächst in Pilotstudien, auch die Oberflächenbeschaffenheit von neuen und gebrauchten Epiduralkathetern zu untersuchen.

Die Notwendigkeit zu derartigen Untersuchungen wird durch die Tatsache unterstrichen, daß bisher weder Befunde über die Oberflächenbeschaffenheit derartiger Katheter noch über Veränderungen, die nach längerer Verweildauer möglicherweise auftreten, vorliegen.

Material und Methode

Ungebrauchte Polyamidkatheter verschiedener Hersteller (Braun-Melsungen, Portex) wurden unter gleichen Bedingungen den Originalpackungen entnommen, und es wurde dabei streng darauf geachtet, daß weder die Katheterspitze noch der sonstige, zur Untersuchung vorgesehene Katheterbereich berührt wurde.

Die für die rasterelektronenmikroskopische Analyse ausgesuchten Katheterstücke wurden entweder ohne Vorpräparation mit Leitsilber auf Messingträger montiert und in einer Kathodenzerstäubungsanlage (Polaron) mit 20 nm Gold beschichtet oder aber, um evtl. bei der Präparation von gebrauchten Kathetern auftretende Artefakte auszuschließen, nach einer für die Untersuchung von Biomaterialien bewährten Methode (vgl. [7] und [10]) aufgearbeitet. Die Fixierung erfolgte dabei in einer 1%igen phosphatgepufferten Glutaraldehydlösung (pH 7,4).

Die gebrauchten Katheter wurden nach einer Liegedauer von 4 Tagen ohne Berührung der Katheterspitze und der zu untersuchenden Schaftteile den Patienten entnommen, sofort in die Fixierungslösung gelegt und nach einer Fixationszeit von 16 h 2mal in Phosphatpuffer (pH 7,4) und 2mal in Aqua dest. je 10 min gespült. Nach Dehydratisierung in Dimethoxypropan-HCL [6] und Critical-point-Trocknung aus CO_2, Präparatmontage mit Leitsilber auf Messingträger wurden die Proben zur Herstellung der Leitfähigkeit mit 20 nm Gold beschichtet.

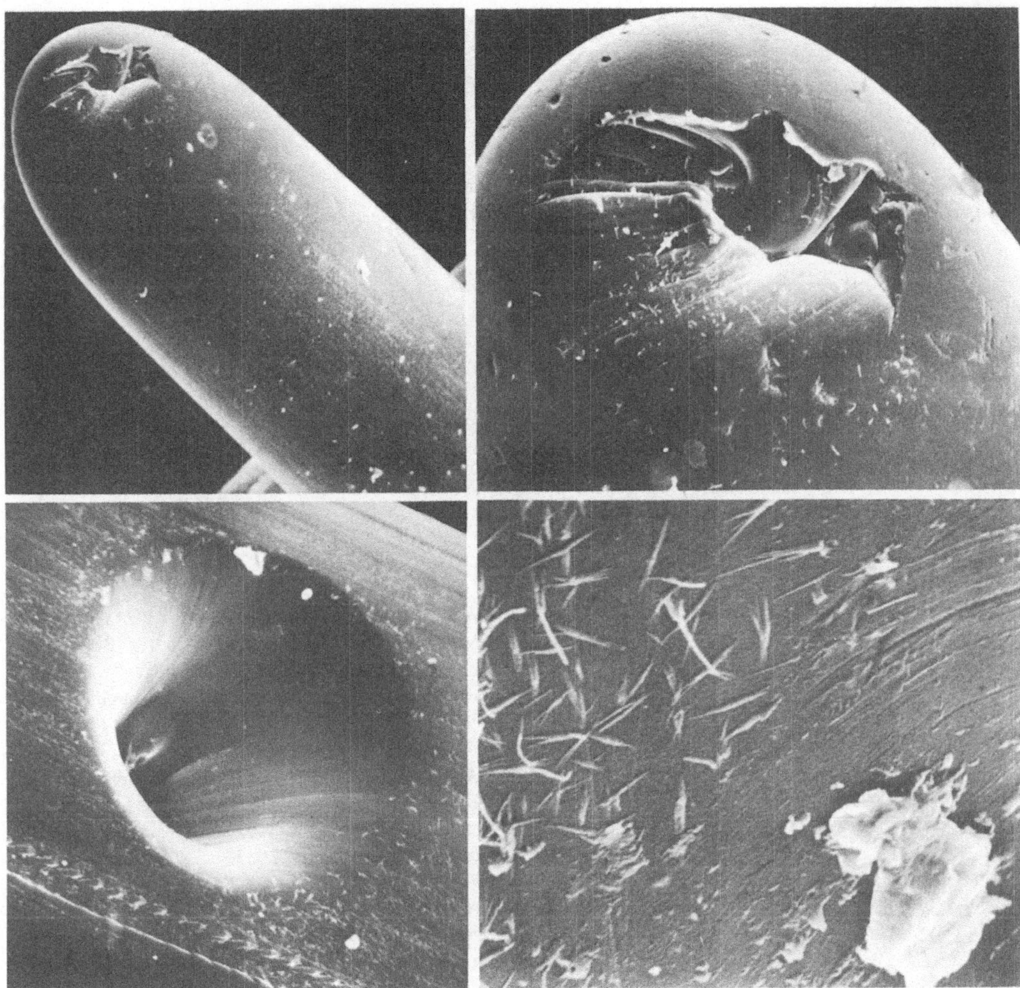

Abb. 1 (*oben links*). Spitze eines ungebrauchten Portex-Epiduralkatheters aus Polyamid. Grober Herstellungsdefekt an der Katheterspitze und bereits bei dieser Vergrößerung sichtbare Rauhigkeit der Katheterwand. Vergr. 47 : 1

Abb. 2 (*oben rechts*). Gleiches Präparat wie in Abb. 1 bei stärkerer Vergrößerung. Neben dem massiven Herstellungsdefekt werden kleinere, lochartige Artefakte und Rißbildungen sichtbar. Vergr. 126 : 1

Abb. 3 (*unten links*). Umgebung einer seitlichen Wandöffnung in einem Portex-Epiduralkatheter. Die seitliche Katheterwand weist einen, an eine Nahtstelle erinnernden Oberflächendefekt auf, der durch ein nicht optimales Herstellungswerkzeug bedingt sein dürfte. Vergr. 197 : 1

Abb. 4 (*unten rechts*). Bei stärkerer Vergrößerung finden sich auf einem Portex-Katheter kristalloide Strukturen. Außerdem ist eine nicht identifizierbare Auflagerung sowie Riefenbildung in der Katheterwand sichtbar. Vergr. 1181 : 1

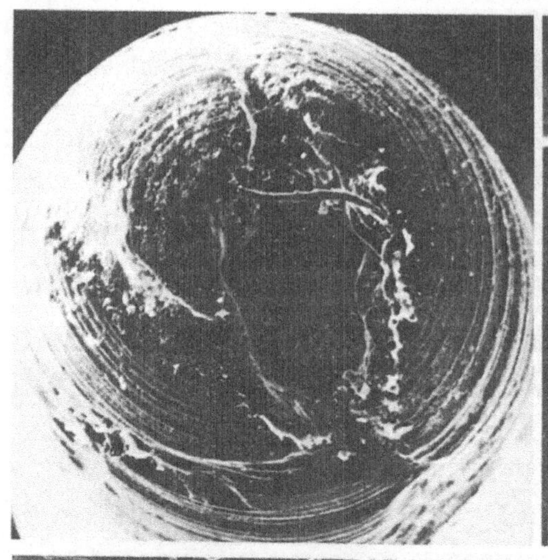

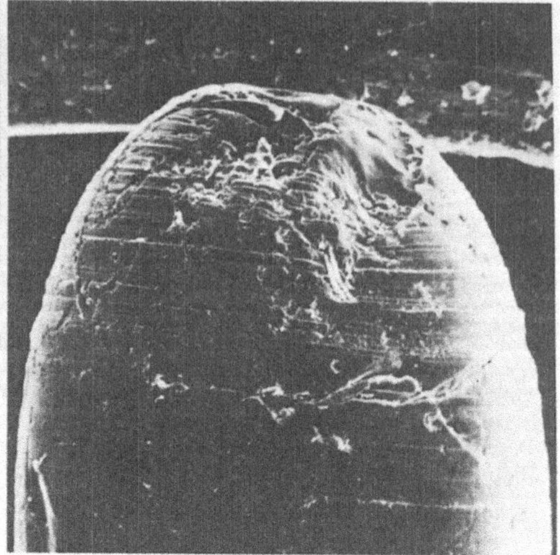

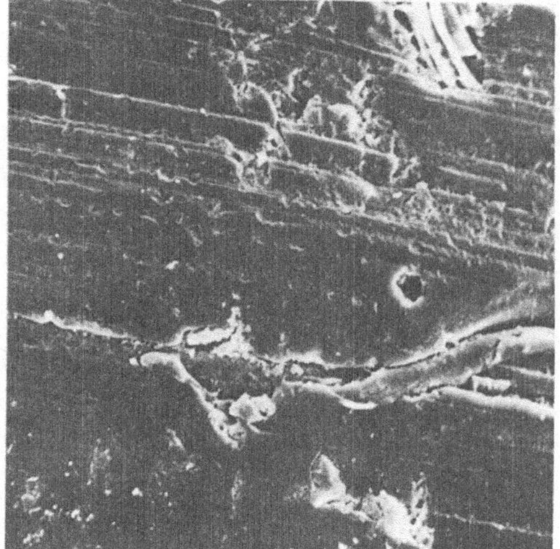

Abb. 5 (*oben links*). Ungebrauchter Braun-Melsungen-Polyamidepiduralkatheter. Bereits bei schwachen Vergrößerungen zeigt die Katheterspitze starke Riefen- und Rißbildungen. Vergr. 20:1

Abb. 6 (*oben rechts*). Spitze eines ungebrauchten Braun-Melsungen-Epiduralkatheters. Starke herstellungsbedingte Oberflächendefekte und Riefenbildungen. Vergr. 20:1

Abb. 7 (*unten*). Ungebrauchter Braun-Melsungen-Epiduralkatheter. Bei einer stärkeren Vergrößerung sind Kratzer und Riefen in der Wand des Katheterschaftes zu erkennen. Vergr. 150:1

Ergebnisse

Obwohl alle Katheter mit äußerster Vorsicht behandelt und Beschädigungen der Katheteroberfläche mit Sicherheit vermieden wurden, lassen sich sowohl an deren Spitzen als auch an den Wandoberflächen beider Fabrikate z. T. sehr gravierende Herstellungsdefekte nachweisen (Abb. 1–7). Neben Rißstellen (s. Abb. 5) und Kerben (s. Abb. 2, 5) finden sich auch lochartige Defekte (s. Abb. 2).

Nach einer Liegedauer von 4 Tagen sind an der Katheteroberfläche flächenhaft ausgebreitete Ablagerungen erkennbar, die aus denaturierten Eiweißen bestehen dürften (Abb. 8a, b, 9). Gelegentlich sieht man adhärente Epithelzellen oder einzelne Erythrozyten (Abb. 10, 12).

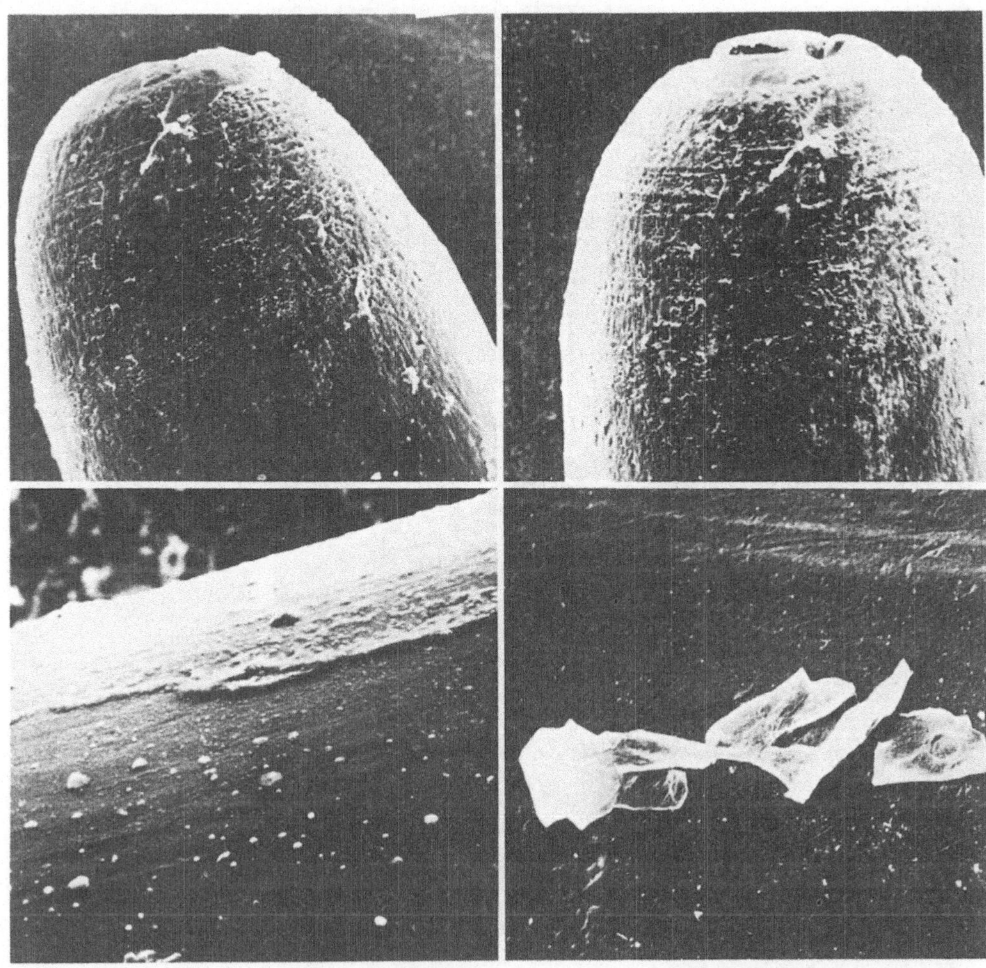

Abb. 8a, b (*oben*). Flächenhaft ausgebreitete Ablagerungen auf der Oberfläche eines gebrauchten Epiduralkatheters. Vergr. 58:1

Abb. 9 (*unten links*). Niederschläge auf der Wand eines gebrauchten Epiduralkatheters. Vergr. 58:1

Abb. 10 (*unten rechts*). Plattenepithelzellen auf der Wand eines gebrauchten Epiduralkatheters. Vergr. 170:1

Diskussion

Die rasterelektronenmikroskopische Oberflächenanalyse von Epiduralkathetern zweier Hersteller hat bei beiden Fabrikaten z. T. sehr erhebliche Herstellungsdefekte aufgedeckt. Derartige Defekte sind nach den Untersuchungen von Rosenbauer [7, 9] prospektive Schwachstellen für Katheterbrüche oder aber, wie dies auch für Membranoxygenatoren [11] oder Herzklappenprothesen [8] nachgewiesen wurde, Prädispositionsstellen für die Entstehung

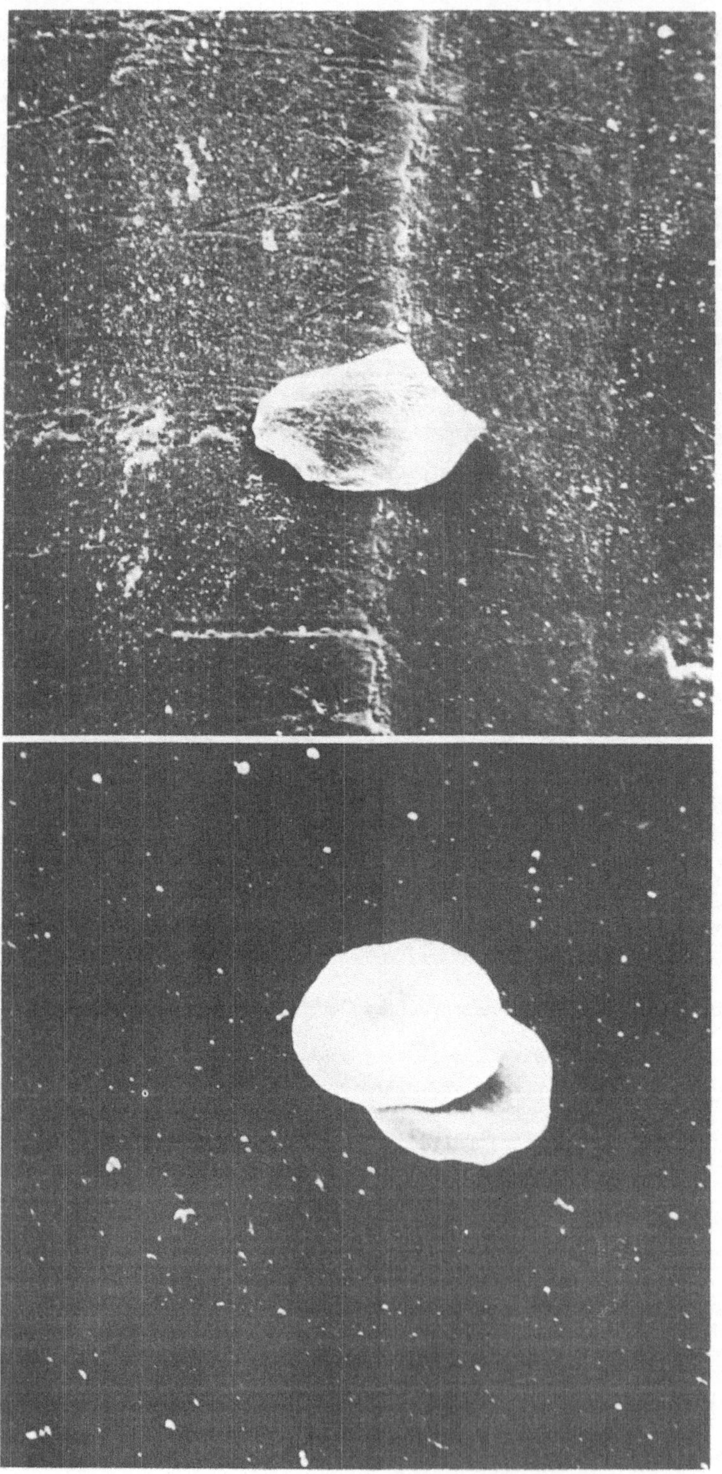

von Thromben. Auch denaturierte Plasmaproteide lagern sich bevorzugt an Oberflächenrauhigkeiten ab.

In der jetzigen Studie fanden sich ebenfalls hauptsächlich Auflagerungen überall dort, wo Oberflächendefekte, Unebenheit oder Rauhigkeit in der Katheterwandung waren. Ob bei den Epiduralkathetern Reaktionen des umgebenden Gewebes oder Reaktionen mit Lokalanaesthetika, deren pH-Wert bei 5,8–6,0 liegt, eine zusätzliche Rolle spielen, müssen weitere Untersuchungen ergeben.

Zusammenfassung

Rasterelektronenmikroskopische Pilotstudien an Epiduralkathetern zweier Hersteller haben erhebliche Herstellungsdefekte gezeigt. An gebrauchten Kathetern fanden sich bes. im Bereich dieser Defekte Auflagerungen. Eine Aussage über die Bedeutung dieser Befunde mit Hinblick auf mögliche neurologische Komplikationen bei der kontinuierlichen Epiduralanaesthesie lassen sich zumindest zum gegenwärtigen Zeitpunkt nicht machen. Hierzu sind Untersuchungen an einem größeren Material notwendig. Es ist aber zu fordern, daß bei der Herstellung eines vielleicht belanglos erscheinenden Details der Epiduralanaesthesie, wie z. B. des Katheters, die Fertigungsmethoden verbessert werden und die Sicherheit des Materials erhöht wird.

Literatur

1. Bourassa MG, Cantin M, Sandborn EB, Peterson E (1976) Scanning electron microscopy of surface irregularities and thrombogenesis of polyurethane and polyethylene coronary catheters. Circulation 53:992
2. Libsack CV, Kollmeyer K (1979) Role of catheter surface morphology on intravascular morphology on thrombosis of plastic catheters. J Biomed Mater Res 13:459
3. Löffler B, Bauer H (1980) Untersuchungen zur Thrombogenität verschiedener Kathetermaterialien. In: Müller-Wiefel H, Barras JB, Ehringer H, Krüger M (Hrsg) Mikrozirkulation und Blutthreologie. Therapie der peripheren Verschlußkrankheiten. Witzstrock, Baden-Baden Köln New York, S 244–248
4. Müller KM, Blaschke R, Steinmaier F (1977) Oberflächenstrukturen von Venenkathetern. Med Welt 28:2055
5. Müller KM, Friemann J, Hartenauer U, Blaschke R (1981) Frühstadien der Oberflächenablagerungen auf zentralen Venenkathetern nach 24 stündigem intravasalem Blutkontakt. Med Welt 32:1362
6. Muller LL, Jacks TJ (1975) Rapid chemical dehydration of samples for electron microscopic examinations. J Histochem Cytochem 23:107
7. Rosenbauer KA (im Druck) Light microscopic and sem findings on intravenous polyurethane catheters. Scan Electron Microsc

◀ **Abb. 11** (*oben*). Plattenepithelzelle und Niederschläge aus denaturierten Eiweißen auf der Wand eines gebrauchten Epiduralkatheters. Vergr. 234 : 1

Abb. 12 (*unten*). Erythrozyten auf der Wand eines gebrauchten Epiduralkatheters nach 4tägiger Liegedauer. Vergr. 1463 : 1

8. Rosenbauer KA, Herzer JA (1980) Further electron microscopic studies of different types of prosthetic heart valves which were in place between one and more than ten years. Scan Electron Microsc 3:219–225
9. Rosenbauer KA, Herzer JA (1981) Surface morphology and tensile force at breaking point of different kinds of intravenous catheters before and after usage. Scan Electron Microsc 3:125
10. Rosenbauer KA, Kegel BH (1978) Rasterelektronenmikroskopische Technik. Präparationsverfahren in Medizin und Biologie. Thieme, Stuttgart
11. Rosenbauer KA, Herzer JA, Kojimahara M, Falke K, Jansen B, Schulte HD, Birks W (1976) Langzeitperfusion im Tierversuch unter Anwendung beschichteter und unbeschichteter extrakorporaler Kreislaufsysteme. Licht- und rasterelektronenmikroskopische Untersuchungen. Fachz Lab 20:815

Über die Problematik von Epiduralkathetern mit seitlichen Löchern

O. H. Schulte-Steinberg

Über viele Jahre wurden für die kontinuierliche Epiduralanaesthesie ausschließlich Katheter mit endständiger Öffnung verwendet. Die Gefahr der Gewebs-, Gefäß- und Duraverletzungen durch die scharfen Ränder der zunächst nur mit der Schere von der Rolle abgeschnittenen Epiduralkatheter ließ den Wunsch nach weniger traumatischen Geräten laut werden.

Die Industrie hat in der Folge 2 Versionen entwickelt (Abb. 1): 1. Katheter mit blindverschlossenem rundem Ende und kleinen seitlichen Löchern, 2. Katheter mit endständigem Loch und abgerundetem Rand.

Die Katheter der Version 1 hatten in ihrer Entwicklungszeit besonders mit dem Problem des Abknickens im Bereich der durch Löcher geschwächten Wand zu kämpfen. Dieses

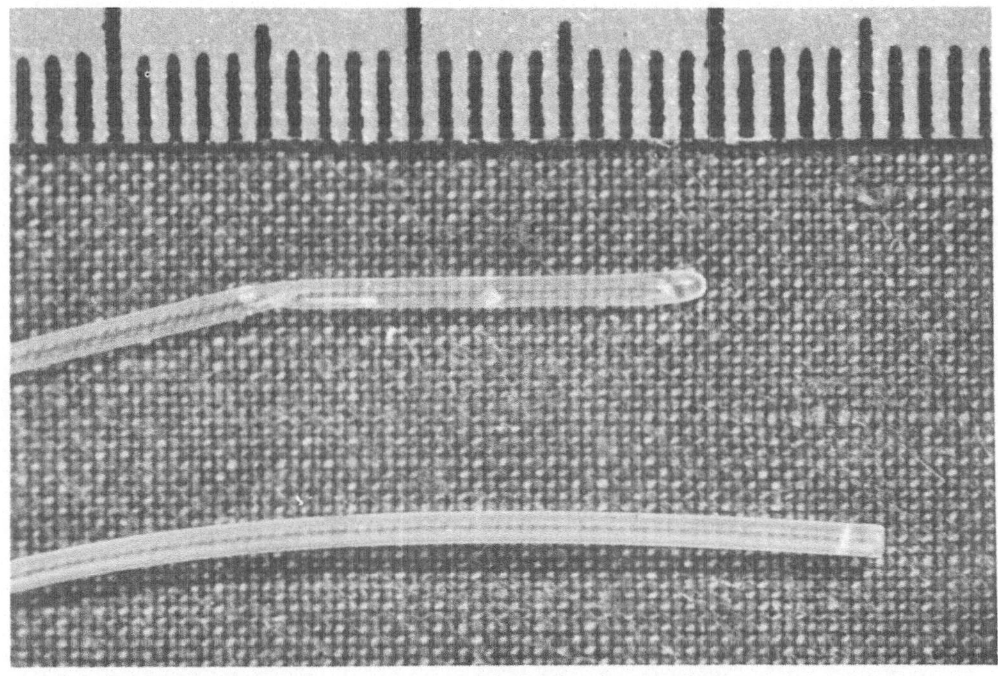

Abb. 1. Katheter mit blindverschlossenem runden Ende und kleinen seitlichen Löchern (*oben*) und Katheter mit endständigem Loch und abgerundetem Rand (*unten*)

Problem scheint im wesentlichen gelöst zu sein. Dagegen besteht immer noch die Gefahr des Abrisses am gelöcherten Teil des Katheters, und uns wurde kürzlich ein solcher Fall bekannt von einem mit der Methodik sehr vertrauten Anaesthesisten. Aber auch andere klinische Eigenheiten dieser Katheter gibt es zu berücksichtigen. Die intravasale Lage eines Katheters zu erkennen, ist zweifellos schwieriger beim Katheter mit seitlichen Löchern und blindem Ende. Mit der Aspiration kommt es eher zu einem Anlegen der Gefäßwand an den Katheter, und es wird zu wenig Blut in das Lumen befördert, um außen sichtbar zu werden. Die kleinlumigen Löcher erschweren auch die Aspiration von Liquor bei einer akzidentellen Durapunktion.

Zur Illustration mag folgender klinischer Fall dienen:

Nach Einlage eines Epiduralkatheters wurde mit negativem Ergebnis auf Blut und Liquor aspiriert. Nach Gabe einer Dosis von über 20 ml 0,5%igem Bupivacain gab die Patientin nach 5 min Parästhesien in den Fingern an. Zu diesem Zeitpunkt war weder eine An- noch eine Hypalgesie klinisch in diesem Bereich festzustellen. 10 min nach der Injektion mußte die Patientin intubiert werden wegen eintretender Ateminsuffizienz und einer nun schließlich erkennbaren totalen Spinalanaesthesie.

Die Erklärung mag in einem teilweisen Durchtritt des Katheters durch die Dura liegen. Die Mehrzahl der seitlichen Löcher lag sicherlich noch im Epiduralraum, wo die Hauptmenge des nach dem Bromage-Schema errechneten Lokalanaesthetikums deponiert wurde. Diese Erfahrung mit der erst nach 10 min deutlich gewordenen totalen Spinalanaesthesie läßt auch den Wert der häufig als absolut notwendig angesehenen Testdosis fragwürdig erscheinen.

Die Verwendung eines Katheters mit endständigem Loch hätte hier die subarachnoidale Lage sicherlich besser erkennen lassen. Wir verwenden nach ausführlichem Gebrauch von Kathetern mit seitlichen Löchern nun ausschließlich wieder die 2. Version mit endständiger abgerundeter Öffnung, wie übrigens auch Bromage, der nach mannigfachen Versuchen wieder zum, selbst von der Rolle abgeschnittenen Katheter zurückgekehrt ist. Eine Verbesserung bedeutet abschließend die von uns angegebene Einführhilfe, die ein Abknicken des Katheters am Ansatz der Nadel vermeidet und die Überwindung der gebogenen Nadelöffnung und späteren Hindernissen erleichtert.

Seit wir diese Einführhilfe benutzen, haben wir nie mehr einen Mandrine zur Stabilisierung am Nadeleingang im Katheter verwenden müssen. Letztlich kann man also sagen, der einfachste Katheter hat am wenigsten Komplikationsmöglichkeiten.

Diskussion

Lanz:
Besteht nicht mit dem endständig offenen Katheter die Gefahr, daß man Gefäße anreißt und dadurch ein epidurales Hämatom setzt?

Schulte-Steinberg:
Aus meiner Montrealer Erfahrung kann ich das nicht bestätigen. Wir haben über lange Zeit auch hier in Deutschland, als noch keine Katheter vorhanden waren, das Kathetermaterial in der Rolle importiert, selber abgeschnitten und markiert. Mit diesem Katheter haben wir nicht häufiger epidurale Blutungen diagnostiziert als wir das heute mit dem anderen Kathetermaterial tun. Aber das ist keine echte Untersuchung, sondern nur ein klinischer Eindruck.

Stanton-Hicks:
Until now there is no sufficient data to support the contention that a catheter with a hole at the end is safer to use than one with sideholes. But from a study on a model, where a subarachnoid sack, it may be suggested that the use of catheters with a hole at the end may be safer. It was shown that the hydrostatic pressure prevented the solution from entering the subarachnoid space when the model was raised to a vertical position and the catheter was injected in this position. Then most of the fluid went out of the proximal hole into the epidural space. But when the model was lain horizontal, then more of the solution went into the subarachnoid space. It is quite a possibility with a catheter that has got side holes.

Wüst:
In my opinion the discussion of whether catheters with a hole at the end or catheters with sideholes is a better way to prevent total spinal anaesthesia or inadvertant intravascular injections is until now only based on suggestions. Moore reported when using catheters with a hole at the end in a series of 3,506 epidural anaesthetics an incidence of total spinal in 0.03% and of an inadvertant intravascular injection of 0.03%. In 24,000 epidural anaesthetics done in Düsseldorf using a catheter with sideholes the incidence of a total spinal and of an inadvertant intravascular injection of a local anaesthetic solution was 0.09%. Thus there is until now no sufficient evidence for the argument to use only catheters with an endhole. Before I see the need to change from catheters with sideholes to the other type it has to be shown by further research that the catheter with a hole at the end is safer than the one with sideholes.

Frage:
What is the maximum single dose of Mepivacaine?

Stanton-Hicks:
In the USA the maximum dose of Mepivacaine is 500 mg without and 600 mg with epinephrine.

I don't know what your limits are here in Germany for bupivacaine. In the USA the maximum dose for this drug is 280 mg.

Lanz:
The maximum dose of Bupivacaine in Germany is 150 mg. The reason or the data, on which these lower doses in our country are based is not known.

Stanton-Hicks:
They are based on animal experiments as are most of these things. Dose response studies of these agents have obviously been done in which the drug has been placed into different tissues. From the resulting blood levels, the levels in the tissues and the sign of toxic reactions in the central nervous system the maximum doses of the local anaesthetic which do not produce central nervous symptoms is determined. These studies were done 15 years ago prior to the availability of gaschromatography and the knowledge of the kinetics of druguptake, distribution and excreation. I believe that many of these limits are going to be changed now, but this will take a long time. In clinical practice the maximum doses are unrealistic but, of course, if you exceed them and, if you get into trouble, then you are the person who will be hung.

III Opiate epidural/intrathekal zur intra- und postoperativen Analgesie

Vorsitz: A. S. Tung, Pittsburgh/USA, M. d'Arcy Stanton-Hicks, Denver/USA und E. Hartung, Düsseldorf

Studies on the Development of Tolerance Following Spinal Analgetics

A. S. Tung, and T. L. Yaksh†

Many biologic responses secondary to opiate receptor interactions, both in vitro and in vivo, are subject to the development of tolerance. Thus, it would not be surprising to observe a decrease in the antinociceptive response to intrathecal or epidural opiates after prolonged use. Indeed, this phenomenon has been observed both clinically and in experimental animals.

In recent experiments on rats with chronic implanted intrathecal catheters, we examined tolerance development to the analgesic response of intrathecal morphine [1]. After measuring their baseline response to 15 μg intrathecal morphine (a dose required to reliably produce a substantial increase in their escape latency in the hot-plate and tail-flick tests), we injected one group of animals intrathecally with 45 μg morphine. A control group was given daily intrathecal saline. On days 5 and 8, each of the groups received the "probe" dose of morphine (15 μg). As shown in Table 1, the results indicate that the analgesic response to intrathecal morphine decreased to about 40% of the original level in 8 days. Similar observations were made previously with intrathecal opiates in primates [2]. As for the analgesic response to epidural opiates, the development of tolerance over a 4–6 day period has also been observed in cats [3].

Intrathecal or epidural opiates have been used extensively for treatment of cancer pain with good results. In spite of animal experiments showing cross tolerance between systemic and spinal opiate analgesia [4], it has been observed that patients tolerant to systemic narcotics will respond to intrathecal morphine [5]. A case of systemic opiate withdrawal syndrome

Table 1. Results of intrathecal (IT) morphine-tolerance study in rats using the hot plate test. The probe dose used was 15 μg. Animals in the morphine group were given 45 μg morpine IT daily, while the saline group received daily IT saline.

Response to Morphine 15 μg IT	Day 1	Day 5	Day 8
Morphine group (% MPE)	93.06 ± 2.13 (n = 25)	60.22 ± 14.72 (n = 8)	33.27 ± 5.22 (n = 25)
Saline group (% MPE)	95.87 ± 4.13 (n = 5)	–	92.07 ± 7.92 (n = 5)

$$\% \text{ MPE} = \frac{\text{Postdrug latency (baseline)}}{\text{cut-off time (baseline)}}$$

was reported after adequate analgesia was obtained with an intrathecal injection of morphine [6]. With regard to tolerance development to intraspinal opiate analgesia, the experience of different investigators has been varied. Ventafridda observed in eight cancer patients that the analgesic response to bolus doses of intrathecal morphine decreased significantly over a 3-day period [7]. On the other hand, Lazorthes and colleagues [8] observed prolonged pain relief after multiple injections of morphine delivered through an indwelling intrathecal catheter in three cancer patients for periods of 30–50 days. Onofrio and colleagues [9] reported the implantation in a cancer patient of a chronic infusion pump connected to an intrathecal catheter inserted via a laminectomy around the T8 level. At an infusion rate of 1.2 mg/3 ml/24 h, the patient had adequate pain relief without systemic narcotic supplementation for 4 months. No other adverse effects were detected. With regard to epidural opiate analgesia, tolerance has also been observed, but at a much slower rate of development when compared with intrathecal injections as in Ventafridda's series. Müller and colleagues [10] reported that, within the first 14 to 30 days in a series of cancer patients, the response to twice daily injections of epidural 2–5 mg morphine was very stable. After this period, patients required an increased dose of epidural opiate to produce adequate pain relief. We failed to detect any decrease in analgesia response to daily caudal morphine injections in patients with pelvic cancer pain after 1 week [11]. Zenz has also observed effective analgesia from epidural opiates for periods of up to 3 weeks [12].

It appears probable that the rate of tolerance development to opiates is dependent in part on the degree of receptor activation. Thus, repeated intrathecal injections produce high local drug levels in the spinal cord, excessive receptor activation, and, subsequently, rapid tolerance development. In contrast, slow intrathecal infusion or epidural injections requiring perhaps diffusion through the dura to cause receptor activation may be less likely to result in tolerance development. It should be noted that the contrast between the results of animal experiments and the growing amount of clinical literature may be due to the nature of the pain. Thus in the animal work, all animals are subjected to an escape or threshold measure, i.e., they do not feel a prolonged discomfort. In chronic pain, the afferent barrage may be less, but it is constant. Whether this may play a role is still under investigation because a similar lack of cross tolerance between the antinociceptive effect of spinal μ and δ receptor agonists has been obtained in morphine-tolerant primates.

The next important question concerning spinal opiate tolerance is the availability of alternative drugs, should a decrease in the opiate analgesia response occur. There has been increasing evidence to support the existence of multiple subpopulations of opiate receptors. The characterization of different opiate-receptor subpopulations is done by correlating the pharmacologic profile observed with different physiologic effects. Thus, Martin and colleagues [13] proposed three classes of opiate receptors (mu, kappa, and sigma) according to the different naloxone-sensitive effects observed in a chronic spinal dog model for three different groups of opiates (represented by morphine, ethylketocyclazocine, and SKF 10047, respectively). Lord and colleagues [14] proposed the existence of mu and delta receptors after observing, first, a different rank order of potency for various opiate alkaloids and peptides in suppressing the electrically induced contractions of the guinea pig ileum versus the mouse vas deferens and, second, a differential ability of these agents to displace naloxone and d-Ala_2-d-Leu_5-enkephalin (DADL) from brain homogenates. The agonists for the mu and delta receptors were represented by morphine and DADL, respectively. Fields and colleagues [15] have shown in binding studies that both mu and delta receptors exist in the spinal cord. Recently, by examining the sensitivity to naloxone sensitivity and cross tolerance

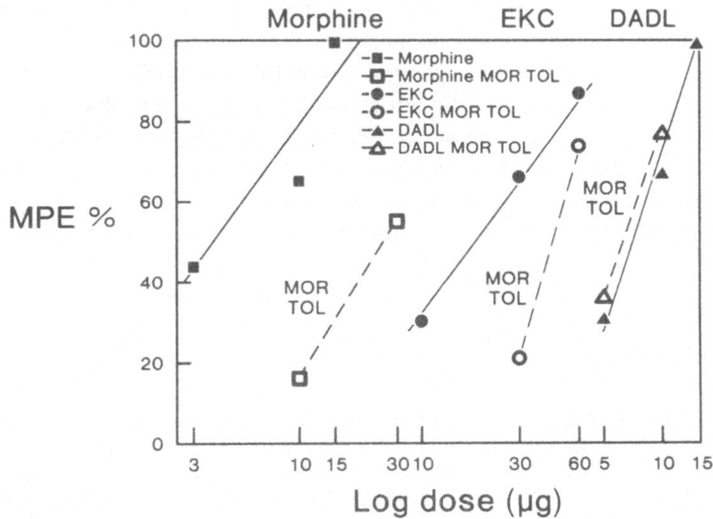

Fig. 1. Dose response curves of intrathecal morphine, ethylketocyclazocine (EKC), and D-ala$_2$-D-leu$_5$-enkephalin (DADL) in naive and morphine tolerant (MOR TOL) rats in the hot-plate test. MPE% = Postdrug latency (baseline) / Cut-off time (baseline)

studies in rats, we were able to show that both mu and delta receptors were involved in the mediation of spinal analgesia [16]. Thus, rats made tolerant by daily injections of systemic morphine showed a sevenfold increase in the ED_{50} for intrathecal morphine. In parallel groups of morphine-treated animals, the ED_{50} for intrathecal DADL was not altered (see Fig. 1). These data suggest that, in patients tolerant to the analgesic effect of a mu agonist such as morphine, a delta agonist such as DADL, if it were clinically approved, could be substituted.

Apart from the opiates, other neurotransmitter systems have been implicated in spinal analgesia. Thus, α-adrenergic, serotonergic, and GABA-like agonists have all been shown to elevate the nociceptive threshold after their intrathecal administration in animals in a variety of pain models [17–19]. More significantly, there is no cross tolerance between rat and primates intrathecal opiates and α-adrenergic agonists, such as clonidine or ST-91, a polar adrenergic agonist [1, 2]. In addition, the coadministration of low doses of intrathecal morphine and ST-91, presumably producing minimal activation of each associated receptor, yielded a highly significant elevation in the nociceptive threshold in rats [20] and primates [2]. This combination of two pharmacologically distinct agents produced an effect which did not result in significant tolerance, in contrast to the rapid tolerance resulting when an equianalgetic dose of intrathecal morphine alone was employed. This suggests that the use of drug mixtures would produce minimal activation of multiple analgesic receptor systems and may be an alternative method for providing prolonged spinal analgesia.

It should be noted that these data showing differential rates of tolerance development with combination therapy or the lack of cross tolerance between mu and delta receptor agonists argue strongly that the loss of drug effect is due to some change in the agonist-effector interaction. Such interpretations are also consistent with the wealth of in vitro bioassay data, where the response patterns of the isolated tissue from a morphine-tolerant animal can clearly be distinguished from those of a control. There is growing evidence, however, that insofar as the behavioral measures of tolerance are concerned, environmental cues and learning may play a consequential role in the development of altered responses to pain in the presence of a drug. Colpaert and colleagues [22, 23] observed that animals subjected to painful stimuli (mechanical or chemical) during the administration of the drug failed to show significant tolerance development to systemically administered opiates in contrast to nonstressed animals. The possibility of altering the development of tolerance by various pharmacologic and behavioral approaches suggests clear directions for future analgetic research.

References

1. Tung AS, Wang JY, Yaksh TL (to be published) Tolerance to intrathecal opiates in the rat
2. Yaksh TL, Reddy SVR (to be published) Studies on the analgetic effects of intrathecal opiates, α-adrenergic agonists and baclofen: their pharmacology in the primate. Anesthesiology
3. Tung AS, Yaksh TL (to be published) Evaluation of epidural opiates in the cat. 8th International congress of pharmacology, Tokyo
4. Yaksh TL, Kohl RL, Rudy TA (1977) Induction of tolerance and withdrawal in rats receiving morphine in the spinal subarachnoid space. Eur J Pharmacol 42:275–284
5. Tung A, Maliniak K, Tenicela R, Winter PM (1980) Intrathecal morphine for intraoperative and postoperative analgesia. JAMA 244:2637–2638
6. Tung AS, Tenicela R, Winter PLM (1980) Opiate withdrawal syndrome following intrathecal administration of morphine. Anesthesiology 53:340
7. Ventafridda V, Figliuzzi M, Tamburini M, Gori E, Parolaro D, Sala M (1979) Clinical observation on analgesia elicited by intrathecal morphine in cancer patients. In: Bonica JJ et al (eds) Adv in pain research and therapy, vol 3. Raven, New York, pp 559–565
8. Lazorthes Y, Gouarderes Ch, Verdie JC, Monsarrat B, Bastide R, Campan L, Alwan A, Cros J (1980) Analgesie par injection intrathecale de morphine etude pharmacocinetique et application aux douleurs irreductibles. Neurochirurgie 26:159–164
9. Onofrio B, Yaksh TL, Arnold PG (to be published) Continous low-dose intrathecal morphine administration in the treatment of chronic pain of malignant origin. Mayo Clin Proc
10. Müller H, Stoyanov M, Dorner U, Hempelmann G (to be published) opiates for relief of cancer pain. In: Yaksh TL, Müller H, Engquist A (eds) Anaesthesia and intensive care medicine. Springer, Berlin Heidelberg New York
11. Tung AS, Tenicela R, Barr G (to be published) Caudal opiates for pelvic cancer pain
12. Zenz M, Piepenbrock S, Hilfrich J, Husch M (to be published) Pain therapy with epidural morphine in patients with terminal cancer. In: Yaksh TL, Müller H, Engquist A (eds) Anaesthesia and intensive care medicine. Springer, Berlin Heidelberg New York
13. Martin WR, Eades CG, Thompson JA, Huppler RD, Gilbert PE (1976) The effects of morphine and nalorphine-like drugs in the non-dependent and morphine dependent chronic spinal dog. J Pharmacol Exp Ther 197:517–532
14. Lord JAH, Waterfield AA, Hughes J, Kosterlitz HW (1977) Endogenous opioid peptides: multiple agonists and receptors, Nature 267:495–499
15. Fields NL, Emson PC, Leigh BK, Gilbert RFT, Iversen LL (1980) Multiple opiate receptors in primary afferent fibres. Nature 214:351–352
16. Tung AS, Yaksh TL (to be published) Involvement of multiple opiate receptors in spinally mediated analgesia. Pain
17. Reddy SVR, Yaksh TL (1980) Antinociceptive effecs of lanthanum, neodymium and europium following intrathecal administration. Neuropharmacology 19:181–185
18. Yaksh TL, Wilson PR (1979) Spinal serotonin terminal system mediates antinociception. J Pharmacol Exp Ther 208:446–453
19. Wilson PR, Yaksh TL (1978) Baclofen is antinociceptive in the spinal intrathecal space of animals. Eur J Pharmacol 51:323–330

20. Wang J-Y, Yasuoka S, Yaksh TL (to be published) Studies on the analgetic effect of intrathecal ST-91 (2-[2,6-diethylphenylamino]-2-imidazoline): antagonism, tolerance and interaction with morphine. Pharmacologist
21. Clineschmidt BV, McGuffin JC, Bunting PB (1979) Neurotensin: antinocisponsive action in rodents. Eur J Pharmacol 54:129–138
22. Colpaert FC, Niemegeers CJE, Janssen PAJ, Maroli AN (1980) The effects of prior fentanyl administration and of pain on fentanyl analgesia: tolerance to and enhancement of narcotic analgesia. J Pharmacol Exp Ther 213:418–424
23. Siegel S, Hinson RE, Krank MD (1980) Morphine-induced attenuation of morphine tolerance. Science 212:1533–1534

Intraoperative peridurale Opiatanalgesie

H. Müller, U. Börner, H. Gips, M. Stoyanov und G. Hempelmann

Die Existenz von Opiatrezeptoren in der Substantia gelatinosa des Rückenmarks ermöglicht eine regionale Schmerzreduktion durch rückenmarksnahe Opiatgabe [1]. Mikroiontophoretische [31] und tierexperimentelle Untersuchungen [33] haben gezeigt, daß niedrige Opiatdosen zwar die späte nozizeptive Entladung in den Rückenmarkshinterhörnern blockieren (dumpfer Schmerz: = C-Fasern), eine Hemmung der frühen Entladung (heller Schmerz: $A\delta$-Fasern) aber nur durch hohe lokale Opiatkonzentrationen möglich ist. So werden chirurgische Eingriffe mit den bei anderen Indikationen (chronischer und postoperativer Schmerz) verwandten Opiatdosen nicht toleriert. Eine weitere Dosissteigerung ist jedoch beim spontanatmenden Patienten durch unvorhersehbare Umverteilungsvorgänge über Liquor und Blut mit konsekutiven zentralen Begleiteffekten nicht vertretbar [18]. Im Rahmen einer intraoperativen Anwendung muß weiterhin beachtet werden, daß die synaptische Transmission dicker Afferenzen ($A\alpha$, $A\beta$) und damit das Tastgefühl unbeeinträchtigt bleiben. Auch ist eine Beeinflussung vegetativer Reaktionen umstritten, obwohl eine Reihe von Untersuchungen Hinweise für Effekte an der vegetativen Afferenz erbracht haben [7, 14, 22]. Die rückenmarksnahe Opiatgabe kann im Rahmen einer Allgemeinanaesthesie den Bedarf an Narkotika senken [7, 17, 30]. Zweckmäßig erscheint auch die Kombination von periduralen Opiaten und Lokalanaesthetika (2, 11, 12, 15, 19, 20, 26, 30, 31). Die dabei zu beobachtende gegenseitige Wirkungsverstärkung kann als Ausdruck der allgemeinen Fähigkeit der intrinsischen spinalen Modulationssysteme zur synergistischen Interaktion angesehen werden [32].

Methodik

Die intraoperative peridurale Opiatanalgesie wurde zunächst im Tierversuch erprobt (Rhesusaffen, n = 7, homologe Tubentransplantation). Kurz vor Operationsbeginn wurde in einer Ketaminbasisnarkose 0,025 mg/kg Fentanyl peridural appliziert. Bei kontrollierter Lachgas-Sauerstoff-Beatmung wurden die Herzfrequenz und der blutig gemessene systemische Druck während dem operativen Eingriff kontinuierlich überwacht. Die hämodynamischen Verhältnisse bei diesen Tieren wurden mit denen einer Kontrollgruppe verglichen (n = 5), die die gleiche Fentanyldosis unter identischen Bedingungen intravenös appliziert erhielt. Beim Mensch wurde die Methode in bislang über 500 Fällen angewandt, und zwar vorwiegend bei lang dauernden gynäkologischen, urologischen und orthopädischen Operationen im Bereich von Unterbauch und untere Extremität (mittlere Operationsdauer: 3,2 h). Nach der peridu-

Tabelle 1. Methodisches Vorgehen bei der kombinierten periduralen Opiatanaesthesie

A. Periduralkatheter:
1. 5 ml Bupivacain 0,5%
2. Fentanyl 0,005 mg/kg, verdünnt mit physiologischer Kochsalzlösung auf 0,1 ml/cm Körperlänge

B. Narkoseeinleitung:
1. Etomidate 0,2–0,3 mg/kg
2. Succinylcholin 1 mg/kg zur Intubation
3. kontrollierte Beatmung mit N_2O-O_2 (2:1)
4. Pancuroniumbromid zur intraoperativen Relaxierung
5. Intraoperative Sedierung mit 10 mg Diazepam oder Halothan 0,2–0,3 Vol.%

C. Peridurale Nachinjektion:
1. Intraoperativ (Nach 3–4 h): 10 ml Bupivacain 0,25%
2. Postoperativ: Morphin 0,05 mg/kg

ralen Applikation einer Testdosis von 5 ml Bupivacain 0,5% wurden 0,005 mg/kg Fentanyl, verdünnt mit physiologischer Kochsalzlösung auf ein Gesamtvolumen von 0,1 ml/cm Körpergröße, peridural appliziert. Nach Schlafinduktion mit Etomidate erfolgte die Intubation und kontrollierte Beatmung mit Lachgas-Sauerstoff unter Relaxation mit Pancuroniumbromid (Tabelle 1). Dieses Anaesthesieverfahren wurde mit der bislang von uns bei Unterbauchlaparotomien bevorzugt angewandten konventionellen Kombinationsnarkose (peridurale Lokalanaesthetikagabe, z. B. 20 ml Bupivacain 0,5%, kontrollierte Lachgas-Sauerstoff-Beatmung) verglichen. Bei beiden Methoden ist eine zusätzliche Sedierung zur besseren Toleranz der Beatmung und lückenlosen Amnesie erforderlich, z. B. mit kleinen Benzodiazepindosen (10 mg Diazepam i.v.) oder sehr niedrigen Halothankonzentrationen (0,2–0,3 Vol.%). Alle Untersuchungen beziehen sich auf Unterbauchlaparotomien (abdominelle Uterusexstirpation) bei Patienten im guten Allgemeinzustand (ASA-Score I).

Bei beiden Anaesthesieverfahren wurden hämodynamische Untersuchungen mit invasiven Methoden vorgenommen (Swan-Ganz-Thermodilutionskatheter, zentralvenöser Katheter, Kanülierung der A. radialis). Bei der nach der oben beschriebenen Methode (Sedierung durch eine einmalige Gabe von 10 mg Valium i.v.) durchgeführten kombinierten periduralen Opiatanaesthesie wurden in festgelegten Abständen vor und während der Operation hämodynamische Messungen vorgenommen (n = 20). Bei der periduralen Applikation von 20 ml Bupivacain 0,5% unter einer Lachgas-Sauerstoff-Beatmung wurden die entsprechenden Messungen vor und 10 min nach der Gabe des Lokalanaesthetikums durchgeführt (n = 10). Trotz Vorgabe von Infusionsvolumen (1000 ml Ringer-Lösung) kam es bei einzelnen Patienten zu erheblichen Blutdruckabfällen. Wegen den im unterschiedlichen Ausmaß erforderlichen Gegenmaßnahmen, insbesondere einer raschen Volumensubstitution, waren vergleichbare Verhältnisse für weitere Meßzeitpunkte nicht mehr gegeben.

Nach beiden Anaesthesieverfahren wurden in der unmittelbar postoperativen Phase für 60 min Atmungs- und Kreislaufparameter (arterieller Mitteldruck, Herzfrequenz, Atemfrequenz, Blutgase in der A. radialis) erfaßt. Sowohl nach kombinierter periduraler Opiatanaesthesie (n = 20 und 10) als auch nach Kombinationsnarkose mit Lokalanaesthetikum (n = 10 und 10) wurde der Einfluß der Sedierungsmethode (10 mg Diazepam i.v. oder Halothan 0,3 Vol.%) auf die postoperativen Verhältnisse verglichen. Bei weiteren 10 Patienten

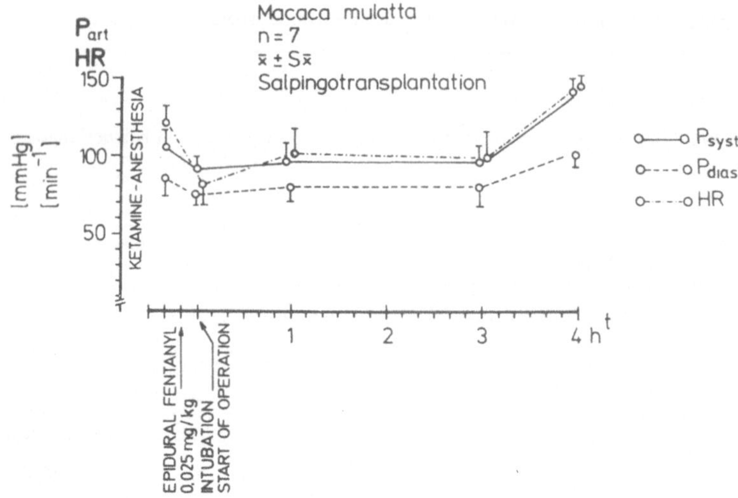

Abb. 1. Verhalten von systemischem Blutdruck (p_{syst}, p_{diast}) und Herzfrequenz (*HR*) nach periduraler Applikation von 0,025 mg/kg Fentanyl während einer Ketaminanaesthesie, Tubentransplantation bei Rhesusaffen, n = 7, $\bar{x} \pm$ sd

wurden entsprechende Parameter nach Neuroleptanalgesie (letzte Fentanyldosis mindestens 30 min vor Operationsende, keine postoperative Naloxonantagonisierung) erfaßt.

Im Verlauf beider Verfahren der periduralen Kombinationsanaesthesie wurden Hormonspiegel im Blut (ADH, ACTH und Kortisol) zur Erfassung von Streßreaktionen bestimmt (n = jeweils 10).

Bei der kombinierten periduralen Opiatanaesthesie wurden Blut- und Liquorproben zur Messung der Fentanylkonzentration entnommen (n = 11). Während die Blutentnahme in vorgegebenen Abständen wiederholt wurde, erfolgte die Durapunktion bei jedem Patienten nur einmal nach 1, 2, 3 oder 4 h.

Ergebnisse und Diskussion

Das hämodynamische Monitoring nach periduraler Fentanylgabe im Tierversuch ergab eine 3–4stündige Phase konstanter Kreislaufparameter unter der Operation (Abb. 1). Dies kann als Ausdruck einer suffizienten Analgesie gewertet werden. Nach der intravenösen Applikation der gleich Fentanyldosis unter sonst identischen Bedingungen war die Phase stabiler Kreislaufverhältnisse wesentlich kürzer (30–50 min). Im klinischen Bereich finden sich Angaben über eine Reduktion des Bedarfs an Allgemeinanaesthetika nach rückenmarksnaher Opiatgabe [9, 17, 30].

Hämodynamische Untersuchungen bei der kombinierten periduralen Opiatanaesthesie während gynäkologischen Unterbauchlaparotomien ergaben ebenfalls konstante Parameter über den gesamten Meßzeitraum. Demnach ermöglicht die Kombination von periduralem Bupivacain and Fentanyl in niedrigen Dosen eine suffiziente Analgesie unter den genannten Bedingungen. Außer einer geringen Abnahme des systemischen Kreislaufwiderstands mit ent-

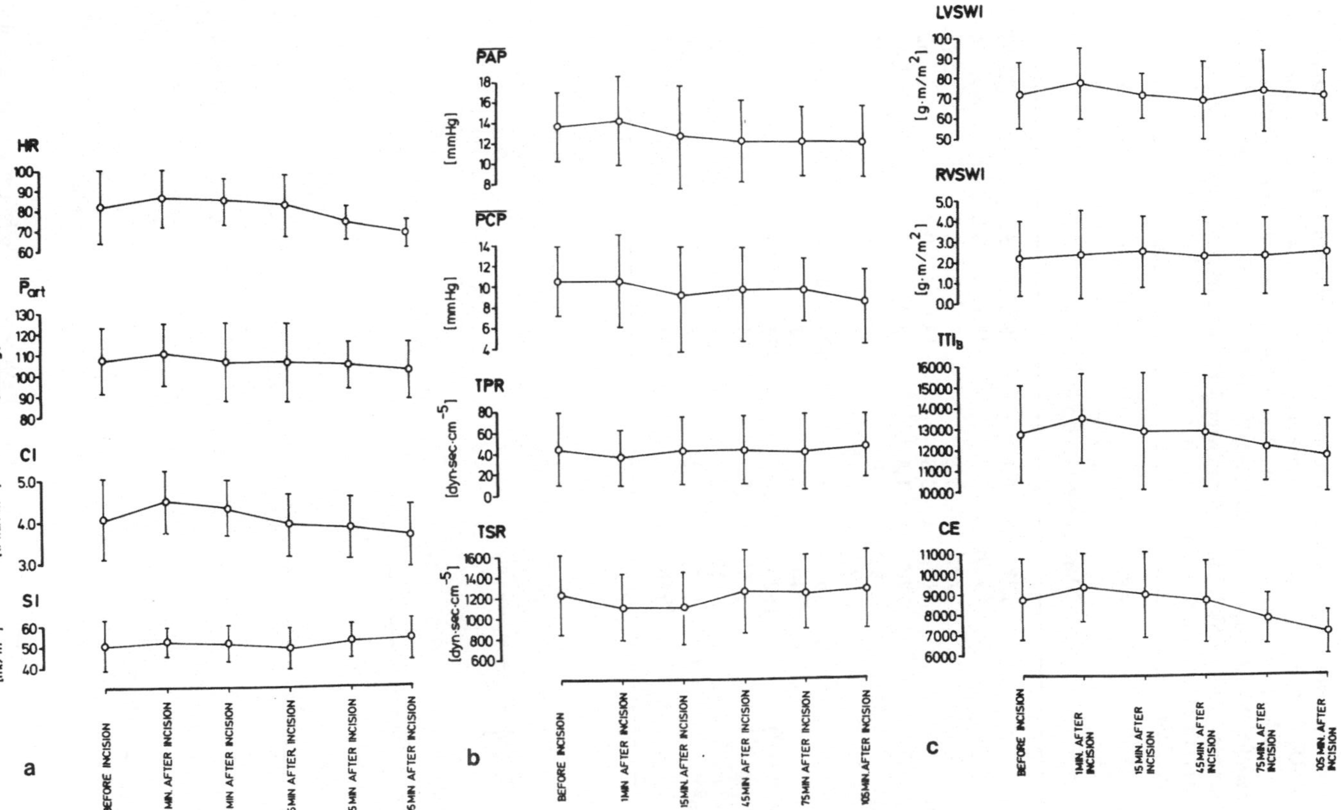

Abb. 2a–c. Hämodynamische Veränderungen bei kombinierter periduraler Opiatanaesthesie. *HR*: Herzfrequenz, $\overline{p}_{art}$: mittlerer systemischer Blutdruck, *CI*: Herzindex, *SI*: Schlagindex, $\overline{PAP}$: mittlerer Pulmonalarteriendruck, $\overline{PCP}$: pulmonaler Kapillardruck, *TPR*: pulmonaler Gefäßwiderstand, *TSR*: systemischer Gefäßwiderstand, *LVSWI*: linksventrikulärer Schlagarbeitsindex, *RVSWI*: rechtsventrikulärer Schlagarbeitsindex, TTI_b: Tension-time-Index nach Brettschneider, *CE*: Cardiac-effort-Index, Unterbauchlaparotomien, n = 20, $\overline{x} \pm sd$

Tabelle 2. Hämodynamische Veränderungen nach der periduralen Applikation von 20 ml Bupivacain 0,5% unter kontrollierter N_2O-O_2-Beatmung; p_{syst}: systolischer Blutdruck, p_{diast}: diastolischer Blutdruck, *HR*: Herzfrequenz, $\overline{PAP}$: mittlerer Pulmonalarteriendruck, $\overline{PCP}$: pulmonaler Kapillardruck, *CVP*: zentralvenöser Druck, *CI*: Herzindex, *SV*: Schlagvolumen, *SI*: Schlagindex, *TSR*: systemischer Gefäßwiderstand, *TPR*: pulmonaler Gefäßwiderstand, *LVSWI*: Linksventrikulärer Schlagarbeitsindex, *RVSWI*: rechtsventrikulärer Schlagarbeitsindex, *CE*: Cardiac-effort-Index, n = 10, $\bar{x} \pm sd$

		vor	10 min nach	[%]
		20 ml Bupivacain 0,5% p. d.		
p_{syst}	(mmHg)	127,4 ± 4,1	98,2 ± 5,5	−22,92
p_{diast}	(mmHg)	91,0 ± 2,9	75,1 ± 3,2	−17,48
HR	(min^{-1})	77,1 ± 1,8	74,2 ± 2,7	− 3,77
$\overline{PAP}$	(mmHg)	16,8 ± 1,5	13,0 ± 0,9	−22,62
$\overline{PCP}$	(mmHg)	12,5 ± 1,5	9,7 ± 1,0	−22,40
CVP	(mmHg)	9,2 ± 1,0	8,0 ± 0,9	−13,05
CI	($1/min \cdot m^2$)	3,10 ± 0,19	2,59 ± 0,15	−16,46
SV	(ml)	67 ± 3	59 ± 4	−11,95
SI	(ml/m^2)	40 ± 2	37 ± 2	− 7,50
TSR	($dyn \cdot s \cdot cm^{-5}$)	1520 ± 108	1433 ± 92	− 5,73
TPR	($dyn \cdot s \cdot cm^{-5}$)	69 ± 8	64 ± 8	− 7,25
LVSWI	($g \cdot m/m^2$)	53 ± 3	39 ± 4	−26,42
RVSWI	($g \cdot m/m^2$)	5,3 ± 1,2	4,1 ± 0,9	−22,65
CE		7948 ± 317	6103 ± 273	−23,22

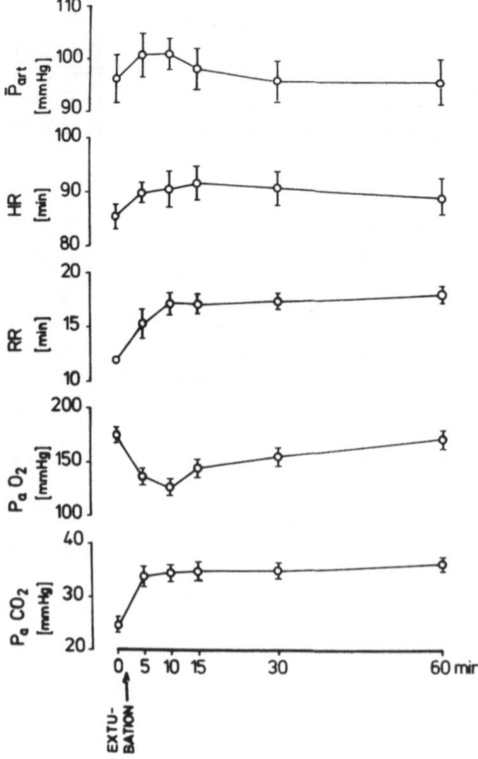

Abb. 3. Postoperatives Verhalten von arteriellem Mitteldruck ($\bar{p}_{art}$), Herzfrequenz (*HR*), Atemfrequenz (*RR*) und arteriellen Blutgasen (p_aO_2, p_aCO_2) nach unterschiedlichen Anaesthesieverfahren: nach kombinierter periduraler Opiatanaesthesie mit einmaliger Gabe von 10 mg Diazepam i.v., (n = 20). Für weitere Angaben s. Tabelle 3

Tabelle 3. Postoperatives Verhalten nach unterschiedlichen Anaesthesieverfahren. *A*: kombinierte peridurale Opiatanaesthesie mit einmaliger Gabe von 10 mg Diazepam i.v. (n = 20), *B*: kombinierte peridurale Opiatanaesthesie mit zusätzlicher Gabe kleiner Halothankonzentrationen (0,2–0,3 Vol.%) (n = 10), *C*: Kombinationsnarkose mit periduraler Bupivacaingabe und einmaliger Applikation von 10 mg Diazepam i.v. (n = 10), *D*: Kombinationsnarkose mit periduraler Bupivacaingabe und zusätzlicher Inhalation von 0,2–0,3 Vol.% Halothan (n = 10), *E*: Neuroleptanalgesie (n = 10), $\overline{x} \pm sd$

		10 min	30 min	60 min
		nach Operationsende		
$\overline{p}_{art}$	A	100,6 ± 3,2	95,1 ± 4,0	95,1 ± 4,5
	B	102,4 ± 4,1	100,0 ± 5,0	98,2 ± 4,8
	C	98,6 ± 3,3	95,0 ± 3,1	93,8 ± 4,7
	D	99,0 ± 3,6	96,6 ± 5,1	94,2 ± 4,3
	E	101,3 ± 3,1	100,1 ± 3,6	100,1 ± 3,7
HR	A	90,3 ± 3,6	90,1 ± 3,5	88,5 ± 3,6
	B	91,0 ± 3,7	90,2 ± 3,6	88,9 ± 3,7
	C	86,3 ± 3,4	86,0 ± 3,1	85,2 ± 3,4
	D	87,0 ± 4,0	86,2 ± 3,5	85,8 ± 3,7
	E	82,6 ± 4,1	78,5 ± 5,3	79,1 ± 4,7
RR	A	17,2 ± 1,2	17,3 ± 0,4	17,9 ± 0,4
	B	17,3 ± 1,0	17,8 ± 0,6	18,2 ± 0,5
	C	17,2 ± 0,9	17,7 ± 0,5	18,0 ± 0,4
	D	17,6 ± 0,6	17,9 ± 0,4	18,4 ± 0,3
	E	12,6 ± 1,0	13,2 ± 0,9	14,3 ± 1,1
p_aO_2	A	126 ± 10	154 ± 10	172 ± 11
	B	128 ± 9	159 ± 10	174 ± 10
	C	127 ± 9	159 ± 10	173 ± 10
	D	129 ± 10	160 ± 10	174 ± 10
	E	124 ± 8	142 ± 10	160 ± 10
p_aCO_2	A	34,9 ± 1,2	35,9 ± 1,0	36,2 ± 0,8
	B	34,7 ± 1,0	35,0 ± 0,8	36,1 ± 0,8
	C	34,7 ± 1,1	35,0 ± 1,1	36,1 ± 0,9
	D	34,6 ± 1,0	35,0 ± 0,9	35,9 ± 0,9
	E	39,3 ± 1,0	42,4 ± 1,2	42,0 ± 0,9

sprechendem Anstieg des Herzindex in den ersten 30 min nach der periduralen Applikation der Lokalanaesthetika-Opiat-Kombination fanden sich keine Zeichen einer Herz-Kreislauf-Beeinträchtigung, z. B. Blutdruckabfall oder adrenerge Stimulation (Abb. 2). Günstige Einflüsse periduraler Opiate im Sinne einer Kreislaufstabilisierung wurden auch bei Tierexperimenten [32] oder bei klinischen Untersuchungen [8] beschrieben.

Im Gegensatz dazu erbrachten hämodynamische Messungen nach der periduralen Applikation von 20 ml Bupivacain 0,5% unter einer Lachgas-Sauerstoff-Beatmung einen deutlichen Blutdruckabfall (Tabelle 2). Dieser laßt sich nicht nur auf eine periphere Gefäßerweiterung, sondern auch auf eine deutlich reduzierte kardiale Leistung zurückführen [27]. Bei Wegnahme des adrenergen Tonus ist die Möglichkeit zu peripheren oder kardialen Kompensationsmechanismen nicht mehr gegeben [13]. Insbesondere bei vorbestehendem Volumen-

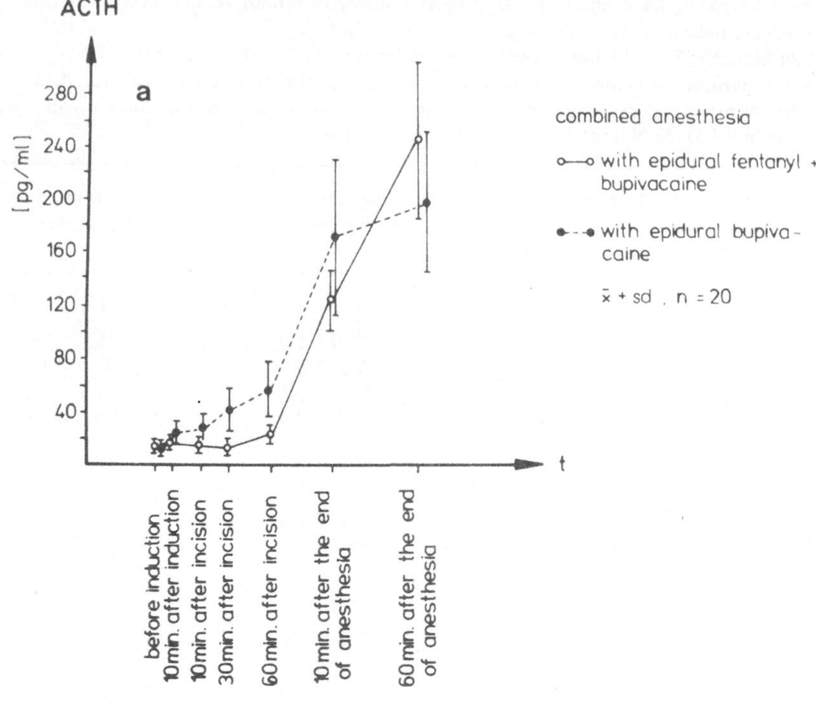
ACTH
a
[pg/ml]
280
240
200
160
120
80
40
t
before induction
10 min. after induction
10 min. after incision
30 min. after incision
60 min. after incision
10 min. after the end of anesthesia
60 min. after the end of anesthesia
combined anesthesia
with epidural fentanyl + bupivacaine
with epidural bupiva-caine
x̄ + sd, n = 20

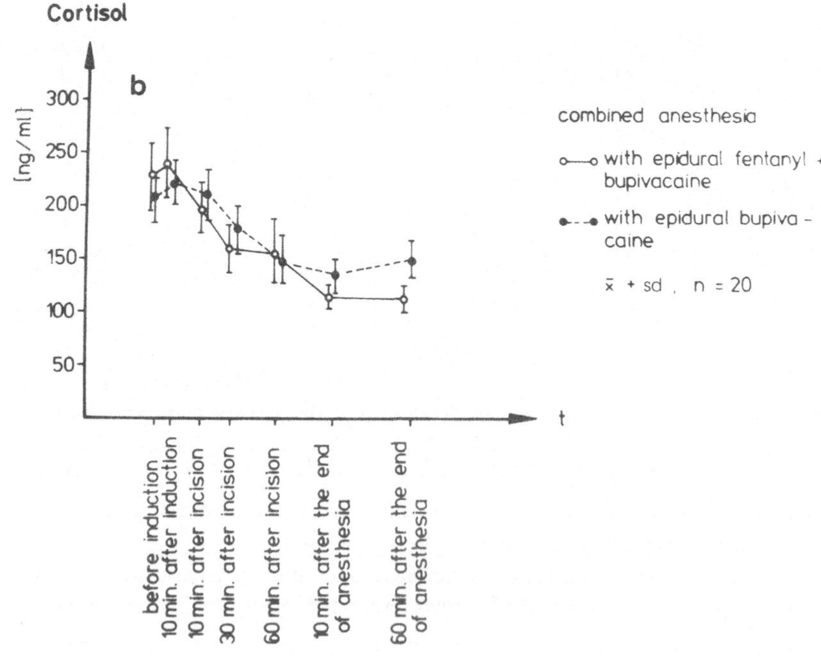
Cortisol
b
[ng/ml]
300
250
200
150
100
50
t
before induction
10 min. after induction
10 min. after incision
30 min. after incision
60 min. after incision
10 min. after the end of anesthesia
60 min. after the end of anesthesia
combined anesthesia
with epidural fentanyl + bupivacaine
with epidural bupiva-caine
x̄ + sd, n = 20

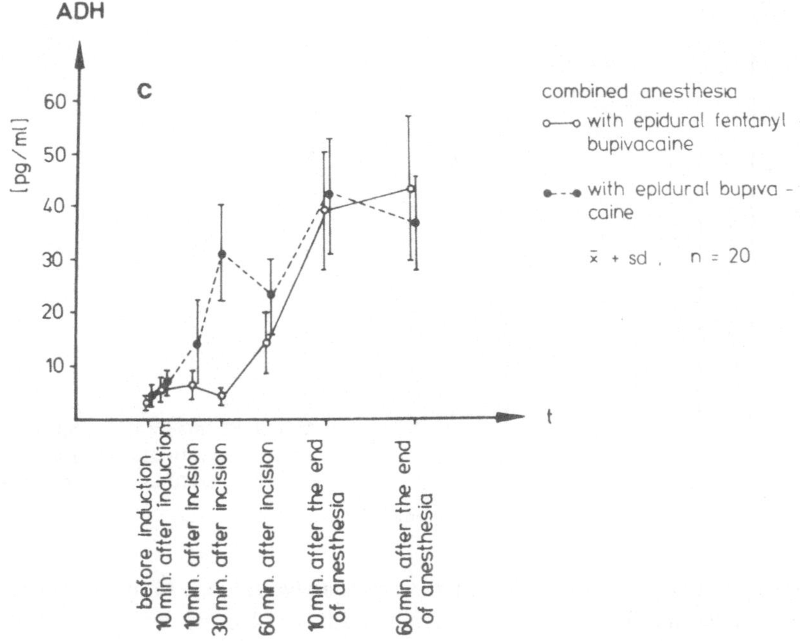

Abb. 4a–c. Plasma-Hormon-Spiegel bei kombinierter periduraler Opiatanaesthesie (n = 10) und Kombinationsnarkose mit periduraler Applikation von 20 ml Bupivacain 0,5% (n = 10). Einmalige intraoperative Gabe von 10 mg Diazepam i.v. **a** ACTH, **b** Kortisol, **c** ADH. Unterbauchlaparotomien, $\bar{x} \pm sd$

mangel kann es zu einer bedrohlichen Minderperfusion lebenswichtiger Organe kommen [3], die rasch behoben werden muß.

In der postoperativen Phase sind beide Anaesthesieverfahren durch eine rasche Kooperationsfähigkeit der Patienten ohne Schmerzen gekennzeichnet. Die kombinierte peridurale Opiatanaesthesie hat zudem gegenüber der Kombinationsnarkose mit alleiniger Lokalanaesthetikagabe den Vorteil einer postoperativ ungestörten Motorik, was nicht nur für den Patienten angenehmer ist, sondern auch den Erfordernissen der Thromboembolieprophylaxe zugute kommt. Beim Vergleich der postoperativen Veränderungen von Blutgasen und Atemfrequenz ergaben sich bei beiden Methoden keine Hinweise für eine Atmungsbeeinträchtigung. Die respiratorischen Verhältnisse waren in jedem Fall günstiger wie nach der systemischen Fentanylgabe bei der Neuroleptanalgesie. Auch beim Vergleich von unterschiedlichen Sedierungsmethoden im Rahmen beider periduraler Analgesieverfahren waren keine signifikanten Unterschiede vorhanden, obwohl grundsätzlich die Verhältnisse nach der kontinuierlichen Verabreichung niedriger Halothanvolumina etwas besser ausfielen wie nach intraoperativer Benzodiazepingabe (Abb. 3, Tabelle 3).

Die Bestimmung von Streßhormonen ergab bei beiden Methoden eine suffiziente Unterdrückung von endokrinen Reaktionen auf die Operation, wobei die intraoperativen Verhältnisse für ADH und ACTH, wohl als Ausdruck einer deutlicheren zentralen Komponente, bei der kombinierten periduralen Opiatanaesthesie signifikant besser waren. Beim ACTH (Normalbereich des verwandten Radioimmunassays: bis zu 50 pg/ml bei Erwachsenen unter Ruhebedingungen) kam es nach einer intraoperativ stabilen Phase zu einem Anstieg in der

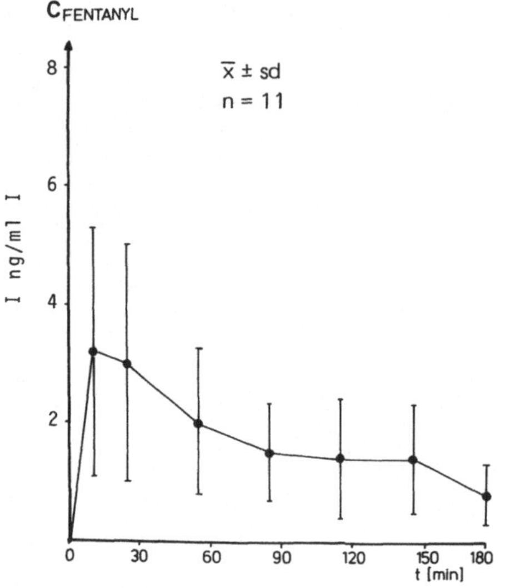

Abb. 5. Plasma-Fentanyl-Spiegel im Verlauf der kombinierten periduralen Opiatanaesthesie (0,005 mg/kg Fentanyl peridural). n = 11, $\overline{x}$ ± sd

postoperativen Periode nach beiden Anaesthesieverfahren. Ähnliche Verhältnisse finden sich nach anderen Formen einer Allgemeinanaesthesie [21, 25]. Wie erwartet, blieb die adrenokortikale Reaktion (Normalbereich des verwandten Radioimmunassays für Kortisol: bis zu 200 ng/ml bei Erwachsenen unter Ruhebedingungen) nach konventioneller Periduralanaesthesie aus (PDA) [6, 10]. Entsprechende Verhältnisse waren auch bei der kombinierten periduralen Opiatanaesthesie vorhanden. Eine Beeinflussung der operationsbedingten Kortisolreaktion wurde von Welchew u. Thornton [29] bei alleiniger periduraler Opiatgabe nicht festgestellt. Es handelt sich dabei jedoch um Untersuchungen bei Thorakotomien, wo auch die konventionelle PDA in dieser Hinsicht keine ausreichende Effektivität aufweist [5]. Die in unserer Untersuchung bei beiden Methoden reduzierte Kortisolreaktion sprach auch auf die postoperativ durch zentralen Streß erhöhten ACTH-Spiegel nicht mehr an. Die Ursache kann in der adrenokortikalen Blockade oder in Störungen der hypophysär-adrenokortikalen Steuerung durch die Anaesthesie oder das chirurgische Trauma [24] liegen (Abb. 4).

Im Hinblick auf die streßinduzierte ADH-Reaktion waren die intraoperativen Verhältnisse bei der kombinierten periduralen Opiatanaesthesie deutlich günstiger wie bei der Kombinationsnarkose mit alleiniger Lokalanaesthetikagabe (Normalbereich des verwandten Radioimmunassays: bis zu 20 pg/ml bei Erwachsenen unter Ruhebedingungen). Während von Bormann et al. [4] nach Kombination einer alleinigen periduralen Fentanylgabe mit einer oberflächlichen Neuroleptanalgesie bei einem gemischten Patientenkollektiv mit z. T. auch thoraxchirurgischen Eingriffen keine ausreichende Unterdrückung der ADH-Reaktion beobachtete, entsprachen die von uns bei Unterbauchlaparotomien gefundenen Verhältnisse am ehesten denen nach einer Kombination von PDA und Neuroleptanalgesie [28]. Aus den hormonellen Befunden der kombinierten periduralen Opiatanaesthesie bei Unterbaucheingriffen ergeben sich demnach sowohl Hinweise auf eine suffiziente Analgesie als auch auf eine ausreichende Narkosetiefe (s. Abb. 4).

Dennoch fanden sich bei dieser Methode Plasma-Fentanyl-Konzentrationen, die deutlich unter denen einer Neuroleptanalgesie liegen (J. Heykants, On the pharmacokinetics of fentanyl, unveröffentlicht) [16]. Sie entsprachen weitgehend denen einer entsprechend dosierten intramuskulären Injektion (J. Heykants, On the pharmacokinetics of fentanyl, unver-

Tabelle 4. Vergleich der Plasma- und Liquorkonzentrationen (ng/ml) nach periduraler Fentanylgabe (0,005 mg/kg), n = 11, $\bar{x} \pm$ sd

Zeit nach periduraler Applikation [h]	Plasmakonzentration (ng/ml)	Relation	Liquorkonzentration (ng/ml)
1	2,0	× 17,0	34
2	1,4	× 21,4	30
3	0,8	× 37,5	30
4	0,3	× 83,3	25

öffentlicht). Maximale Plasma-Fentanyl-Konzentrationen wurden sehr schnell erreicht und nahmen bereits nach 10 min wieder ab. Im Gegensatz dazu lagen die Liquorkonzentrationen weit oberhalb den bei einer Neuroleptanalgesie erreichten Liquorspiegeln [23] und zeigten auch im weiteren Verlauf wenig Tendenz zur Abnahme (Abb. 5, Tabelle 4).

Während bei langdauernden Operationen in kombinierter periduraler Opiatanaesthesie nach 3–5 h Puls- und Blutdruckanstiege auftraten, die durch die Nachinjektion einer kleinen Lokalanaesthetikamenge (10 ml Bupivacain 0,25%) wieder aufgehoben werden konnten, wurden postoperative peridurale Nachinjektionen in einem Interval von 5,9 ± 1 h zur Erstinjektion erforderlich.

Im weiteren Verlauf kann die Analgesie durch peridurale Lokalanaesthetika- oder Opiatgabe aufrecht erhalten werden. Wegen der langen Wirkungsdauer erscheint die peridurale Morphingabe am zweckmäßigsten. Im allgemeinen genügen 1–3 postoperative peridurale Morphingaben (2–5 mg, mit physiologischer Kochsalzlösung verdünnt), um die gesamte postoperative Schmerzphase zu überbrücken [19].

Zusammenfassend läßt sich feststellen, daß die peridurale Fentanylgabe (Dosierung etwa entsprechend der halben intravenösen Dosis zur Neuroleptanalgesie) in Ergänzung mit gegenüber der konventionellen PDA reduzierten Lokalanaesthetikadosen sowohl im Hinblick auf hämodynamische als auch hormonelle Reaktionen eine ausreichende Analgesie bei Unterbauchoperationen unter kontrollierter Lachgas-Sauerstoff-Beatmung ergibt.

Zusammenfassung

Kleine peridurale Dosen von Lokalanaesthetika und Opiaten führen über eine gegenseitige Wirkungsverstärkung zu einer ausreichenden chirurgischen Analgesie. Die peridurale Kombination von Bupivacain (5 ml 0,5%) und Fentanyl (0,005 mg/kg) wurde während Unterbauchoperationen unter Lachgas-Sauerstoff-Beatmung mit der konventionellen PDA (5 und 15 ml Bupivacain 0,5%) verglichen. Im Gegensatz zur letztgenannten Methode (Blutdruckabfall um 22%) war die kombinierte peridurale Opiatanaesthesie durch eine bemerkenswerte hämodynamische Stabilität gekennzeichnet. Im Verlauf beider Anaesthesieformen ergab sich eine ausreichende Unterdrückung intraoperativer endokriner Reaktionen (ACTH, Kortisol und ADH). Weiterhin zeigte sich nach beiden Methoden keine Beeinträchtigung der postoperativen Atmung. Die Liquorkonzentrationen waren nach periduraler Fentanylgabe 17–83mal höher wie die Plasmaspiegel.

Im Vergleich zur PDA mit Lokalanaesthetika ergaben sich bei der kombinierten periduralen Opiatanaesthesie eine längere Analgesiedauer, kein Risiko der Intoxikation selbst bei versehentlicher intravenöser Injektion, geringere hämodynamische Auswirkungen durch Sympathikusblockade und eine verminderte Beeinträchtigung der postoperativen Motorik.

Summary

Mutual enhancement of analgesic action after small epidural doses of local anesthetics and opiates results in sufficient surgical analgesia. During lower abdominal surgery and controlled ventilation with oxygen-nitrous oxide a combination of epidural Bupivacaine (5 ml 0,5%) and Fentanyl (0.005 mg/kg) was compared with conventional epidural analgesia (5 and 15 ml Bupivacaine 0.5%). In contrast to the latter method (decrease in blood pressure by 22%) combined epidural opiate anesthesia was characterized by a remarkable hemodynamic stability. During both types of epidural analgesia there was a sufficient depression of intraoperative endocrine responses (ACTH, cortisol and ADH). In addition, both methods did not lead to significant impairment of postoperative respiration. After epidural Fentanyl application *CSF* concentrations were 17 to 83 times higher than plasma levels.

Compared to epidural anesthesia with local anesthetics combined epidural opiate anesthesia offered a longer duration of analgesia, no risk of intoxication even after inadvertant direct intravenous injection, less hemodynamic reactions by sympathetic blockade and less interference with postoperative motor function.

Literatur

1. Atweh SF, Kuhar MJ (1977) Autoradiographic localization of opiate receptors in rat brain, spinal cord and lower medulla. Brain Res 124:53
2. Birkhan HJ, Rosenberg B, Simon K, Moskowitz B (1982) Epidural morphine. A new approach to postoperative analgesia in urologic surgery. In: Yaksh TL, Müller H (eds) Spinal opiate Analgesia, vol 144, Anaesthesiology and intensive care medicine. Springer, Berlin Heidelberg New York, p 37
3. Bonica JJ, Kennedy WF, Akamatsu TJ (1972) Circulatory effects of peridural block: III. Effects of acute blood loss. Anesthesiology 36:219
4. von Bormann B, Weidler B, Dennhardt R, Frings N, Lennhartz H, Hempelmann G (im Druck) Plasma-ADH-Spiegel unter kombinierter Neuroleptanalgesie-peridurale Opiatanalgesie. Anaesthesist
5. Bromage PR, Shibita HR, Willoughby HW (1971) Influence of prolonged epidural blockade on blood sugar and cortisol responses to operations upon the upper part of the abdomen and the thorax. Surg Gynecol Obstet 132:1051
6. Cosgrove DO, Jenkins JS (1974) The effects of epidural anaesthesia on the pituitary-adrenal response to surgery. Clin Sci Mol Med 46:403
7. Cousins MJ, Glynn CJ, Wilson PR, Mather LE, Graham JR (1979) Aspects of epidural morphine. Lancet II:584
8. De Castro J, D'Inverno E, Lecron L, Levy D, Toppet-Belatoni E (1980) Perspectives d'utilisation des morphinoides en anesthésie locorégionale. Anesth Analg Reanim 37:17
9. Dirksen R, Nijhuis GMM (1980) Epidural opiate and perioperative analgesia. Acta Anaesth Scand 24:367
10. Engquist A, Brandt MR, Fernandes A, Kehlet H (1977) The blocking effect of epidural analgesia on the adrenocortical and hyperglycaemic responses to surgery. Acta Anaesth Scand 21:330

11. Handjis GP, Liolios A, Anagnostakos A, Vailas G, Tsantakis CE (1982) Epidural morphine for 24 hours of postoperative analgesia. In: Yaksh TL, Müller H (eds) Spinal opiate Analgesia, vol 144, Anaesthesiology and intensive care medicine. Springer, Berlin Heidelberg New York, p 47
12. Kawashima Y, Uchida N, Kawahira S, Meguro K, Nampo T, Fujita Y (1982) A step to complete pain relief after surgery. In: Yaksh TL, Müller H (eds) Spinal opiate Analgesia, vol 144, Anaesthesiology and intensive care medicine. Springer, Berlin Heidelberg New York, p 53
13. Krebs R (1978) Pharmakologie und Toxikologie der Lokalanästhetika. In: Ahnefeld FW, Bergmann H, Burri C, Dick W, Halmágyi M, Hossli G, Rügheimer E (Hrsg) Lokalanästhesie, Bd. 18, Klinische Anästhesiologie und Intensivtherapie. Springer, Berlin Heidelberg New York, p 32
14. Leslie J, Camporesi E, Urban B, Bromage P (1979) Selective epidural analgesia. Lancet II:151
15. Manolescu R, Elian I, Lehmann JM (1982) Peridural bupivacain and morphine for residual pain after peripheral vascular surgery. In: Yaksh TL, Müller H (eds) Spinal opiate Analgesia, vol 144, Anaesthesiology and intensive care medicine. Springer, Berlin Heidelberg New York, p 58
16. Michiels M, Hendriks R, Heykants J (1977) A sensitive radioimmunoassay for fentanyl. Plasma levels in dogs and man. Eur J Clin Pharmacol 12:153
17. Müller H, Börner U, Stoyanov M, Hempelmann G (1980) Intraoperative peridurale Opiatanalgesie. Anaesthesist 12:656
18. Müller H, Börner U, Stoyanov M, Hempelmann G (1982) Theoretical aspects and practical considerations concerning selective opiate-analgesia. In: Yaksh TL, Müller H (eds) Spinal opiate Analgesia, vol 144, Anaesthesiology and intensive care medicine. Springer, Berlin Heidelberg New York, p 9
19. Müller H, Börner U, Stoyanov M, Hempelmann G (1982) The perioperative use of epidural opiates. In: Yaksh TL, Müller H (eds) Spinal opiate Analgesia, vol 144, Anaesthesiology and intensive care medicine. Springer, Berlin Heidelberg New York, p 67
20. Müller H, Stoyanov M, Börner U, Hempelmann G (1982) Epidural opiates for relief of cancer pain. In: Yaksh TL, Müller H (eds) Spinal opiate Analgesia, vol 144, Anaesthesiology and intensive care medicine. Springer, Berlin Heidelberg New York, p 125
21. Oyama T (1980) Influence of anaesthesia on the endocrine system. In: Stöckel H, Oyama T (eds) Endocrinology in anaesthesia and surgery. Springer, Berlin Heidelberg New York
22. Rieder W, Müller H, Klug N, Kling D, Lüben V, Stoyanov M, Hempelmann G (1981) Neurologische Untersuchungsbefunde bei periduraler Opiatgabe. In: Hempelmann G, Müller H (Hrsg) Peridurale Opiatanalgesie. Bibliomed, Köln S. 61
23. Schleimer R, Benjamini E, Eisele J, Henderson G (1978) Pharmacokinetics of fentanyl as determined by radioimmunoassay. Clin Pharmacol Ther 23:188
24. Thoren L (1974) General metabolic response to trauma including pain influence. Acta Anaesthesiol Scand 55:9
25. Traynor C, Hall GM (1981) Endocrine and metabolic changes during surgery: Anaesthetic implications. Br J Anaesth 53:153
26. Varga L (1982) Continuous epidural analgesia in the perioperative period. In: Yaksh TL, Müller H (eds) Spinal opiate Analgesia, vol 144, Anaesthesiology and intensive care medicine. Springer, Berlin Heidelberg New York, p 99
27. Ward RJ, Bonica JJ, Frennd FG, Akamatsu T, Danzinger F, Englesson S (1965) Epidural and subarachnoid anesthesia: Cardiovascular and respiratory effects. JAMA 191:275
28. Weidler B, von Bormann B, Dennhardt R, Hempelmann G (im Druck) Plasma-ADH-Spiegel als perioperativer Streßparameter. Anaesthesist
29. Welchew EA, Thornton JA (1982) The control of postoperative pain by thoracic epidural fentanyl and its effect upon the stress response. In: Yaksh TL, Müller H (eds) Spinal opiate Analgesia, vol 144, Anaesthesiology and intensive care medicine. Springer, Berlin Heidelberg New York, p 103
30. Yakashita Y, Fukuda K, Morioka T, Kano T, Araki Y (1979) Intrathecal application of morphine. I. As a supplement of anesthesia and a prolonged relief of postoperative pain. Jpn J Anesth 12:1584
31. Yaksh TL (1978) Inhibition by etorphine of the discharge of dorsal horn neurons: Effects upon the neuronal response to both high- and low-threshold sensory input in the decerebrate spinal cat. Exp Neurol 60:23
32. Yaksh TL (1981) Analgesia and the spinal action of opiates. In: Hempelmann G, Müller H (Hrsg) Peridurale Opiatanalgesie. Bibliomed, Köln S. 43
33. Yaksh TL (1982) Animal studies on the spinal action of opiates in analgesia. In: Yaksh TL, Müller H (eds) Spinal opiate Analgesia, vol 144, Anaesthesiology and intensive care medicine. Springer, Berlin Heidelberg New York, p 1

Diskussion

Frage:
Wie haben sie technisch nach epiduraler Fentanylapplikation gleichzeitig die Liquorkonzentrationen gemessen?

Müller:
Es handelt sich dabei immer nur um Einzelmessungen bei jedem Patienten. Wir haben nicht kontinuierlich gemessen, sondern zu einem fest definierten Zeitpunkt, nach 1, 2, 3 oder 4 Stunden, jeweils bei jedem Patienten eine Liquorentnahme vorgenommen. Eine kontinuierliche Liquorentnahme ist nicht zulässig, da es dann zum Übertritt von Fentanyl aus dem Epiduralraum in den Intrathekalraum kommt.

Hack:
Wie erklären Sie die Diskrepanz der postoperativen ACTH-Sekretion zu den weiterhin niedrigbleibenden Kortisolspiegeln? Dies ist ein ganz ungewöhnlicher Befund. Wir haben bei herkömmlicher Epiduralanaesthesie mit Lokalanaesthetika, auch die ACTH- und die Kortisolspiegel in den postoperativen Verlauf hinein verfolgt und haben zeigen können, daß beide Hormone über die eigentliche Operationsphase, bei Anwendung der Kathetertechnik, auch postoperativ erniedrigt bleiben.

Müller:
In älteren Untersuchungen aus dem Jahre 1974, in denen die Spiegel von ACTH und ADH bestimmt wurden, wurde diese Diskrepanz ebenfalls gefunden. Man kann dies entweder durch die Blockade selbst oder durch eine Störung im Rückmeldesystem erklären.

Stanton-Hicks:
Brandt, Enquist and Kehlet have found that the levels of cortisol and ACTH are low as long as the epidural block was kept above T 5. If the level was below T 5 they did not get the same depression and I think your epidural blocks must have been below this level.

Müller:
Wir haben eine fixe Dosis von 20 ml lumbal bei L 3/L 4 appliziert. Nach dieser Dosis reichte der Block nicht in jedem Fall bis T 4.

Dennhardt:
Unter einer ausreichend hohen epiduralen Blockade bleiben die ADH-Konzentrationen im physiologischen Bereich. Ohne Epiduralanaesthesie hingegen steigen die Konzentrationen in den gezeigten Bereich an, so daß ich glaube, daß bei den von Herrn Müller gezeigten Patienten eine nicht ganz adäquate Analgesie bzw. Blockierung der sympathischen Afferenzen vorhanden war und dementsprechend die ADH-Sekretion stimuliert wurde.

Müller:
Intraoperativ haben wir keine Anstiege der ADH-Werte beobachtet. Während der Unterbauchlaparotomien konnten wir anhand dieser Parameter keine Zeichen einer Streßreaktion nachweisen.

Stanton-Hicks:
It is important to appreciate that the stimulation from this particular surgical procedure is much lower segmentaring than would be the case in upper abdominal surgery.

Verlich:
Mixing local anaesthetics with other drugs might be dangerous and could be noxious to the nerves and to the medulla spinalis. If you dilute morphine with glucose, the pH of glucose 5% is usually after sterilization 3,5 or less and injeting this mixture hurts the patient and, I believe, this might damage the spinal roots. There are permanent neurological sequalae reported after chloroprocaine, whose pH is about 3.1. If this solution is injected in the intrathecal space, which might happen if you perforate the dura, then permanent damage may occur. So the pH of the solutions which you applicate epidurally must be in the range of 6,0 to 7,5.

Müller:
We never mix opiates with local anesthetics. We inject one after the other. We have measured the pH of every solution alone and the pH of the mixture. The pH values were quite normal. They are between 4,8 and 7. It depends on the solutions which are used for solution.

Anger:
Sie haben nach Fentanyl postoperativ keine Atemdepression gesehen. Ist das eine Frage der Dosierung? Und haben Sie überhaupt einmal eine Atemdepression gesehen?

Müller:
Es ist bislang keine späte Atemdepression nach Fentanyl beschrieben worden, und das ist auch einer der Gründe, weshalb wir Fentanyl genommen haben für diesen Zweck. Das hängt sicher mit den physikochemischen Eigenschaften der Substanz zusammen. Fentanyl ist sehr lipoidlöslich und hat somit keine lange Verweildauer im Liquor, wie dies bei Morphin der Fall ist. Die Häufigkeit der Atemdepression wird darauf zurückgeführt.

Anger:
Ich könnte mir doch vorstellen, daß nach entsprechend hohen Fentanyldosen es auch akut zu Atemdepressionen kommt.

Müller:
Das spielt aber intraoperativ keine Rolle, wenn wir beatmen.

Comparison of pH Values in CSF after Spinal Administration of Various Hyperbaric Opiates

C. B. Devaux, F. Alibert, E. Clavier, and J. Thiebot

Spinal analgesia with opiates was first used for treatment of intractable pain [15]. At present this is still the main indication worldwide, followed by postoperative pain [2, 5, 6], and labor. All authors found some respiratory effects depending on the dosage and the level of the block.

The aim of this study was to investigate a possible central action on the medulla by means of cerebrospinal fluid (CSF) variations due to physico-chemical modifications induced by variations in the acid-base equilibrium of the CSF. We attempted to answer a simple question: Is there a correlation between arterial blood pH and HCO_3^- and CSF pH and HCO_3^- ? In order to elucidate this problem, we studied five groups of patients suffering from chronic pain from a metastatic carcinoma (gastric metastasis).

Patients and Methods

Patients were included in the study, if they gave written consent, and if there was no evidence of hemodynamic disturbances, abdominal distention, or local infections in the lumbar area; 40 men and 35 women participated in this study. The male group was older and taller than the female group which was heavier (Table 1).

Preparation of the Hyperbaric Opiate Solution

A 20% dextrose solution in water was mixed with an equal volume of opiate prepared in equipotent dosages: Morphine HCl was considered to have the potency of 1, phenoperidine of 10, fentanyl the potency of 100, R 39,209 the potency of 700, and buprenorphine the potency of 40. An aqueous solution was used to avoid a stereospecific interaction of agonist-antagonist receptors by saline. The solutions were drawn from autoclaved ampules and prepared in glass syringes immediately before injection.

Experimental Procedure

The spinal canal was punctured at the L3–L5 level with a 20-g gauge Tuohy needle. An epidural catheter was threaded through the needle both for injection of the opiates and for sam-

Table 1. Biometric data from the five groups of patients

Group	Age (years)	Weight (kg)	Height (cm)
Morphine HCl	57,31	63,16	165.30
n = 15	3.15	2.67	2.74
	NS	NS	NS
Phenoperidine	45.39	57.61	163.82
n = 15	5.73	1.90	3.13
	NS	NS	NS
Fentanyl	63.39	61.27	165.71
n = 15	3.18	2.25	1.25
	NS	NS	NS
R 39,209	58.82	59.33	161.83
n = 15	7.35	2.37	2.31
	NS	NS	NS
Buprenorphine	58.09	67.13	169.35
n = 15	2.29	1.75	1.34
	NS	NS	NS
Males	59.65	63.17	170.23
n = 15	2.85	1.82	1.49
	**	NS	**
Females	51.47	69.81	160.21
n = 15	1.63	1.13	2.10
	NS	**	NS

NS, not significant ($P > 0.05$); * $0.05 > P > 0.01$; ** $P < 0.01$

pling of the CSF. The opiates were injected without barbotage. Simultaneously, respiration (TV, RF and RV) was registered and arterial blood samples were taken; CSF free flow sampling was performed in glass syringes before and after maximal analgesia. The samples were collected through a thin layer of paraffin oil to avoid contamination with ambient room air. In the different groups, mean values were calculated, the *t* test for unpaired data was used to compare the effects of the various opiates on respiration and CSF pH, and the *t* test for paired data was used to test the effects within the groups.

Results

For all opiates tested, a decrease of pH and bicarbonate in the CSF at the time of maximal analgesia was found. The control values of pH in the CSF were in general higher than commonly reported in the literature [1, 5, 6]. Furthermore, a significant increase of pCO_2 in CSF was found for all opiates. There were no significant changes of the pO_2 in the CSF (Table 2).

After injection of the different opiates, the pH decreased in CSF and arterial blood. These changes were highly significant when phenoperidine, R 39,209, and buprenorphine

Table 2. pH, pO_2, pCO_2, HCO_3^- in CSF before and after injection of the opiates

Drugs	pH		pO_2 mmHg		pCO_2 mmHg		HCO_3^- mmol/l	
	Before	After	Before	After	Before	After	Before	After
Morphine HCl	7.493	7.433	27.37	23.06	2.61	3.25	19.83	17.86
n = 15	0.031	0.045	1.53	6.02	0.11	0.09	4.21	0.81
	NS	*	NS	NS	NS	*	NS	**
Phenoperidine	7.429	7.332	24.81	22.66	3.12	3.21	22.40	18.94
n = 15	0.027	0.043	1.62	1.73	0.04	0.39	0.53	0.44
	NS	**	NS	NS	*	*	**	**
Fentanyl	7.395	7.364	23.39	19.96	2.69	3.17	22.91	19.39
n = 15	0.039	0.025	0.70	1.13	0.06	0.12	0.57	0.35
	NS	*	NS	NS	*	*	*	*
R 39,209	7.409	7.379	27.54	25.26	2.61	2.88	19.25	15.26
n = 15	0.023	0.012	1.44	0.82	0.10	0.09	0.07	0.03
	*	*	NS	NS	*	*	**	**
Buprenorphine	7.381	7.348	22.04	20.50	2.96	3.18	21.67	16.41
n = 15	0.020	0.011	0.95	0.64	0.06	0.01	0.09	0.07
	**	**	NS	NS	*	*	**	**

See footnotes to Table 1

Table 3. Changes of pH in CSF and arterial blood before and after injection of opiates

Drugs	pH CSF		pH Arterial blood	
	Before	After	Before	After
Morphine HCl	7.493	7.433	7.513	7.451
n = 15	0.031	0.045	0.015	0.030
	NS	*	NS	*
Phenoperidine	7.429	7.332	7.447	7.349
n = 15	0.027	0.043	0.017	0.001
	NS	**	*	**
Fentanyl	7.395	7.364	7.421	7.372
n = 15	0.039	0.025	0.013	0.010
	NS	*	NS	*
R 39,209	7.409	7.379	7.439	7.391
n = 15	0.023	0.012	0.020	0.018
	*	*	**	**
Buprenorphine	7.381	7.348	7.457	7.363
n = 15	0.020	0.011	0.031	0.011
	**	**	**	**

See footnotes to Table 1

Table 4. Changes induced in pH of the cerebral spinal and arterial blood by phenoperidine, R 39,209 and buprenorphine. These drugs induced highly significant changes of the pH in the two compartments

Drugs	CSF Δ pH	Arterial blood Δ pH
Phenoperidine	– 0.087	– 0.098
R 39,209	– 0.030	– 0.048
Buprenorphine	– 0.033	– 0.094

Table 5. Changes of the HCO_3^- in CSF and arterial blood before and after drug administration

Drugs	HCO_3^- CSF mmol/l		HCO_3^- Arterial blood mmol/l	
	Before	After	Before	After
Morphine HCl	19.83	17.86	24.32	21.61
n = 15	4.21	0.81	1.19	2.15
	NS	**	*	**
Phenoperidine	22.40	18.94	24.52	20.35
n = 15	0.53	0.44	0.28	0.36
	**	**	*	**
Fentanyl	22.91	19.39	23.81	20.19
n = 15	0.57	0.35	0.15	0.07
	*	*	*	*
R 39,209	19.25	15.26	22.74	19.57
n = 15	0.07	0.03	1.10	0.90
	**	**	*	**
Buprenorphine	21.67	16.41	23.65	20.14
n = 15	0.09	0.07	0.23	0.65
	**	**	*	**

See footnotes to Table 1

were injected (Tables 3 and 4). The HCO_3^- and the CSF and arterial blood decreased significantly after drug administration (Table 5), showing a much greater change in the CSF than in arterial blood (Table 5).

Discussion

The aim of this study was to find out how opiates injected into the CSF cause changes of the acid-base status and, furthermore, to find out whether there are specific effects of different drugs or solutions. When discussing these problems, one must keep the differences of pH in the examined solutions in mind. As Table 6 clearly shows, there are changes of the pH and HCO_3^- mainly related to the dilution with dextrose. The change in pH is significantly

Table 6. Mean values of pH, pO_2, pCO_2, and HCO_3^- in CSF diluted either with the solution or the hyperbaric preparation of the drug

Drugs	pH	pO_2 mmHg	pCO_2 mmHg	HCO_3^- mmol/l
Morphine HCl				
Solution	7.631	26.61	2.58	19.31
	0.003	1.10	0.73	1.05
	**	NS	NS	**
Hyperbaric solution	7.462	28.72	3.34	17.15
	0.010	1.32	0.25	3.13
	**	NS	NS	*
Phenoperidine				
Solution	7.352	24.10	2.02	8.31
	0.031	0.15	0.53	0.35
	**	NS	NS	*
Hyperbaric solution	7.201	25.73	1.57	4.57
	0.085	0.27	0.61	0.29
	**	NS	**	**
Fentanyl				
Solution	7.523	21.20	1.81	11.31
	0.037	0.31	0.27	0.59
	**	NS	*	**
Hyperbaric solution	7.412	21.73	1.78	8.42
	0.059	0.52	0.19	0.27
	**	NS	*	**
R 39,209				
Solution	7.030	21.25	3.31	10.42
	0.018	0.18	0.01	0.18
	**	*	*	**
Hyperbaric solution	6.772	21.73	2.25	9.15
	0.025	0.27	0.10	0.13
	**	NS	*	**
Buprenorphine				
Solution	7.599	24.81	1.47	11.00
	0.021	0.03	0.03	0.01
	**	NS	*	**
Hyperbaric solution	7.263	23.63	1.12	10.84
	0.015	0.17	0.09	0.13
	**	NS	*	**

See footnotes to Table 1

Table 7. Early effects of different opiates on the pH in CSF and in arterial blood

Drugs	CSF pH		pH arterial blood	
	Before	5′	Before	5′
Morphine HCl	7.491 0.015	7.490 0.010	7.510 0.009	7.507 0.016
Phenoperidine	7.417 0.010	7.419 0.013	7.450 0.007	7.447 0.005
Fentanyl	7.413 0.011	7.417 0.015	7.490 0.015	7.487 0.027
R 39,209	7.415 0.009	7.413 0.012	7.454 0.025	7.453 0.031
Buprenorphine	7.387 0.015	7.389 0.011	7.441 0.033	7.445 0.037

greater with R 39,209 and buprenorphine (Table 6). We ask to what extent our measurements are influenced at maximal analgesia by a direct effect of opiates on the respiratory center. This would be the case if the dose of morphine were higher than 50 $\mu g \times kg^{-1}$ of body weight. In the present study not more than 35 $\mu g \times kg^{-1}$ was injected.

In contrast to the results of the present study, we found in a pilot study no effects of the opiates used in this study on pH in the CSF and in arterial blood (Table 7). However, we have to consider, as pointed out by Pappenheimer [10] and Plum [12] [11] that chemoreceptors located in the medulla oblongata are sensitive to changes of the $[H^+]$ or pH. Leusen [7] reported 10 years ago the direct action on ventilation when perfusing the cerebral ventricles with acid solutions. Mitchell [9] made the same observations, which were confirmed by Pappenheimer [10] in goats and by Fencl [3, 4] in man. The ventilatory responses due to changes in CSF pH offer a powerful mechanism for the homeostatic regulation of CSF acid-base balance in many situations associated with non-respiratory acidosis or alkalosis [8, 13, 14].

When looking at the results of Mitchell [9] and Plum [12] obtained by collection of CSF in normal subjects, different patterns are apparent. If bicarbonate concentrations are the same in the cisternal and lumbar CSF, the pH in the lumbar CSF is higher and the pH in the cisternal CSF significantly lower. The values are greatly reduced under conditions such as meningitis, carcinomatosis, or subarachnoid hemorrhage. Under these circumstances, local glycolysis in the lumbar sac rises and the regional lactate concentration increases, thereby decreasing the pH in the lumbar CSF.

Conclusion

On the basis of these data and the results obtained in our study, it is possible to say that the changes of the pH and the HCO_3^- seen with different hyperbaric solutions are primarily related to the initial changes of the pH of lumbar CSF induced by direct effect chemoreceptors in the medulla and, secondarily, are due to the depressant effects of opiates on respiration.

References

1. Bradley RD, Semzle SJG (1962) A comparison of certain acid-base characteristics of arterial blood, jugular veinous blood and cerebro spinal fluid in man and the effect on them of some acute and chronic acid-base disturbances. J Physiol 160:381
2. Crawford RD (1978) CSF pH and ventilation acclimatization to altitude. J Appl Physiol 45:275
3. Fencl V, Miller TB, Pappenheimer JR (1966) Studies on the respiratory response to disturbances of acid-base balance, with deductions concerning the ionic composition of cerebral interstitial fluid. Am J Physiol 210:459
4. Fencl V, Vale JR, Broch JA (1969) Respiration and cerebral blood flow in metabolic acidosis and alkalosis in humans. J Appl Physiol 27:67
5. Fisher RG (1975) The cerebro-spinal fluid. Mayo Clin Proc 50:482
6. Lassen MA, Christensen MS (1976) Physiology of cerebral blood flow. Br J Anesth 48:719
7. Leusen I (1970) Regulation of cerebrospinal fluid composition with reference to breathing. Physiol Rev 52:1
8. Marem JH (1972) Bicarbonate formation in cerebrospinal fluid: role in sodium transport and pH regulation. Am J Physiol 222:885
9. Mitchell RA, Loeschke HH, Maisson WH et al. (1963) Respiratory responses mediated through superficial chemosentitive aeros on the medulla. J Appl Physiol 18:523
10. Pappenheimer JR (1967) The ionic composition of cerebral extracellular fluid and its relation to control of breathing. The Harvey lectures. Academic, New-York, p 71
11. Plum F, Posher JB (1973) Acid-base balance of cisternal and lumbar. CSF in hospital patients. N Engl J Med 289:1346
12. Plum F, Siesjo BK (1975) Recent advances in CSF physiology. Anesthesiology 42:708
13. Siesjo BK (1968) The regulation of cerebrospinal fluid pH. Kidney Int 1:360
14. Swanson AG, Rosengren H (1962) Cerebrospinal fluid buffering during acute experimental respiratory acidosis. J Appl Physiol 17:812
15. Wang JK, Nauss LA, Thomas JE (1979) Pain relief by intrathecally applied morphine in man. Anesthesiology 50:149

Patient-controlled Analgetics Therapy with Epidural Pethidine for Postoperative Pain Relief

A Preliminary Report

B. Zarén, P. Hartvig, and A. Tamsen

For some 4 years, we have used patient-controlled analgesics therapy (PACAT) for clinical and pharmacologic studies on narcotic analgesics. The philosophy behind this is that only the suffering patient knows how severe the pain is and when the pain relief is effective. From this point of view, it seemed logical to entrust the patient in pain with the means of relieving it. Basically, PACAT implies the use of a drug-dispensing system which can administer a preset dose of analgesic when the patient requires pain relief by activating a press-button switch. This method has been used for intravenous administration in postoperative patients and has been shown to be useful for studies of individual analgesic requirements, analgesic plasma concentration, and equianalgesic dosage ratios of narcotic analgesics [1, 2]. In this investigation, this method was used for epidural administration of pethidine in order to study: (a) the analgesic dose requirements among patients and to establish an equianalgesic dose of intravenous pethidine; (b) the plasma concentration of analgesics after this route of administration; and (c) the distribution of pethidine in relation to cerebrospinal fluid (CSF) in subjective optimal pain relief.

Material and Methods

Eleven patients took part in this study, seven were studied following major abdominal surgery and four following thoracic surgery. There were five men and six women with a mean age of 45 years. All were in good general condition. On the day before surgery, the patients were informed of the nature and the purpose of the investigation and were also instructed how to use a press-button-triggered programmable drug injector to self-administer doses of pethidine epidurally to relieve postoperative pain. Individual patient data are listed in Table 1.

A modified form of neuroleptanesthesia with mechanical ventilation was used in all patients. During anesthesia, analgesia was augmented with fentanyl as required to suppress signs of surgical stress. After induction of anesthesia, the patient was turned onto the left side and an epidural catheter was introduced at the Th10–11 or Th11–12 interspace and at the Th5–6 interspace in abdominal and thoracic surgery, respectively. After surgery, muscle relaxation was reversed with atropine and synstigmine and the patients were extubated and transferred to the intensive care unit. As soon as the patients complained of pain, they were allowed to start self-administration of 10-mg doses of pethidine in a volume of 1 ml. The drug injector was programmed to allow a maximum of one dose in every 15-min

Table 1. Clinical data for 11 patients self-administering pethidine epidurally

No.	Initials Age-sex	Body weight	Diagnosis/surgical procedure	Intake of pethidine, mg/h	Mean measured plasma concentration	Measured CSF concentration of pethidine
1	GL-m-56	70	Ulcerative colitis/proctocolectomy	7.0	100	–
2	SW-m-42	77	Ulcerative colitis/colectomy	11.9	220	10,000
3	AH-f-39	101	Cancer of sigmoid colon/resection of sigmoid colon	7.4	127	1,210
4	MK-f-31	53	Crohn's disease/resection of small intestine	4.8	60	1,565
5	VV-m-50	80	Ulcerative colitis/proctocolectomy	16.9	166	3,070
6	LL-f-54	81	Cancer of the rectum/anterior resection of the colon	4.1	72	365
7	CE-f-32	60	Crohn's disease/resection of ileum and caecum	15.6	260	898
8	ML-m-50	77	Tumor of the right lung/segment resection	15.6	167	625
9	SS-m-38	101	Emphysema/lobectomy	16.7 (0–24 h) 22.6 (0–44.5 h)	284	660
10	GB-f-62	62	Tumor of the right lung/extirpation of the tumor	4.4	150	270
11	BL-f-39	62	Tumor of the right lung/resection of the middle and upper lobes	12.9	139	2,242
	Mean ± SD	75 ± 16		10.7 ± 5.2	157.6 ± 72.8	

period. No other analgesic drug was given during the PACAT period which lasted for 17–44.5 h. Postoperative monitoring was carried out according to the routines of the intensive care unit. In addition, arterial blood gases during air breathing were checked several times during the PACAT period.

The CSF samples were obtained just after induction of anesthesia and at the end of the self-administration period. The pethidine concentration in plasma and CSF was assayed by gas chromatography with electron capture detection and concentrations are expressed as concentration of pethidine base [3, 4].

Results and Discussion

The clinical course was uneventful in all patients. The pain relief was very good in all patients as evaluated by a questionnaire distributed 2–4 days after PACAT. Four patients experienced drowsiness and two patients felt nausea or vomited during the PACAT period. In none of the patients was respiratory depression observed and no patient complained of itching. Observations of urinary retention were not possible as most of the patients required catheterization due to the operative procedures.

The hourly intake of pethidine among patients varied from 4.4 to 22.6 mg with a mean of 10.7 ± 5.2 mg. The group of patients who underwent abdominal surgery required somewhat less than the other group (9.7 ± 5.2 as compared to 12.4 ± 5.5 mg h^{-1}). There was a tendency for higher intake during the 1st h of self-administration but, thereafter, the mean hourly intake remained fairly constant between 7.5 and 12 mg. Intake per hour could not be related to age or body weight. In one patient, SS-m-38, who was allowed to self-administer for 44.5 h, the intake was higher during the last 20.5 h; 29.6 mg h^{-1} as compared to 16.7 mg h^{-1} during the first 24 h. The mean hourly intake of 11 mg can be compared to a mean consumption of 26 mg h^{-1} pethidine given intravenously to a similar patient group [2].

Pethidine rapidly appeared in plasma after a 10 mg epidural dose and, after 15 min, measurable concentrations could be determined. The mean measured plasma concentration varied from 60 to 284 ng ml^{-1} among patients. The mean measured plasma concentration was correlated to the hourly administered dose. The average mean measured plasma concentration of 157 ng ml^{-1} may be compared to 551 ng ml^{-1} measured after intravenous self-administration [2]. It is obvious that the large interindividual variation in intake and in plasma concentration of pethidine after intravenous self-administration also persists after epidural administration. The CSF concentration of pethidine varied more than 40-fold among patients and, in all of them, the CSF concentration also exceeded that of the plasma concentration. This observation is in sharp contrast to the situation after intravenous administration, where a constant ratio of the CSF to plasma concentration of 0.40 : 0.55 was measured [5]. The CSF concentration of pethidine could not be related to the intake per hour or to the total pethidine dose taken during the PACAT period. There was an inverse correlation between the CSF concentration and the length of time between the last pethidine dose and the moment of CSF sampling. The time varied from 23 to 146 min (Fig. 1). These data suggest that an accumulation of pethidine in CSF is unlikely during a short period (24 h) of multiple-dose epidural administration of pethidine.

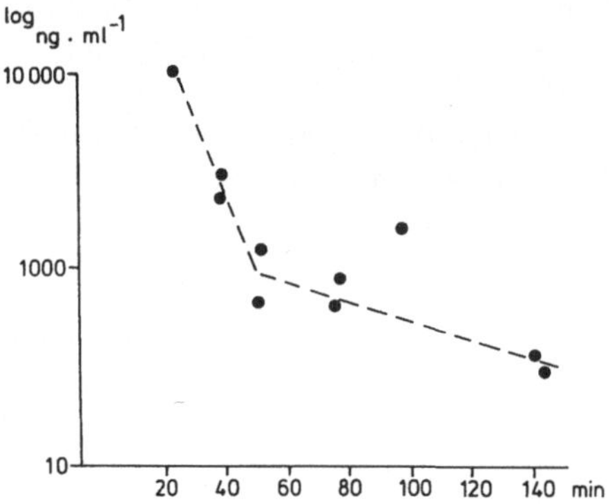

Fig. 1. CSF concentration of pethidine

The dose of pethidine used for epidural administration has varied among different authors from 10 [6] to 100 mg [7]. In the present investigation, we found a large interindividual variations in intake. This variation was also seen after intravenous self-administration of pethidine and, in that case, the intake could be related to the levels of Fraction I endorphins in the CSF [5]. The number of patients has hitherto been too small to draw any definite conclusions about the clinical advantage in offering patients self-administration of epidural narcotic analgesics. In this investigation the method has worked well and seems to be a useful tool for further studies.

References

1. Tamsen A, Hartvig P, Fagerlund C, Dahlström B (1982) Patient-controlled analgesic therapy, Part I: pharmacokinetics of pethidine in the preoperative and postoperative periods. Clin Pharmacokinet 7: 149
2. Tamsen A, Hartvig P, Fagerlund C, Dahlström B (1982) Patient-controlled analgesic therapy, Part II: individual analgesic demand and analgesic plasma concentrations of pethidine in postoperative pain. Clinical Pharmacokinet 7:164
3. Hartvig P, Karlsson K-E, Lindberg C, Johansson L (1976) Determination of pethidine in plasma by electron capture gas chromatography after reaction with trichloroethylchloroformate. J Chromatogr 121:235
4. Hartvig P, Karlsson K-E, Lindberg C, Boréus LO (1977) Simultaneous determination of therapeutic plasma concentrations of pethidine and nor-pethidine in man by electron capture gas chromatography. Eur J Clin Pharmacol 11:65
5. Tamsen A, Sakurada T, Wahlström A, Terenius L, Hartvig P (1982) Postoperative demand for analgesics in relation to individual levels of endorphins and substance P in cerebrospinal fluid. Pain 13:171
6. Bapat AR, Kshirsagar NA, Bapat RD (1980) Extradural pethidine. Br J Anaesth 52:637
7. Cousins MJ, Mather LE, Glynn CJ, Wilson PR, Graham JR (1979) Selective spinal analgesia. Lancet 1:1141

Morphin epidural zur postoperativen Analgesie – eine Doppelblindstudie

E. Lanz, W. Rieß, D. Theiss und U. Sommer

Um die Wirksamkeit von epiduralem Morphin für die postoperative Analgesie festzustellen, führten wir eine Doppelblindstudie durch. Dabei verglichen wir Wirkung und Nebenwirkungen der gleichen Morphindosis epidural und intramuskulär sowie die eines Plazebos.

Methodik

199 Patienten erhielten für orthopädische Operationen der unteren Extremitäten eine lumbale Katheterperiduralanaesthesie (KPDA) mit Mepivacain 2% bzw. Bupivacain 0,5%.

Im voraus wurden die nach ihrer Reihenfolge numerierten Patienten 3 Gruppen randomisiert zugeteilt:

1. Morphin epidural,
2. Morphin i.m.,
3. NaCl-Plazebo epidural (Tabelle 1).

Die Injektionen erfolgten am Ende der Operation.

Die Patienten wurden auf Station im Raum für Frischoperierte für 20 h sorgfältigst überwacht. Bei Bedarf erhielten sie Analgetika, gelegentlich kombiniert mit einem Sedativum. Es wurde ein postoperatives Überwachungsprotokoll geführt. Die Gruppenzugehörigkeit der Patienten war auf Station unbekannt.

Tabelle 1. Doppelblindstudie mit 3 randomisierten Gruppen

I. Morphin epidural
Morphin 0.1 mg/kg KG in 15 ml NaCl epidural (und NaCl 0.01 ml/kg KG i.m.)

II. Morphin intramuskulär
Morphin 0.1 mg/kg KG i.m. (und 15 ml NaCl epidural)

III. NaCl-Placebo
NaCl 15 ml epidural und NaCl 0.01 ml/kg KG i.m.

Injektion am Ende der Operation

Tabelle 2. Patientendaten und Morphindosierung

		Morphin epidural (n = 57)	Morphin i.m. (n = 57)	NaCl-Plazebo (n = 50)
Durchschnittsalter	[Jahre]	50,3	46,8	48,8
Geschlecht – männlich	[n]	26	25	17
weiblich		30	31	33
Durchschnittsgewicht	[kg]	70,4	69,3	63,2
Durchschnittliche Morphindosis	[mg]	7,0	6,9	

Tabelle 3. Daten zur Periduralanaesthesie, zum Operationsgebiet und zur Morphin- bzw. Plazeboinjektion

		Morphin epidural (n = 57)	Morphin i.m. (n = 57)	NaCl-Plazebo (n = 50)
Durchschnittliche Uhrzeit des PDA-Beginns	[Uhr]	10,2	10,6	10,7
Mepivacain 2% zur PDA	[%]	61	67	56
Bupivacain 0,5% zur PDA	[%]	39	33	44
Operationsgebiet:	[n]			
Hüfte		15	18	18
Oberschenkel		2	2	2
Knie		25	21	24
Unterschenkel, Fuß		15	15	16
Durchschnittliche Uhrzeit der Morphin- bzw. Plazeboinjektion	[Uhr]	12,0	12,6	12,3
Vollständige Analgesie bei Morphin- bzw. Plazeboinjektion	[%]	93	95	98

Am 1. postoperativen Tag befragte immer derselbe Anaesthesist die Patienten. Auch er kannte die Gruppenzugehörigkeit der Patienten nicht.

Die Daten wurden auf Lochkarten übertragen und statistisch ausgewertet.

Ergebnisse

Die Patienten der 3 Gruppen waren vergleichbar bezüglich Alter, Geschlecht, Gewicht und somit verabreichter Morphindosis (Tabelle 2). Die mittlere epidurale Morphindosis betrug 7,0 mg, die mittlere i.m. Dosis 6,9 mg.

Ebenfalls vergleichbar waren (Tabelle 3): Die Uhrzeit des Anlegens der KPDA, die Wahl der zur KPDA verabreichten Lokalanaesthetika Mepivacain 2% und Bupivacain 0,5%, die

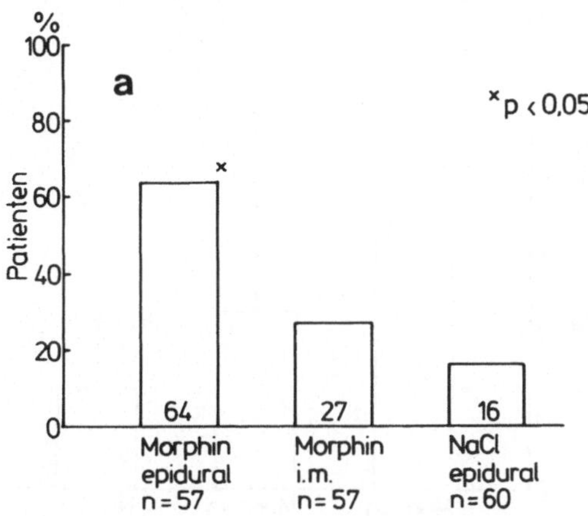

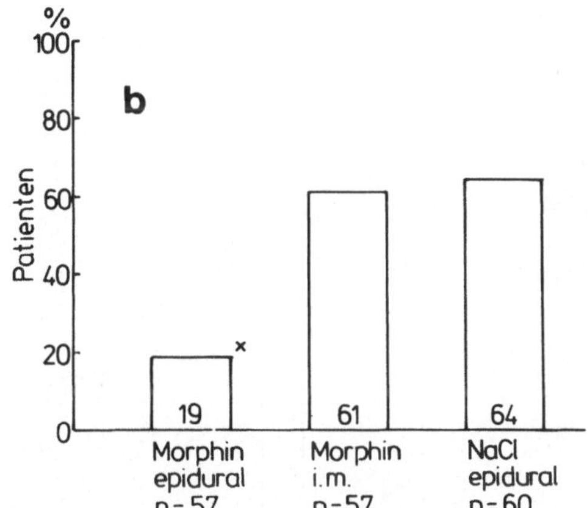

Abb. 1. **a** Keine, **b** starke Schmerzen während 24 h nach der Operation

Operationsgebiete, die Uhrzeit der Morphin- bzw. Plazeboinjektion und die Analgesie zu diesem Zeitpunkt.

Postoperative Analgesie

Nach Morphin epidural hatten 2/3 der Patienten während 24 h nach der Operation *keine Schmerzen*; nach Morphin i.m. und NaCl blieben nur etwa 1/4 bzw. 1/6 schmerzfrei (Abb. 1a).

Nach Morphin epidural berichtete nur etwa 1/5 der Patienten über *starke postoperative Schmerzen*, nach Morphin i.m. und NaCl waren dies jeweils etwa 3/5 (Abb. 1b).

Bei den Patienten, die postoperative Schmerzen hatten, traten diese *nach Morphin epidural später* auf als nach Morphin i.m. und NaCl (Abb. 2).

Nach Morphin epidural verlangte etwa 1/4 der Patienten *Analgetika*, nach Morphin i.m. und NaCl jeweils etwa 2/3 (Abb. 3). Ein *Sedativum* erhielt etwa 1/10 der Patienten nach Morphin epidural, etwa 1/4 bzw. 1/3 nach Morphin i.m. bzw. NaCl.

Nach Morphin epidural *schliefen* in der 1. postoperativen Nacht mehr Patienten gut und weniger Patienten schlecht als in den beiden Vergleichsgruppen (Abb. 4).

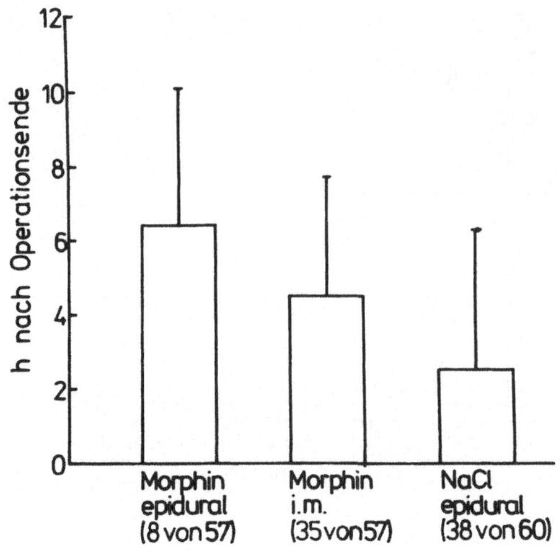

Abb. 2. Auftreten des starken postoperativen Schmerzes in h nach Operationsende

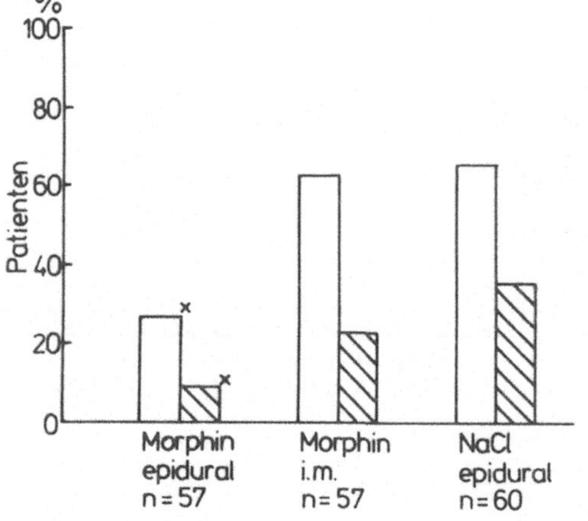

Abb. 3. Postoperativer Verbrauch an Analgetika und Sedativum

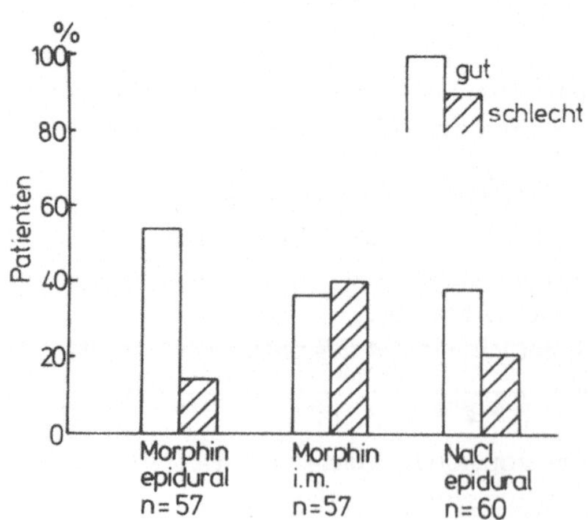

Abb. 4. Schlaf während der 1. postoperativen Nacht

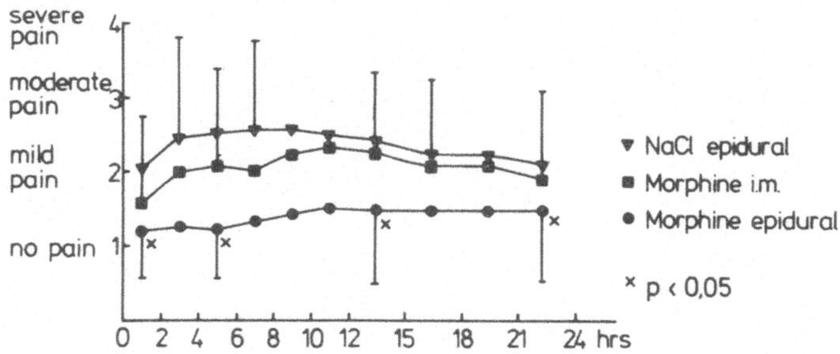

Abb. 5. Verlauf des durchschnittlichen Schmerzes während 24 h nach Operationsende

Die Patienten stuften den Schmerz in die 5 *Schweregrade* kein, leichter, mäßiger, starker und sehr starker Schmerz ein (Abb. 5).

Nach Morphin epidural blieb der *durchschnittliche Schmerz* über die gesamte Beobachtungszeit gering und niedriger als in den beiden Vergleichsgruppen, obwohl die Kontroll- und Plazebogruppe mehr Analgetika und Sedativum erhielten.

Informativer ist die *Häufigkeit der Einstufungen des Schmerzes* während der ersten 24 h nach der Operation (Abb. 6a–c). Nach Morphin epidural wurden keine oder leichte Schmerzen von knapp 90% der Patienten angegeben. Aber auch nach Morphin epidural klagten etwa 10% der Patienten über mäßige bis starke Schmerzen. Nach Morphin i.m. gaben etwa 60% der Patienten keine oder leichte Schmerzen an, ca. 40% mäßige, starke oder sogar sehr starke Schmerzen.

Nach Morphin epidural stuften etwa 4/5 der Patienten das *postoperative Allgemeinempfinden* als gut ein; nach Morphin i.m. waren es 2/3 und nach NaCl etwa die Hälfte (Abb. 7).

Um Unterschiede des postoperativen Schmerzes nach verschiedenen Operationsarten auszuschalten, wurde die postoperative Analgesie *nach Totalendoprothese des Hüftgelenks* verglichen. Auch bei dieser homogenen Gruppe war die Schmerzfreiheit nach Morphin epidural überlegen.

Um den *Einfluß der Dosis von Morphin* epidural zu prüfen, wurden 2 Dosierungsgruppen gebildet, eine oberhalb und eine unterhalb von 6,6 mg, was dem Median der Morphindosierung entsprach (Tabelle 4). Die durchschnittliche Dosierung in den beiden Gruppen unterschied sich um 2,3 mg Morphin. Die Patienten mit der höheren Dosierung hatten eine bessere Analgesie.

Frauen wogen durchschnittlich ca. 14 kg weniger und erhielten somit im Mittel 1,4 mg Morphin epidural weniger als Männer. Ihre postoperative Analgesie war weniger ausgeprägt als die der Männer.

Um den *Einfluß des Alters* auf die Wirkung der epiduralen Morphingabe zu prüfen, wurden die Patienten in eine Gruppe unter und eine andere über 50 Jahre unterteilt. Die Altersmittelwerte dieser beiden Gruppen unterschieden sich um 33 Jahre. Die epidurale Morphindosis war etwa gleich. Die postoperative Analgesie war in beiden Gruppen vergleichbar.

Nach KPDA mit Bupivacain wurden häufiger keine postoperativen Schmerzen angegeben als nach Mepivacain (Tabelle 5). Nach Bupivacain war die durchschnittliche Einstufung des Schmerzes über 24 h niedriger, der Schlaf besser, der Analgetikaverbrauch geringer und das postoperative Allgemeinbefinden besser benotet.

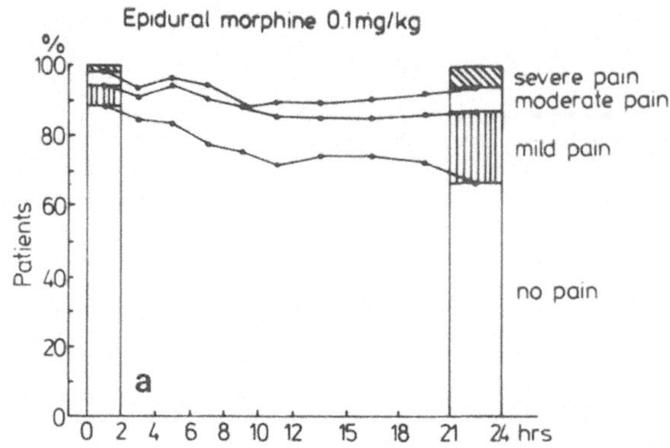

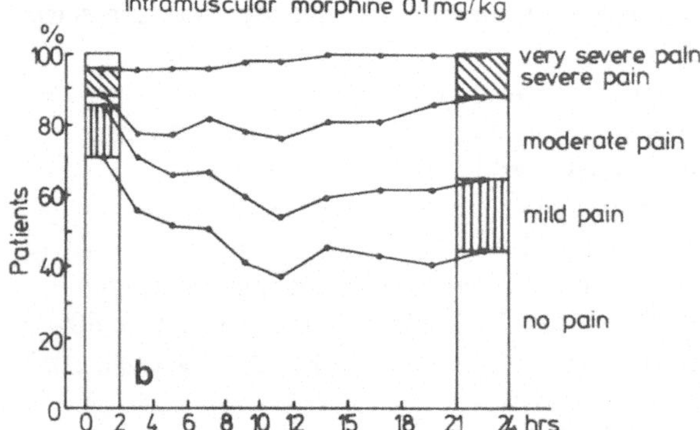

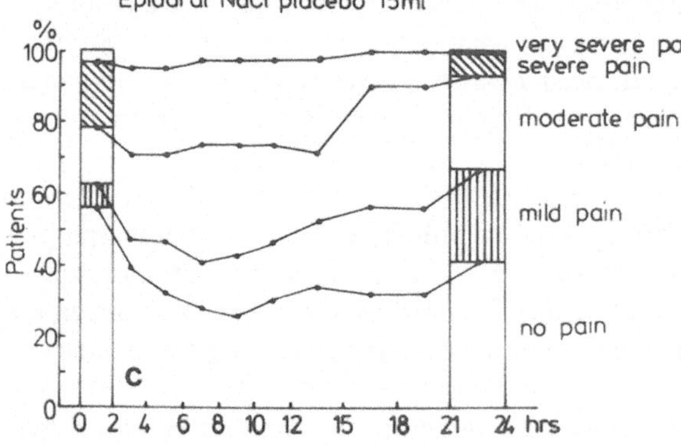

Abb. 6a–c. Häufigkeiten der Schmerzeinstufungen während 24 h nach Operationsende. a Morphin epidural, b Morphin i.m., c NaCl-Plazebo epidural

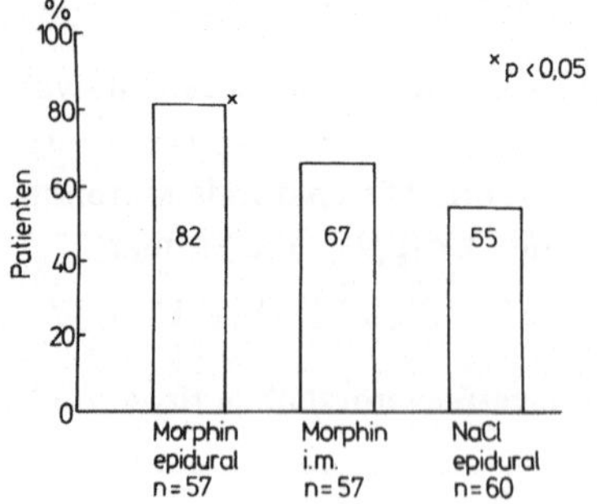

Abb. 7. Beurteilung des postoperativen Allgemeinempfindens „gut“

Tabelle 4. Einfluß der epiduralen Morphindosis

		Niedrigere Dosis ⩽ 6,6 mg	Höhere Dosis > 6,6 mg
Durchschnittsdosis	[mg]	5,8	8,1
Schmerzen während 24 h	[%]		
keine		63	66
stark		25	14
Durchschnittliche Einstufung des Schmerzes über 24 h	[%]		niedriger
Schlaf während der 1. Nacht gut	[%]	48	59
Analgetikaverbrauch	[%]	50[a]	25
Postoperatives Allgemeinbefinden	[%]		
gut		77	86
schlecht		9	0

[a] p = < 0,05

Tabelle 5. Postoperative Analgesie nach Bupivacain bzw. Mepivacain

		Bupivacain 0,5% (n = 35)	Mepivacain 2% (n = 22)
Durchschnittliche Morphindosis	[mg]	7,2	7,0
Schmerzen während 24 h	[%]		
keine		76	56
stark		10	25
Durchschnittliche Einstufung des Schmerzes über 24 h	[%]	niedriger	
Schlaf während der 1. Nacht			
gut		70	43
schlecht		5	20
Analgetikaverbrauch	[%]	15	41
Postoperatives Allgemeinbefinden	[%]		
gut		95	72
schlecht		0	7

Nebenwirkungen

Störungen der Blasenentleerung waren am häufigsten. Nach Morphin epidural wurde ca. 2 h später erstmals spontan Wasser gelassen als in den Vergleichsgruppen (Abb. 8). Nach Morphin epidural war der Harndrang häufiger auffällig und unangenehm, Carbachol (Doryl) wurde häufiger verabreicht und eine Katheterisierung war häufiger erforderlich (Abb. 9).

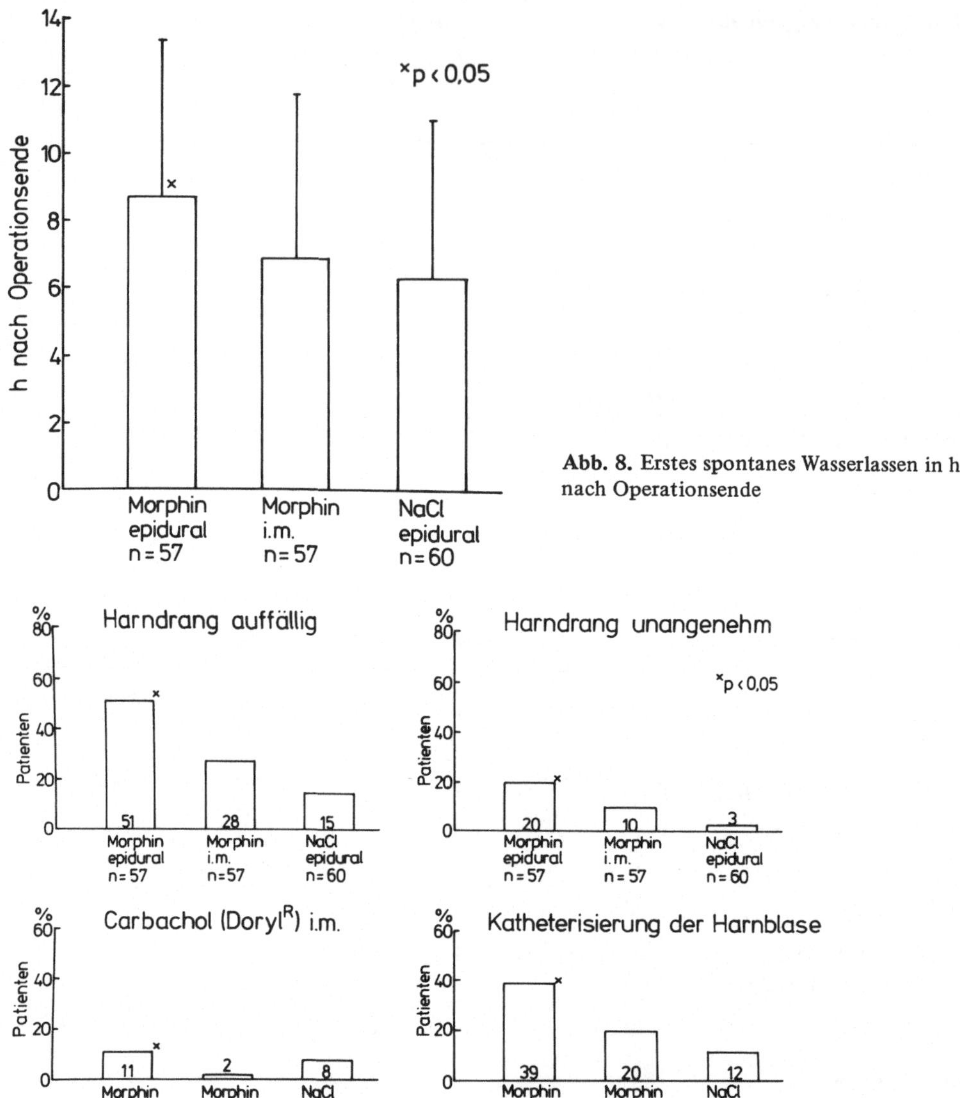

Abb. 8. Erstes spontanes Wasserlassen in h nach Operationsende

Abb. 9. Häufigkeit von Miktionsstörungen

Bei höherer Dosierung des epiduralen Morphins ergaben sich mehr Miktionsprobleme. Männer hatten mehr Schwierigkeiten als Frauen. Ältere Patienten boten nicht mehr Probleme als jüngere.

Juckreiz – selten generalisiert, meist nur am Körperstamm, den Extremitäten, nur im Gesicht oder der Genitalgegend – trat am häufigsten nach Morphin epidural auf, seltener nach Morphin i.m. und nie nach NaCl (Abb. 10).

Sonstige Beschwerden wie Übelkeit, Erbrechen, Müdigkeit und Kopfschmerzen wurden in den 3 Gruppen etwa gleich häufig beobachtet (Abb. 11).

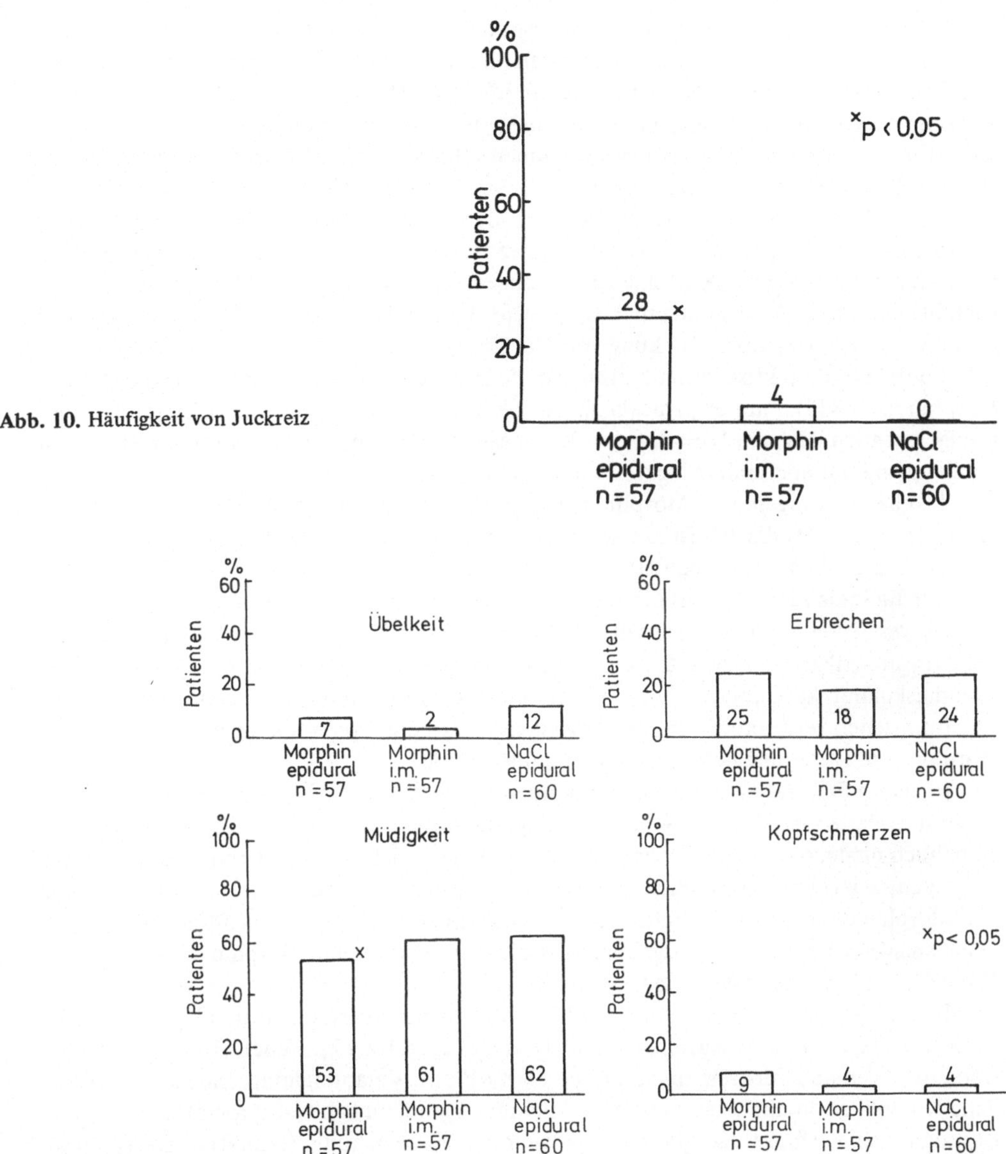

Abb. 10. Häufigkeit von Juckreiz

Abb. 11. Häufigkeit sonstiger Beschwerden

Diskussion

Durch die epidurale NaCl-Plazebogruppe wurde deutlich, daß nach ortopädischen Operationen etwa 1/3 der Patienten keine bzw. nur geringe postoperative Schmerzen empfand. Die i.m. Injektion von Morphin brachte nur eine geringe Verbesserung der postoperativen Analgesie während der ersten 8 h. Die epidurale Morphinapplikation jedoch war beiden Vergleichsgruppen überlegen. Sie war aber nicht bei allen Patienten erfolgreich.

Die epidurale Morphindosis von durchschnittlich 7,0 mg wählten wir, da wir bei Voruntersuchungen mit 2–4 mg lange Latenzzeiten und Versager beobachteten. Dies stimmt mit den Ergebnissen anderer Untersucher überein [2, 5, 9, 10, 12, 14, 15, 17]. So benötigten auch Bromage et al. [2] für ausreichende Analgesie nach Unterbauchoperationen durchschnittlich 7,6 mg, nach Oberbauchoperationen 10,3 mg. Viele Autoren erreichten allerdings gute Analgesie mit Dosen unter 5 mg [1, 6, 7, 9, 11, 13, 14, 18, 19, 20].

Unsere Untersuchung gab Hinweise dafür, daß höhere Dosen Morphin die postoperative Analgesie verbessern [2, 15, 18]. Die niedrigere Dosis bei Frauen könnte die Ursache für deren schlechtere Analgesie sein. Eine gewichtsbezogene Dosierung von Morphin scheint demnach bei epiduraler Anwendung nicht gerechtfertigt [2]. Das Alter der Patienten hatte keinen Einfluß auf die analgetische Wirkung von Morphin [2].

Von klinisch-praktischer Bedeutung ist die intensivere postoperative Analgesie von Morphin nach KPDA mit Bupivacain als mit Mepivacain. Dies kann nicht nur mit der um wenige Stunden längeren Wirkung von Bupivacain erklärt werden. Bupivacain sollte im Zusammenhang mit epiduralem Morphin bevorzugt werden.

2 Nebenwirkungen nach Morphin stehen im Vordergrund: Miktionsstörungen und Juckreiz [14]. Unsere Studie gab Hinweise dafür, daß es sich bei den Miktionsstörungen um ein dosisabhängiges Phänomen handelt.

Der Juckreiz scheint ebenfalls eine dosisabhängige Wirkung des Morphins zu sein. Das von uns verwendete Morphin enthält keine Zusätze [14]. Die begrenzte Lokalisation, das Fehlen von urtikariellen Symptomen und das häufigere Auftreten nach epiduraler als nach intramuskulärer Applikation könnten gegen eine allergische Reaktion auf Morphin sprechen.

Inzwischen verfügen wir über Erfahrung mit etwa 600 epiduralen Applikationen von Morphin. Die Dosierung betrug zwischen 2 und 10 mg.

In einem Fall trat eine Atemdepression auf [3, 8, 13–15, 17]. Es handelte sich um einen 73jährigen Patienten, der 10 mg Morphin epidural erhielt. 8 h nach der Injektion wurde er allmählich müde, somnolent bis bewußtlos, 2 h danach fiel eine Bradypnoe und schließlich Apnoe auf sowie ein Blutdruckabfall. Der Patient wurde rechtzeitig intubiert und beatmet.

Morphin epidural ist zweifellos stärker wirksam als nach i.m. Anwendung [14, 16, 18]. Seine analgetische Wirkungsdauer übertrifft die von systemischer Morphinverabreichung, ein Hinweis für die Wirkung auf spinalem Niveau.

In der hier verabreichten Dosis, die höher als die der meisten Autoren lag, wirkt es jedoch nicht in allen Fällen ausreichend analgetisch [2, 9, 10, 12]. Nebenwirkungen wie Miktionsstörungen und Juckreiz sind häufiger als nach i.m. Verabreichung. Eine lebensbedrohliche Komplikation, die Atemdepression mehrere Stunden nach Gabe von Morphin epidural, ist möglich und erfordert sorgfältige langdauernde Überwachung. Reduktion der epiduralen Morphindosis vermindert die Nebenwirkungen, aber auch die analgetische Wirkung. Deshalb sollten weitere Substanzen mit zuverlässigerer analgetischer Wirkung und geringeren Nebenwirkungen gesucht und geprüft werden [4].

Literatur

1. Asari H, Inoue K, Shibata T, Soga T (1981) Segmental effect of morphine injected into the epidural space in man. Anesthesiology 54:75
2. Bromage PR, Olshwang D, Magora F, Davidson JT (1980) Epidural narcotics for postoperative analgesia. Anesth Analg (Cleve) 59:473

3. Christensen V (1980) Respiratory depression after extradural morphine. Br J Anaesth 52:841
4. De Castro J, Lecron L (1981) Peridurale Opiat-Analgesie. Verschiedene Opiate. Komplikationen und Nebenwirkungen. In: Zenz M (Hrsg) Peridurale Opiat-Analgesie. Fischer, Stuttgart New York, S 103–128
5. Ebert J, Varner PD (1980) The effective use of epidural morphine sulfate for postoperative orthopedic pain. Anesthesiology 53:257
6. Engquist A (1981) Grundlagen der periduralen Opiat-Analgesie und klinische Erfahrungen. In: Zenz M (Hrsg) Peridurale Opiat-Analgesie. Fischer, Stuttgart New York S 1–17
7. Graham JL, King R, McGaughey W (1980) Postoperative pain relief using epidural morphine. Anesthesia 35:158
8. Gustafsson LL, Feychting B, Klingstedt C (1981) Late respiratory depression after concomitant use of morphine epidurally and parenterally. Lancet I:892
9. Magora F, Olswang D, Eimerl D (1980) Observations on extradural morphine analgesia in various pain conditions. Br J Anaesth 52:247
10. McClure JH, Chambers WA, Moore E, Scott DB (1980) Epidural morphine for postoperative pain. Lancet I: 975
11. Müller H, Börner U, Stoyanov M, Hempelmann G (1980) Intraoperative peridurale Opiatanalgesie. Anaesthesist 29:656
12. Muller A, Straja A, Dupeyron JP, Franckhauser D, Dumeny E (1980) Postoperative hypoalgesia by epidural morphine after abdominal surgery Excerpta Med Int Congr Ser 533:380
13. Piepenbrock S, Zenz M, Otten G (1981) Peridurale Opiat-Analgesie in der postoperativen Phase. In: Zenz M (Hrsg) Peridurale Opiat-Analgesie. Fischer, Stuttgart New York S 47–67
14. Reiz S, Ahlin J, Ahrenfeldt B, Andersson M, Andersson S (1981) Epidural morphine for postoperative pain relief. Acta Anesthesiol Scand 25:111
15. Scott DB, McClure J (1979) Selective epidural analgesia. Lancet I:1410
16. Torda TA, Pybus DA, Liberman H, Clark M, Crawford M (1980) Experimental comparison of extradural and i.m. morphine. Br J Anaesth 52:939
17. Weddel SJ, Ritter RR (1981) Serum levels following epidural administration of morphine with relief of postsurgical pain. Anesthesiology 54:210
18. Yu CM, Youngstrom PC, Cowan RI, Spagnuolo SET, Sutheimer C, Eastwood DW (1980) Post-cesarean epidural morphine: Doubleblind study. Anesthesiology 53:216
19. Zenz M, Hüsch M, Otten G, Otten B (1981) Peridurale Morphin-Analgesie. Anaesthesist 30:28
20. Zenz M, Piepenbrock S, Otten B, Otten G, Neuhaus R (1981) Peridurale Morphin-Analgesie. I. Postoperative Phase. Anaesthesist 30:77

Diskussion

Bahner:
Bei dem Patienten, von dem Herr Lanz den Atemstillstand berichtet hat, dürfte es sich um meinen Schwiegervater handeln. Ich muß leider Herrn Lanz sagen, daß der Patient immer noch neurologische Störungen hat. Er kann nicht mehr Golf spielen. Er hat Sensibilitätsstörungen und ist insgesamt verlangsamt. Er lebt zwar und läuft auch herum, aber ich glaube deshalb kaum, daß man so harmlos sagen kann, daß er rechtzeitig intubiert und beatmet worden ist.

Lanz:
Wir waren selbstverständlich durch diesen Fall an unserem Klinikum schwer geschockt, weshalb ich Ihnen diesen Fall gesondert darstellte. Die Dosis von 10 mg Morphin epidural war sicherlich eine Dosis an der oberen Grenze, wie wir sie zwischen März und Dezember letzten Jahres appliziert haben. Im Dezember 1980 haben wir dann die Dosis auf die Hälfte reduziert. Zur Zeit wird untersucht, ob auch niedrigere Dosen von Morphin, d. h. weniger

als 5 mg, zu einer ähnlichen guten Analgesie ausreichen oder ob damit die erreichte Schmerzfreiheit weniger zufriedenstellend ist.

Theiss:
Nachdem wir diesen Zwischenfall in der Unfallchirurgie nach Morphinapplikation gehabt haben, haben wir mit dieser Analgesietechnik ganz aufgehört. Wir waren uns zu diesem Zeitpunkt über die Gefahren einer späten Atemdepression, d. h. 8–10 h nach Gabe des Morphins, nicht bewußt. Es waren zu diesem Zeitpunkt in der Literatur derartige Fälle noch nicht beschrieben worden. Der Zwischenfall hat sich an einem Wochenende ereignet. Ich bin selbst nicht hinzugezogen worden und kann deshalb nur wiedergeben, was mir von Kollegen berichtet worden ist. Um 20.00 Uhr fiel bei dem Schichtwechsel auf der Normalstation eine Müdigkeit des Patienten auf, die aber das übliche Maß der Müdigkeit eines postoperativen Patienten nicht überschritten habe. Um 22.00 Uhr sei der Kollege auf die Station gerufen worden, da der Patient nicht mehr ansprechbar war. Mit Hinblick auf Kreislauf und Atmung wurden keine Auffälligkeiten bemerkt. Man hat zunächst einen Apoplex oder einen Herzinfarkt in Erwägung gezogen und den Patienten auf die chirurgische Wachstation verlegt. Dort habe er zwar eine Schnarchatmung geboten, die aber ausreichend erschien. Bei dem Versuch, einen Wendeltubus in die Nase zu stecken, habe der Patient akut die Spontanatmung eingestellt, worauf man ihn sofort intubiert und beatmet habe.

Bahner:
Es gibt eine Reihe von Berichten, in denen gezeigt wurde, daß die Atemdepression durch intravenöse Gabe von Naloxon sehr schnell behoben werden kann, ohne daß die Analgesie aufhört.

Stanton-Hicks:
This case is an excellent example for this audience and for any audience. We are evaluating a new technique and we are bound to see this sort of occurence. Dr. Boas and Dr. Scott have described similar reactions to the use of morphine or demerol given either intrathecally or epidurally. We have learned that obviously, when one puts such a large dose of narcotic close to the central nervous system, we will see the same side effects that one sees from parenteral administration, except that these events will occur at a much lower dose. They occur with a dose level which is much smaller than that which would be given parenterally. Respiratory depression has been shown from intraspinal subarachnoid absorption of the narcotic and that postural changes in the patient can cause the narcotic to reach the fourth-ventrical, where it produces respiratory depression. The higher doses of 8 to 10 mg morphine are probably an upper limit for its use. But even if one considers that it is a valuable technique, it means that one should only do it when adequate observation is available.

Müller:
Dürfen wir Morphin oder Morphinderivate epidural anwenden, wenn die Patienten auf Allgemeinstation kommen oder müssen sie auf die Intensivstation? Wie müssen die Patienten überwacht werden, und wer darf nachspritzen?

Stanton-Hicks:
While this technique is an experimental one the drugs should only be given in areas where there is much more intensive nursing. It should be given only in the recovery rooms or postoperative rooms at least where monitoring of the cardiorespiratory system is done more frequently than the normal nursing staff on an open ward are capable of.

Schumacher:
Für die Klinik erscheint mir nach dem, was wir heute gehört haben, von sehr großer Bedeutung zu sein, ob es noch zu verantworten ist, einen Patienten, der in Epiduralanaesthesie operiert worden ist und zur postoperativen Analgesie Morphin erhalten hat, auf eine normale Station zu verlegen.

Dennhardt:
Von meiner Warte aus möchte ich ganz klar sagen, daß jeder Patient, der epidural Opiate bekommen hat, nicht auf eine Allgemeinstation verlegt werden darf.

Zenz:
Alle Patienten, die bei uns epidural Opiate bekommen, bleiben bis 12 h nach der letzten Opiatgabe auf der Intensivstation. Damit ist die Indikation für diese Methode schon gesagt. Es ist bei uns strikt verboten, bei einem Leistenbruch, der in kontinuierlicher Epiduralanaesthesie operiert wurde, für den postoperativen Komfort des Patienten Morphin zu spritzen. Wir beschränken diese Technik auf ausgedehnte Bauchoperationen. In den letzten 2 Jahren haben wir 470 Patienten, die zum einen Opiate systemisch und zum anderen Opiate epidural erhalten hatten, untersucht und festgestellt, daß die Pneumonierate bei systemischer Opiatgabe 9% betrug und durch epidurale Morphininjektion auf 2,7% signifikant gesenkt wurde. Das ist ein klinisch faßbares Ergebnis. Ich meine nicht, daß es bei Leistenbrüchen oder gar bei Meniskusoperationen darzustellen ist.

Müller:
In unserer Klinik werden bei Patienten nach epiduraler Morphinapplikation regelmäßig viertelstündlich Kontrollen von Atemfrequenz und Blutdruck durchgeführt, und wir hatten bisher bei mehreren 1000 Anwendungen keine Atemdepression.
Die Indikation für die epidurale Morphinanwendung besteht auch bei Karzinompatienten. Sie und Herr Zenz haben berichtet, daß Sie Karzinompatienten ambulant mit epiduralem Morphin behandeln.

Zenz:
Wir verwenden epidurale Opiate bei ambulanten Karzinompatienten und haben dabei bisher überhaupt keine Nebenwirkungen gesehen. Diese Ergebnisse stimmen mit den Berichten in der Literatur überein, in der schwerwiegende Nebenwirkungen nur in der postoperativen Phase berichtet wurden, oder wenn mit zentral wirkenden, systemisch verabreichten Opiaten kombiniert wurde. Der Karzinompatient ist in den meisten Fällen wesentlich mobiler und hat damit andere Verhältnisse im Epiduralraum als der postoperative Patient. Man muß außerdem die Alternative sehen. Die Alternative zu der epiduralen Opiatgabe ist nach Untersuchungen von Twycross 600 mg Morphin intramuskulär oder parenteral appliziert. Ich meine, wenn wir dann 10 mg Morphin in den Epiduralkatheter geben, bedeutet dies in jedem Fall für den Patienten eine geringe Gefahr.

Stanton-Hicks:
Obviously at some centers these techniques are being used on an outpatients basis. The people that are using narcotics for this purpose have already had a considerable amount of experience. The doses that are used in these patients are considerably higher than those used by other investigators in the out patient clinic. The main point is obviously that, if anyone of us uses intraspinal opiates we are aware of the side effects and that a rule should be that these patients are watched postoperatively very closely. The old patient and the patient who has respiratory problems will be more susceptible to the onset of respiratory depression and other side effects. Chronic pain patients have a high tolerance to narcotics. They take high doses of narcotics anyway. The acute ingestion of narcotics postoperatively a very different situation from the foregoing one.

Haag:
Sind nach epiduraler Buprenorphinapplikation Atemdepressionen beobachtet worden, und würden Sie nach epiduraler Buprenorphingabe die Patienten ähnlich intensiv überwachen wie nach Morphin?

Zenz:
Auch im Falle von Buprenorphin ist eine intensive Überwachung der Patienten erforderlich. Ein Fall einer Atemdepression nach Buprenorphin ist mir aus der Literatur nicht bekannt.

Devaux:
You might get postoperative analgesia with saline epidurally alone. Terenius showed that there is a competition with sodium on the δ-receptors in the dorsal spinal horn. If you want to exclude this effect, you have to dilute the morphine with glucose 5%. You can dilute morphine in this way very easily without changing the pH of the solution.

Lanz:
I am aware of the difference between administering glucose or sodium chloride to morphine. Schneider was the first who postulated that glucose improves the effect of morphine at the receptor side. However, I don't know of any double blind study comparing glucose and saline. I think that is till open for further investigation.

Müller:
We have compared the effects of diluting morphine either with glucose or with saline on analgesia and the side effects in chronic pain patients as well as for postoperative pain. We did not find any difference in the effects of the 2 preparations and it is the question if this sodium index plays any role for in vivo conditions.

Stanton-Hicks:
When a narcotic is combined with a local anaesthetic, we are now starting to interfere with 2 systems. We are interfering with the morphinergic system and the normal afferent visceral and somatic systems, that the local anaesthetic effects. Therefore one can expect a certain amount of synergism when the 2 are used with a consequent reduction in the need for a higher dosis of narcotics that have been used to produce their equivalent.

Frage:
When we are doing epidural analgesia with local anaesthetics, we try to correlate the dose with the extend of analgesia. Are there any data showing a dose related extention for the analgesia with opiates?

Stanton-Hicks:
It has been shown that there is a certain segmental effect of narcotics. It is not exactly equivalent to the same segmental effect for volume or dose of local anesthetic. That is, the number of mg or volume needed to carry those mg of local anaesthetic which produce a certain number of blocked segments. One can definitely establish that, by changing the volume of the narcotic in the epidural space, we get a greater or lesser number of spinal segments involved.

Lanz:
It has been shown that there is a real segmental analgesia with morphine: the higher you insert and inject narcotic the higher is your extention of analgesia.

Stanton-Hicks:
It is quite obvious from the discussion of today that we have got a hot issue. The prospective clinical use of intraspinal narcotics has very wide reaching effects. There is no question that in chronic pain patients these techniques will be used and one isn't going to be worried about the non-suppression of the endocrine response in those patients. In certain patients, however, where one expects a large stress response, as after lower abdominal surgery, the use of local anesthetics for postoperative pain would be the method of choice. But the narcotics will have other applications. I think, for example, that one will see the combination of local anaesthetics and narcotics for postoperativ pain where the inclusion of both components may also reduce the potential side effects of the sympathetic block and the respiratory depression by the narcotics to the point where this technique will be more clinically useful. The thing that we haved to carry away from here is that there are problems associated with the use of opiates which we have known for years and the epidural route just happens to be another route of administration. The dose is relatively large compared to the dose which would be used systematically, and I think that this should really sound the note of caution.

Buprenorphin als Monoanaesthetikum und in Kombination mit Bupivacain zur kontinuierlichen Epiduralanaesthesie

W. Haag, C. Louis, E. Hartung und E. Freye

Buprenorphin, ein Abkömmling aus der Oripavinreihe (Abb. 1), interagiert als partieller Agonist-Antagonist [10] mit den Opiatrezeptoren, so daß die Substanz Analgesie auslösen kann. Pharmakologisch ist es etwa 40mal potenter als Morphin und zeichnet sich durch eine lange Analgesiedauer aus, die durch eine extrem langsame Dissoziation vom Opiatrezeptor zu erklären ist [9, 14].

Ausgehend von der Vorstellung, daß die von Yaksh [16] auf spinaler Ebene beim Tier nachgewiesenen Opiatbindungsstellen auch in der menschlichen Substantia gelatinosa des Rückenmarkes vorhanden sind, schien das Opiat wegen seiner intensiven Struktur-Wirkungs-Beziehung und seiner hohen Lipophilie für die peridurale Analgesie besonders geeigent zu sein.

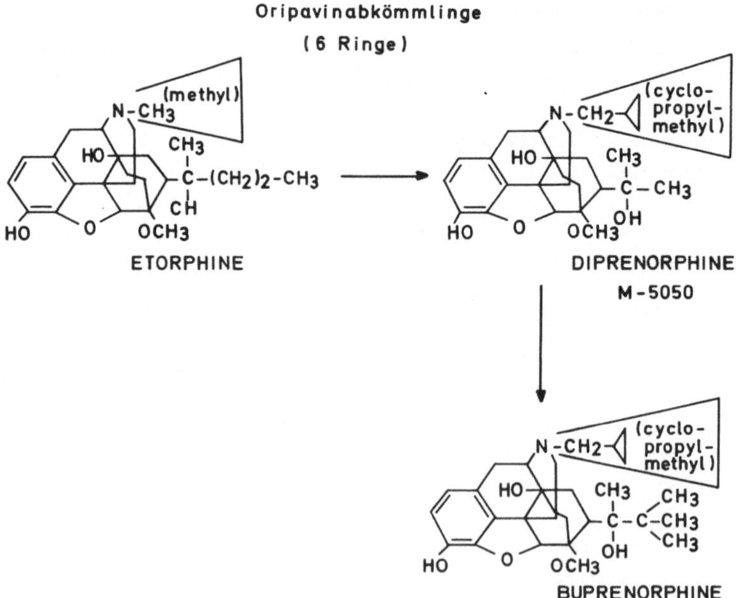

Abb. 1 Orivapinabkömmlinge (6 Ringe)

Tabelle 1. Gruppe 1 (n = 10); 0,3 mg Buprenorphin in 20 ml Kochsalz, bei unzureichender Operationsanalgesie peridurale Nachinjektion von 15–30 ml 0,5% Bupivacain

Patient	Geschlecht	Alter [Jahre]	Größe [cm]	Gewicht [kg]	ASA	Operationsart	Operationsdauer [min]
St. K.	m	37	184	80	1	Meniskektomie in Blutleere	85
B. A.	w	19	164	52	1	Meniskektomie in Blutleere	50
K. W.	m	24	173	78	1	Metallentfernung, Sehnenverlängerung	75
F. P.	m	25	189	93	1	Arthroskopie, Narbenkorrektur	50
T. T.	w	50	159	57	2	Metallentfernung	45
K. B.	m	59	170	79	2	Totalendoprothese, rechts	130
W. P.	m	25	181	67	1	Knochenprobeexzision, rechter Unterschenkel	70
T. B.	w	18	161	55	1	Meniskektomie, Bandplastik	120
St. T.	m	49	183	88,5	2	Synovektomie, rechtes Knie	105
P. G.	m	48	163	60	3	Meniskektomie	70

Folgende Fragen waren hierbei von Interesse:

1. Genügt die alleinige Buprenorphinapplikation, um eine operative Analgesie zu erreichen?
2. Hat Buprenorphin in Kombination mit Bupivacain – im Gegensatz zur reinen Bupivacaininjektion – einen Einfluß auf die Analgesiedauer?
3. Welche Nebenwirkungen treten nach der periduralen Applikation von Buprenorphin auf?

Material and Methodik

30 Patienten der ASA-Gruppen 1–3, die sich orthopädischen Operationen unterziehen mußten, wurden randomisiert in 2 Gruppen aufgeteilt:

Gruppe 1: alleinige peridurale Injektion von Buprenorphin, gefolgt von Bupivacain,

Gruppe 2: peridurale Injektion von Buprenorphin in Kombination mit 15–30 ml 0,5% Bupivacain.

Tabelle 2. Gruppe 2 (n = 20); 0,3 mg Buprenorphin in 15–30 ml 0,5% Bupivacain peridural injiziert

Patient	Geschlecht	Alter [Jahre]	Größe [cm]	Gewicht [kg]	ASA	Operationsart	Operationsdauer [min]
v. A. E.	m	61	177	81	2	Synovektomie, linkes Knie	90
K. H.	w	56	166	65	3	Totalendoprothese	135
B. W.	m	18	178	79	1	Fadenabszeß	45
B. E.	m	17	177	64	1	Exostose	30
P. S.	w	20	165	58	1	Arthoskopie, linkes Sprunggelenk	25
M. U.	m	18	178	62	1	Operation nach Roux	90
H. D.	m	29	178	93	3	Innenmeniskus, rechts	40
v. R. D.	m	29	180	65	1	Metallentfernung nach Bombelli	105
K. G.	m	50	183	80	2	Metallentfernung nach Umstellungsosteotomie	40
S. L.	w	20	179	62	1	Achillotenotomie, rechts	75
M. E.	m	39	160	65	2	Arthrotomie, linkes Kniegelenk	80
S. L.	m	78	179	95	3	Totalendoprothese rechts	180
S. B.	w	26	135	39	2	Hallux valgus, beidseitig	75
K. P.	m	71	180	72	3	Schaftwechsel	120
N. W.	m	24	190	85	1	Arthroskopie	30
M. M.	w	21	170	60	1	Metallentfernung, linkes Knie	40
B. U.	m	22	165	76	1	Meniskektomie, rechts	45
G. R.	m	24	183	80	1	Osteomausräumung, linke Hüfte	95
S. H.	m	50	182	90	1	Totalendoprothese – Keramik	170
D. W.	m	77	169	55	3	Totalendoprothese, rechts	270

Die Verteilung der Patienten hinsichtlich ihres Alters, des Geschlechtes, der Größe, des Gewichtes sowie der Operationsart und -dauer ist aus Tabelle 1 und 2 ersichtlich.

Nach Aufklärung der Patienten über die Narkoseart wurde ein Periduralkatheter entsprechend der Operationshöhe und den anatomischen Gegebenheiten zwischen L2/L3, L3/L4 bzw. L4/L5 vorgeschoben.

Bei der 1. Patientengruppe (n = 10) wurde Buprenorphin 0,3 mg peridural als Monoanaesthetikum in 20 ml 0,9% NaCl verdünnt injiziert. Im Abstand von 5 min wurde anschließend mit einer Nadel die Höhe der Schmerzempfindung geprüft (Pricktest). War in der 40. min nach der Buprenorphininjektion der Pricktest noch positiv, wurden zusätzlich 15–30 ml 0,5% Bupivacain peridural injiziert.

Bei der 2. Patientengruppe (n = 20) wurden 0,3 mg Buprenorphin in 20 ml 0,5% Bupivacain peridural appliziert. Anschließend wurde auch hier im Abstand von 5 min der Pricktest durchgeführt.

Bei beiden Gruppen wurde die Anschlagzeit bis zum Erreichen einer kompletten Analgesie (negativer Pricktest) gemessen und die Dauer der operativen und postoperativen Analgesie bestimmt. Letztere war durch das Auftreten von Schmerzen terminiert, so daß die erneute Gabe eines Analgetikums notwendig wurde.

Der Blutdruck wurde nach Riva-Rocci, die Pulsfrequenz mit einem EKG-Monitor bestimmt. Bei 5 Patienten wurden die arteriellen Blutgase und der Säure-Basen-Status (ABL2-Radiometer Copenhagen) und bei 11 Patienten prä- sowie postoperativ die Atemfrequenz und die Atemvolumina mit einem Wright-Spirometer bestimmt.

Für die Beurteilung der pharmakoencephalographischen Wirkung von Buprenorphin auf zentralnervöse Reaktionen wurde über One-line bei 4 Patienten das EEG abgeleitet. Hierzu wurden bipolar Ag/AgCl stick-on-Elektroden mit Kollodium über 2 Hirnarealen (Frontal- und Zentralregion) nach dem 10/20-System in den Positionen F_1-F_3 und C_3-P_3 fixiert.

Zur Analyse der Wirkeffekte wurden die spektralen Leistungsanteile mit Hilfe der Fast-Fourier-Transformation, unter Berücksichtigung der klassischen EEG-Frequenzbänder, herangezogen. Ein Berg-Fourier-Analysator (Fa. OTE Biomedica) Modell 1263 mit automatischer Artefaktunterdrückung ermöglichte alle 30 s die Erstellung eines Leistungsspektrums. Dieses wurde nach A-D-Wandlung bei einer Abtastrate von 128/s und 8 bit Auflösung jede Sekunde in "real-time" mit Hilfe der Fast-Fourier-Analyse aus einer 8 s langen Epoche mit 64 Frequenzpunkten im Bereich von 0,5–32 Hz errechnet. Nach Mittelwertbildung über 30 Kurvenzügen wurde das resultierende Powerspektrum alle 30 s auf einen Plotter ausgegeben. Diese kontinuierliche Spektraldarstellung bot die Möglichkeit, in übersichtlicher und komprimierter Form die Grundaktivität und die dominierenden Frequenzen im EEG in zeitlicher Folge sofort zu erfassen.

Bei eingeschränkter präoperativer Lungenfunktion wurde den Patienten Sauerstoff über eine Maske angeboten. Opiate oder andere Analgetika wurden zur Komplettierung der Analgesie nicht verwandt. Am 1. postoperativen Tag wurden die Patienten mit Hilfe eines Fragebogens nach ihren subjektiven Empfindungen in der postoperativen Phase befragt.

Ergebnisse

Bei der Gruppe 1 ließ sich eine operative Analgesie durch die alleinige Buprenorphingabe bis zur 40. min nicht erzielen. 2 Patienten gaben nach Buprenorphin deutliche Hyperaesthesien der unteren Extremitäten an. Erst die zusätzliche Bupivacaininjektion führte nach einer Latenzzeit von 11,4 min zur operativen Analgesie (Tabelle 3). Die durchschnittliche Operationsdauer dieser Patientengruppe betrug 75,5 min. 3 der insgesamt 10 Patienten benötigten während der Operation erneut Bupivacain, da beginnende Schmerzempfindungen angegeben wurden; 4 Patienten erhielten zur Sedierung 5–10 mg Diazepam bzw. 0,2–0,5 mg Flunitra-

Tabelle 3. Vergleich der Gruppe 1 (Buprenorphin mit nachfolgender Gabe von Bupivacain) und Gruppe 2 (Buprenorphin-Bupivacain-Kombination)

	Anschlagzeit bis zur chirurgischen Analgesie [min] x̄ + sd	Nachinjektion intraoperativ erforderlich [%]	Dauer der Operation [min] x̄ + sd	Postoperative Analgesiedauer für 24 h [%]
Gruppe 1 (n = 10)	11,9 ± 3,1	30	75,5 ± 29,0	60
Gruppe 2	14,5 ± 4,3	20	89,0 ± 62,2	60

Tabelle 4. Beobachtete Nebenwirkungen in %

	Gruppe 1	Gruppe 2
Hypotonie	20	15
Sedierung	70	45
Nausea	0	10
Erbrechen	0	10
Schwindelgefühl	10	5
Miktionsbeschwerden	10	15

zepam. Der Blutdruck der Patienten blieb nach der Buprenorphininjektion stabil; die zusätzliche Bupivacaininjektion bewirkte einen geringen Blutdruckabfall um durchschnittlich 20–30 mmHg. Bei 2 Patienten war die hypotone Reaktion so ausgeprägt, daß Akrinor (0,3–0,5 ml) sowie 500–1000 ml Plasmasteril gegeben werden mußten (Tabelle 4). Die Herzfrequenz fiel nach der Bupivacaingabe nur bei 4 Patienten im Mittel um 15 Schläge/min ab. Die an 5 Patienten der Gruppe 1 durchgeführten spirometrischen Messungen entsprachen sowohl intra- als auch postoperativ den Ausgangsbefunden. Der bei 2 Patienten bestimmte arterielle Sauerstoffpartialdruck entsprach bis zur 120. min nach der Buprenorphininjektion dem Ausgangswert. Einer der Patienten zeigte in der 60. min einen Anstieg des arteriellen CO_2-Partialdruckes von 34 auf 43 mmHg. Der Säure-Basen-Status änderte sich während des gesamten Beobachtungszeitraumes nicht.

Die seriellen EEG-Powerspektren zeigen in einem repräsentativen Beispiel nach Buprenorphinapplikation über der Zentralregion (rechtes Powerspektrogramm) eine zunehmende Stabilisierung der im Kontrollzustand schon bestehenden dominanten Aktivitäten im α-Bereich (8–16 Hz) (Abb. 2). Die ehemals eingestreute schnelle Hintergrundaktivität im β-Bereich (16–24 Hz) während der Kontrolle ist unter Buprenorphin deutlich vermindert. Diese Nebenpeaks können bei dem 49jährigen Patienten als eine habituell vorhandene Aktivitätsform gedeutet werden.

35 min nach Buprenorphin findet sich ähnlich wie in der Zentralregion auch im Frontalbereich (linkes Powerspektrogramm) eine Zunahme der Leistungsanteile im niedrigen α-Bereich.

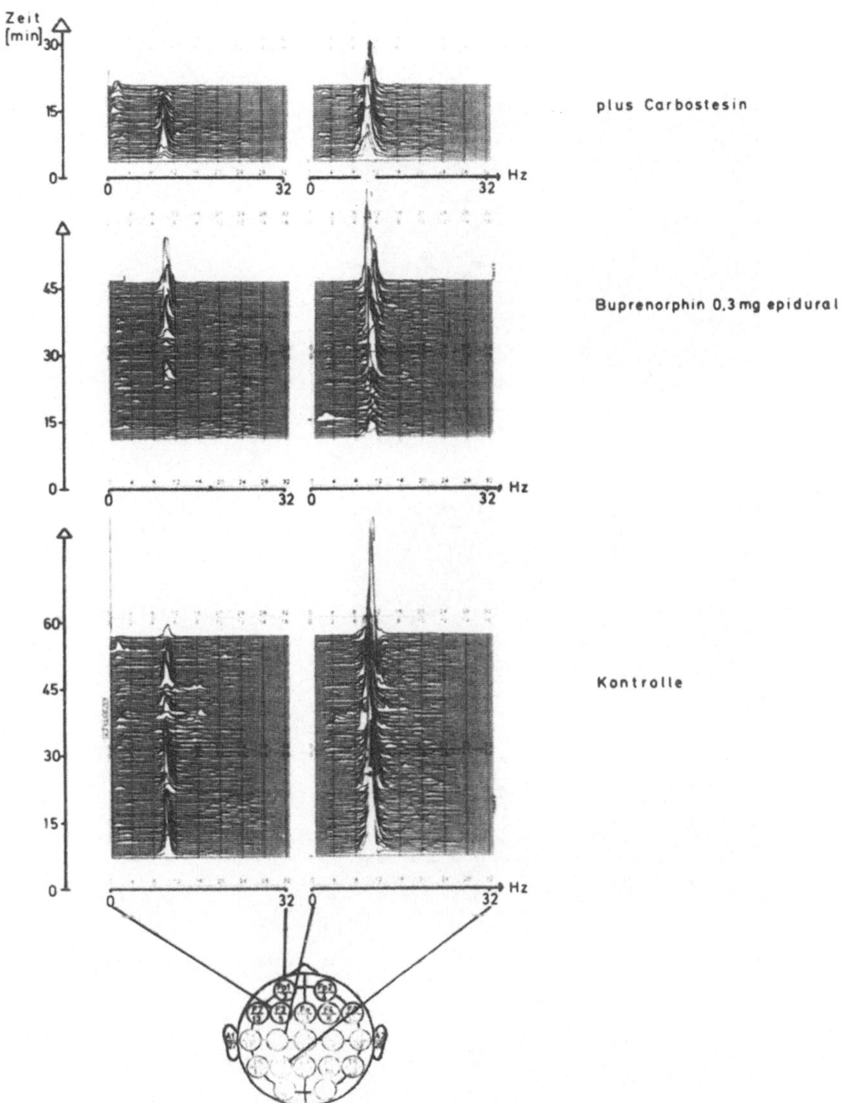

Abb. 2. Veränderungen der Leistungsspektren im EEG in Abhängigkeit von der epiduralen Applikation von Buprenorphin und Carbostesin (Patient 49 Jahre)

Diese Leistungszunahme über beiden Hirnregionen kann als Zeichen einer mäßigen Sedierung gewertet werden.

Die zusätzliche Bupivacaingabe führt zu keiner nennenswerten Zunahme der rhythmischen Aktivitäten; insbesondere ist eine Verschiebung der Poweranteile in den δ-ϑ-Bereich, (0,5–8 Hz), wie er für den Schlafzustand charakteristisch wäre, nicht nachzuweisen.

Die postoperative Schmerzfreiheit war bei 7 der 10 Patienten so ausgeprägt, daß keine weiteren Schmerzmittel benötigt wurden. Die kürzeste postoperative Analgesiedauer betrug 7 h.

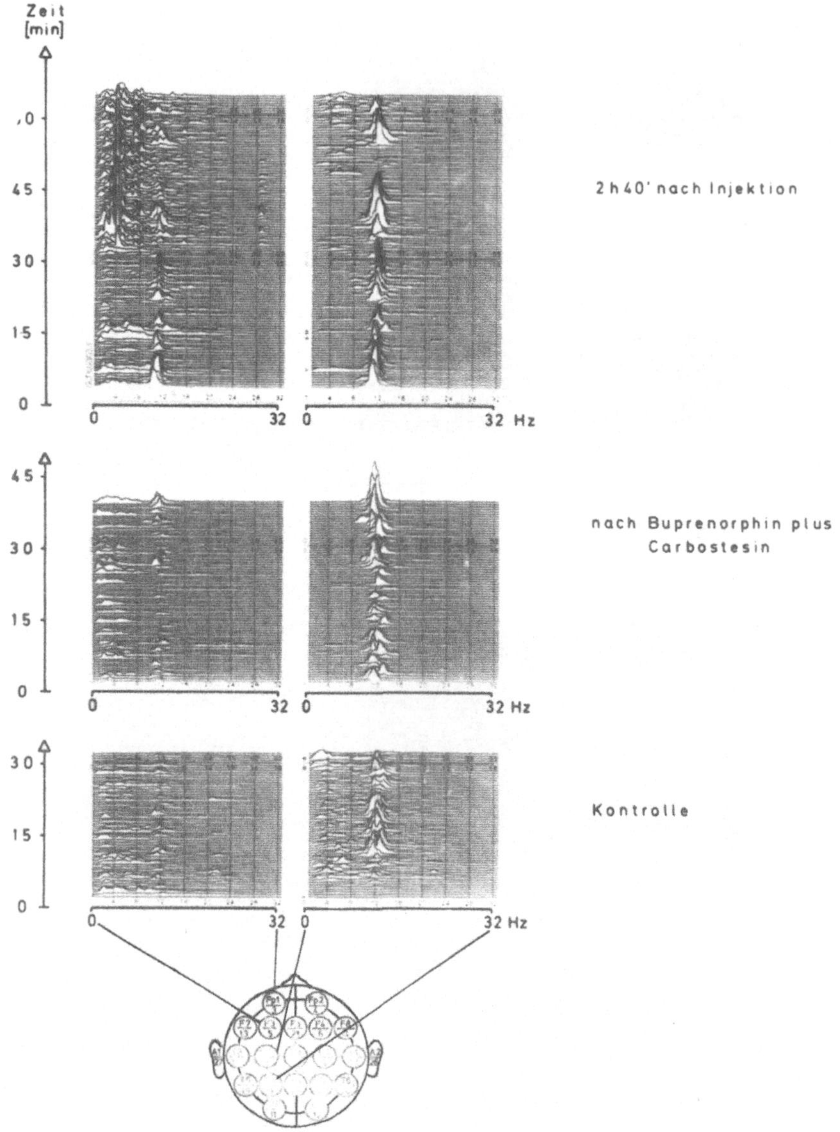

Abb. 3. Veränderungen der Leistungsspektren im EEG (Fast-Fourier-Transformation) in Abhängigkeit von der epiduralen Applikation von Buprenorphin plus Carbostesin (Patient 77 Jahre)

Die 2. Gruppe (Buprenorphin in Kombination mit Bupivacain) zeigte eine mittlere Anschlagzeit bis zur operativen Analgesie von 14,5 min (s. Tabelle 3). Bei einer durchschnittlichen Operationsdauer von 89 min war die Initialdosis von 0,3 mg Buprenorphin plus 15–30 ml 0,5% Bupivacain bei 16 Patienten für die gesamte Operationsdauer ausreichend. Bei 1 Patientin traten allerdings bereits 35 min nach der Initialdosis Schmerzen im Operationsgebiet auf, so daß Bupivacain nachinjiziert werden mußte. Außer bei 3 Patienten mit einem Blutdruckabfall um mehr als 25% und einer Bradykardie (weniger als 50 Schläge/min) zeichnete sich der Kreislauf durch stabile Verhältnisse aus (s. Tabelle 4). Die spirometrischen Messungen an 6 Patienten der Gruppe 2 zeigten während des gesamten Operationsverlaufes eine konstante Atemfrequenz und eine nicht signifikante Abweichung des Atemminutenvolumens vom Ausgangswert. Bei 3 Patienten dieser Gruppe wurden blutgasanalytische Untersuchungen vorgenommen. An 2 Patienten war eine Veränderung des arteriellen Sauerstoffpartialdruckes allerdings nicht festzustellen, da ihnen intraoperativ Sauerstoff über eine Maske gegeben wurde. Bei einem Patienten ohne intraoperative Sauerstoffapplikation entsprachen die per- und postoperativen Blutgaswerte dem Ausgangsbefund. Bei 2 Patienten stieg der arterielle CO_2-Partialdruck auf 46 bzw. 40 mmHg an. Der Säure-Basen-Status aller 3 Patienten war unauffällig.

Ein repräsentatives im On-line-Verfahren erhobenes serielles EEG-Spektrum der linken Frontal- (F_1–F_3) und Zentralregion (C_3–P_3) bei einem 77jährigen Patienten zeigte folgenden Befund (Abb. 3):

Im Kontrollzustand fand sich initial in der Zentralregion (rechtes Powerspektrogramm) eine stabile Dominanz im α-Bereich (um 12 Hz) mit eingestreuter langsamer Hintergrundaktivität im ϑ-Bereich (um 4 Hz).

30 min nach der periduralen Gabe von Buprenorphin 0,3 mg in Bupivacain 0,5% 15 ml trat als Zeichen einer Synchronisierung eine Leistungszunahme dominanter Poweranteile im α-Bereich auf. Diese zentralnervöse Zustandsänderung in Form einer harmonisierenden, rhythmischen Aktivitätsausprägung im α-Band entspricht einem Zustand der Sedierung.

3 h nach der Periduralanaesthesie erfolgte eine Umstrukturierung der EEG-Aktivitäten im Frontalbereich (linkes Powerspektrogramm) in diffuse δ- bis ϑ-Anteile (0,5–8 Hz). Bei gleichzeitigem Zusammenbruch der ehemals dominanten α-Aktivität im Zentralbereich (rechtes Powerspektrogramm) entsprach dies einer Leistungsverminderung zugunsten frontaler Hirnabschnitte wie er für den Schlafzustand charakteristisch ist.

12 Patienten der Gruppe 2 benötigten im postoperativen Verlauf keine weiteren Schmerzmittel. Bei einem Patienten betrug die kürzeste postoperative Schmerzfreiheit allerdings nur 1 h während die übrigen Patienten zwischen 3,5 und 24 h schmerzfrei waren.

Die häufigsten Nebenwirkungen während des Operationsverlaufes und in der postoperativen Phase waren eine – erwünschte – Sedierung und Miktionsstörungen (s. Tabelle 4).

Diskussion

Die alleinige Injektion von Buprenorphin (Gruppe 1) war in keinem unserer Fälle in der Lage, eine ausreichende Analgesie zu gewährleisten. Möglicherweise ist die von uns angenommen Latenzzeit des Buprenorphins von 40 min bis zur Ausbildung eines maximalen Wirkeffektes als zu kurz anzusehen. Allerdings muß aber auch berücksichtigt werden, daß aufgrund der gleichzeitig verabreichten physiologischen Kochsalzlösung eine Konformationsänderung des Opiatrezeptors induziert wurde. Schon Pert u. Snyder [12] und Simon et al. [15] konnten nämlich in vivo demonstrieren, daß aufgrund der allosterischen Form der Opiatbindungsstellen ein natriumreiches Milieu der antagonistischen From des Rezeptors Vorschub leistet, während bei einer natriumarmen Umgebung die anonistische Rezeptorform dominiert. Dies erscheint insofern von Bedeutung, als Buprenorphin ein gemischter Agonist-Antagonist ist, so daß natriumreiches Milieu eher die antagonistische Form zur Bindung führt und eine ausreichende Analgesie nicht induziert werden kann. Allen Patienten mußte deswegen zusätzlich Bupivacain injiziert werden, wonach sich eine deutliche Verkürzung der Bupivacainlatenzzeit, die normalerweise bei 25 min liegt, im Mittel auf 11 min erreichen ließ. Des weiteren war eine Verlängerung der operativen und postoperativen Analgesiedauer nachweisbar. Auch bei der Gruppe 2 ließ sich eine Verkürzung der Anschlagzeit bis zum maximalen Wirkeffekt sowie eine deutliche Verlängerung der operativen und postoperativen Analgesie erreichen. Die Ursache für den langen Wirkeffekt ist mit pharmakodynamischen Wechselbedingungen zwischen dem Opiat und den Morphinrezeptoren in der Substantia gelatinosa zu erklären. Obwohl Buprenorphin ein lipophiles Medikament ist und man daher sowohl eine kurze Latenzzeit als auch eine kurze Analgesiedauer erwarten würde [8], ist die lange Wirkzeit (bis zu 48 h) durch die äußerst langsame Dissoziation des Opiates vom Rezeptor zu erklären [5].

Bei periduraler Applikation ist Buprenorphin ca. 7mal stärker analgetisch wirksam als Morphin [4]; dies erklärt sich aus der größeren "intrinsic activity" des Buprenorphin [13] am Rezeptor. Aufgrund dieser ausgeprägten Rezeptorinteraktion wäre ein atemdepressiver Effekt zu erwarten, wie er auch von Orwin und Mitarbeitern [11] nach systemischer Applikation beobachtet wurde und sich in einer Verminderung der CO_2-Antwortkurve bemerkbar machte.

Intraspinale und epidurale Injektion von Opiaten beinhalten immer die Gefahr einer noch nach Stunden auftretenden Atemdepression [1, 2, 3]. Während lipidlösliche Opiate wie Fentanyl und Buprenorphin durch die Lipide des Rückenmarkes schwammartig aufgesaugt werden, ist Morphin als wasserlösliche Substanz ein Depot in der Spinalflüssigkeit von wo aus es zu den basalen Zisternen und den Ventrikelräumen entsprechend den Strömungsverhältnissen hin transportiert wird und, im IV. Ventrikel angelangt, zur späten Atemdepression führt [7]. Diese physikochemischen Eigenschaften der Opiate sind maßgeblich an den nach Stunden auftretenden lebensbedrohlichen Ateminsuffizienzen beteiligt, ein Effekt, der beim Buprenorphin aufgrund seiner hohen Lipophilie und seiner spezifischen Rezeptorbindung nicht zu erwarten ist. In der Tat demonstrieren unsere Blutgas- und spirometrischen Untersuchungen nur eine mäßige Beeinträchtigung der Atmung, wobei offenbleibt, ob dies auf eine direkte Depression des Atemzentrums oder aufgrund der beobachteten Sedierung hervorgerufen wird, die in den EEG-Power-spektrogrammen demonstriert werden konnte. Die besonders bei alten Patienten (über 60 Jahre) in der späten postoperativen Phase auftretende Vigilanzminderung, die von Schlaf begleitet ist, spricht für die Überlegung, daß auch das lipophile Buprenorphin das retikuläre aktivierende System im Hirnstamm [17] erreicht und beeinträchtigt – entweder nach Resorption durch den venösen Rückenmarkplexus über den Kreislauf oder über die spinale Liquorzirkulation. Dieser sedierende Effekt von Buprenorphin ist besonders nach systemischer Applikation bekannt [6] und ohne signifikante Beeinträchtigung der Atmung in der postoperativen Phase nach epiduraler Applikation sogar wünschenswert.

Andere Nebenwirkungen wie Hypotension und Bradykardie, die zu Beginn der Narkose auftraten, als auch die postoperativen Miktionsstörungen sind auf eine bupivacaininduzierte Sympathikusblockade zurückzuführen, da eine alleinige Buprenorphinapplikation (Gruppe 1) zu keinen Kreislaufveränderungen geführt hatte.

Die Frage, ob eine peridurale Buprenorphinapplikation selektiv mit lokalen Opiatrezeptoren im Rückenmark interagiert, kann bejaht werden, da Louis et al. [8a] bei alleiniger periduraler Bupivacaingabe und zusätzlicher intramuskulärer Buprenorphininjektion (0,3 mg) einen wesentlich höheren Analgetikabedarf intra- und postoperativ feststellen konnten.

Der Vorteil einer kombinierten periduralen Buprenorphin-Bupivacain-Applikation im Vergleich zur alleinigen Bupivacaingabe ist in der kürzeren Anschlagzeit und einer verlängerten operativen und postoperativen Analgesie bei ausgeprägter Kreislaufstabilität zu sehen. Morphintypische Nebenwirkungen, wie Schwindel, Zephalgie, Pruritus, Nausea und Erbrechen treten bei periduraler Applikationsform nur vereinzelt auf.

Weitere Untersuchungen erscheinen jedoch notwendig, um mit Sicherheit zu klären, warum die alleinige peridurale Buprenorphingabe für die Unterdrückung akuter operativer Schmerzen nicht ausreicht.

Zusammenfassung

Der Oripavinabkömmling Buprenorphin wurde im Hinblick auf seine analgetische Potenz nach periduraler Applikation bei 30 orthopädischen Operationen untersucht.

Die alleinige peridurale Verabreichung von 0,3 mg Buprenorphin erbrachte bei 10 Patienten keine operative Analgesie. Die kombinierte peridurale Applikation von 0,3 mg Buprenorphin in 15–30 ml 0,5% Bupivacain verkürzte bei 20 Patienten im Gegensatz zur alleinigen Bupivacaininjektion die Anschlagzeit bis zur Ausbildung einer chirurgischen Analgesie im Mittel auf 11 ± 4 min. Des weiteren war durch diese Kombination eine langdauernde per- und postoperative Analgesie gewährleistet, so daß zusätzliche Analgetika nur in wenigen Fällen notwendig wurden.

Außer einer erwünschten Sedierung bei 70% der Patienten waren keine auffälligen Nebenwirkungen feststellbar. Insbesondere konnte in keinem Fall eine klinisch bedrohliche Atemdepression beobachtet werden.

Gleichzeitig durchgeführte EEG-Messungen mit Hilfe der Power-spektralanalyse demonstrierten besonders bei Patienten jenseits des 60. Lebensjahres in der postoperativen Phase eine Verschiebung der maximalen Leistungsspektren vom α-Bereich (8–16 Hz) in niedrige Frequenzbereiche (0,5–8 Hz); letzteres war klinisch durch Schlaf charakterisiert. Jüngere Patienten (< 40 Jahre) zeigten als Zeichen der Sedierung eine Synchronisation im α-Bereich.

Im Hinblick auf Risikopatienten im orthopädisch-chirurgischen Krankengut erscheint die Anwendung der periduralen Buprenorphin-Bupivacain-Kombination u. E. aus folgenden Gründen empfehlenswert:

1. rasch einsetzende und langanhaltende Analgesie,
2. deutliche Einsparung von Analgetika und Sedativa intra- und postoperativ
3. stabile Kreislaufverhältnisse,
4. keine relevante Atemdepression.

Literatur

1. Baskoff JD, Watson RL, Muldoom SM (1980) Respiratory arrest after intrathecal morphine. Anesthesiology 52:280
2. Boas RA (1979) Hazards of epidural morphine. Anaesth Intensive Care 8:377
3. Christensen V (1980) Respiratory depression after extradural morphine Br J Anaesth 52:841

4. De Castro J, Lecron L (1981) Verschiedene Opiate, Komplikationen und Nebenwirkungen. In: Zenz M (Hrsg) Peridurale Opiat-Analgesie. Fischer Stuttgart New York, S. 103
5. Hambrook IM, Rance MI (1976) The interaction of buprenorphine with the opiate receptor kinetics. In: Kosterlitz HW (ed) Opiats and endogenous opioid peptides. Amsterdam, p 295
6. Harcus AW, Ward AE, Smith DW (1979) Methodology of monitored release of a new preparation buprenorphine. Med J II:163
7. Hempelmann G, Müller H (1981) Morphin and Naloxon. Dtsch Med Wochenschr 106/13:411
8. Herz H, Teschenmacher HJ (1971) Activities and sites of antinociceptive action of morphine-like analgesics. Adv Drug Res 6:79
8a Louis CH, Freye E, Hartung E, Haag W (1982) Buprenorphin in der periduralen Leitungsanästhesie. Anaesth Intensivther Notfall med 17:341
9. Manara L, Cerletti C, Luini A, Tavini A (1978) Rat brain levels and subcellular distribution of in vivo administered buprenorphin. In: Van Ree IM, Terenius L (eds) Characteristics and function of opioids. Amsterdam, Elseviers/North-Holland Biomedical Press, p 225
10. Martin WR (1979) History and development of mixed opioid agonists and antagonists, Br J Clin Pharmacol 7:273
11. Orwin IM, Orwin J, Price M (1976) A double blind comparison of buprenorphin and morphine in conscious subjects following administration by the intramuscular route. Acta Anaesthesiol Belg 3: 171
12. Pert CB, Snyder SH (1974) Opiate receptor binding of agonists and antagonists affected differentially by sodium. Mol Pharmacol 10:868
13. Rance MJ (1979) Animal and molecular pharmacology of mixed agonists-antagonist analgesic drugs. Br J Clin Pharmacol 7:281
14. Rance MJ, Dickens IM (1978) The influence of drug receptor kinetics on the pharmacological and pharmacokinetic profiles of buprenorphin. In: Van Ree JM, Terenius L (eds) Characteritics and function of opioids. Elseviers North-Holland Biomedical Press Amsterdam, p 65
15. Simon EJ, Hiller IM, Grothe J, Edelmann J (1975) Further properties of stereospecific opiates binding sites in rat brain: On the nature of the sodium effect, J Pharmacol Exp Ther 197:531
16. Yaksh TL (1978) Analgetic actions of intrathecal opiates in cat and primate. Brain Res 153:205
17. Zanchetti A (1967) Brainstem mechanisms of sleep. Anaesthesiology 29:81

Wirkungen und Nebenwirkungen der morphininduzierten Periduralanalgesie in der Geburtshilfe

H. J. Hartung, W. Wiest, A. Hettenbach, P.-M. Osswald und R. Klose

Die peridurale Morphinapplikation ist bislang zur Therapie verschiedener Schmerzzustände erfolgreich angewandt worden. So wurde Morphin zur Linderung sonst inkurabler Schmerzen bei Tumorpatienten [2, 3, 9, 12, 22], zur postoperativen Schmerzbehandlung [6, 11, 20, 21, 23] sowie nach Rippenserienfrakturen [15] epidural injiziert. Wenig ermutigend scheinen bisher publizierte Erfahrungen zur Anwendung dieser Methode während der Geburt zu sein [1, 5, 14, 17]. Nachfolgend sollen daher unsere Ergebnisse zur Wehenschmerzbekämpfung mit dieser Methode dargestellt werden.

Methodik

Bei 44 Gravida wurde der peridurale Raum nach der Loss-of-resistance-Methode in Höhe L 1/2–L 4/5 in Seitenlage punktiert und ein Katheter 2–3 cm vorgeschoben. 23 Patientinnen erhielten dann 10 mg Morphin in 15 ml, 21 in 10 ml 0,9%iger NaCl-Lösung peridural appliziert. Geprüft wurde die Ausbreitung der Analgesie durch Kältereize, die Qualität der Analgesie gab die Patientin subjektiv selbst an:

1. vollständige Analgesie, d. h. kein Wehenschmerz mehr,

2. gute Analgesie, d. h. der Wehenschmerz ist nur noch minimal zu bemerken,

3. mäßige Analgesie, d. h. die Wehenschmerzen sind weniger als vor der PDA, aber dennoch deutlich vorhanden,

4. keinerlei analgetischer Effekt.

Beginn und Dauer der Analgesie wurden ebenfalls durch Befragen der Schwangeren erhalten. Die Überwachung des maternalen Kreislaufs erfolgte durch engmaschige, d. h. 5minütliche Blutdruckkontrolle nach Riva Rocci und kontinuierliches Pulsmonitoring, des fötalen Zustand durch Ableiten eines internen Kardiotokogramms. Post partum wurde nach 1, 5 und 10 min der Apgar-Score erhoben sowie der Säure-Basen-Haushalt des Föten bestimmt.

Bei einer unausgewählten Gruppe von 10 Patientinnen sind vor und nach maximaler Wirkung der Morphinperiduralanalgesie die Blutgase bestimmt worden.

Tabelle 1. Dauer des Wirkungseintritts nach Morphinapplikation mit 10 ml bzw. 15 ml Trägerlösung

Wirkungseintritt t [min]	10 mg Morphin in 15 ml NaCl (n = 23)	10 mg Morphin in 10 ml NaCl (n = 21)
1– 5	2	4
6–10	4	10
11–30	15	5
∞	2	2

Tabelle 2. Qualität der Analgesie

Analgesie		10 mg Morphin/ 15 ml NaCl (n = 23)	10 mg Morphin/ 10 ml NaCl (n = 21)
1) Vollständig:	keine Schmerzen	3	1
2) Gut:	geringe Schmerzen	12	14
3) Mäßig:	deutliche Schmerzen	6	4
4) Kein Effekt:	Schmerzen unverändert	2	2

Biometrie

Die statistische Sicherung der Beeinflussung bzw. Nichtbeeinflussung der Wehen- und Kreislaufparameter durch das angewandte Verfahren erfolgte durch Erstellen einer Regressionsgeraden $y = a + bx$, wobei dann durch den T-Test für verbundene Stichproben geprüft wurde, inwieweit sich die Steigung b von 1 signifikant unterscheidet, und ob die Lage des Kurvenschwerpunkts symmetrisch, d.h. der Achsenabschnitt sich signifikant von null unterscheidet. Im Idealfall – bei keinerlei Beeinflussung durch das angewandte Verfahren – wird also die Regressionsgerade durch den Ursprung verlaufen unter einem Winkel von 45°.

Die statistische Beurteilung der Blutgasanalysen erfolgte durch den Wilcoxon-Test für verbundene Stichproben ($p = 0{,}05$).

Ergebnisse

Der Wirkungseintritt der Analgesie (Tabelle 1) wurde zwischen 5 und 30 min. angegeben mit einer deutlichen Häufung bei 10 bzw. 20 min.

Die Qualität der Analgesie (Tabelle 2) bezüglich des Wehenschmerzes zeigte in 65 bzw. 71% eine gute bis vollständige Schmerzlinderung. In weiteren 26 bzw. 19% konnte eine nur mäßige analgetische Wirkung beobachtet werden. Knapp 10% der Patientinnen zeigten auf die peridurale Opiatgabe keinerlei Beeinflussung des Wehenschmerzes.

Die Zeitspanne der Wirkungsdauer (Tabelle 3) reichte von Werten unter 60 min. bis zu einer Zeitdauer von $5^1/_2$ h.

Tabelle 3. Dauer der analgetischen Wirkung

t [min]	10 mg Morphin in 15 ml NaCl (n = 23)	10 mg Morphin in 10 ml NaCl (n = 21)
<60	2	8
65–120	10	10
125–180	6	3
180–330	5	0

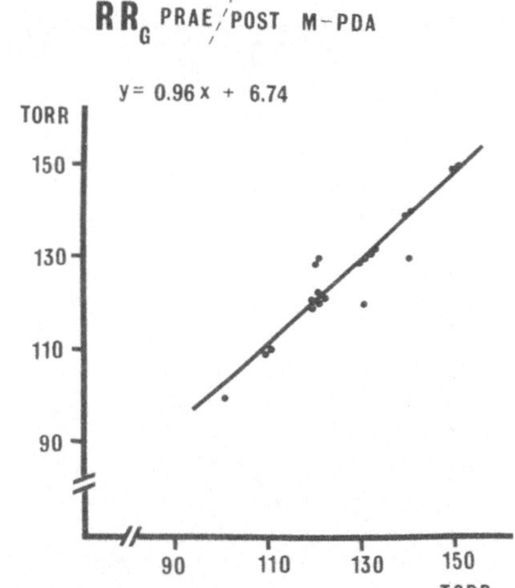

Abb. 1. Systolischer Blutdruck vor und nach epiduraler Morphingabe

Eine dermatomorientierte Ausbreitung der Analgesie konnte klinisch nicht festgestellt werden. Dermale Kälte- und Schmerzreize wurden von fast allen Patientinnen perzipiert.

Unbeeinflußt blieben weiterhin das kardiozirkulatorische (Abb. 1) und respiratorische System (Abb. 2) der Patientinnen. In keinem Fall traten Hypotensionen oder Alterationen des Herzrhythmus auf.

Das intern abgeleitete CTG zeigte sich in allen Parametern – fötale Herzfrequenz (Abb. 3), Wehenfrequenz (Abb. 4), Wehenintensität (Abb. 5), Wehendauer und Basaltonus (Abb. 6) – unverändert.

Die Apgar-Scores (Tabelle 4) ergaben lebensfrische Kinder, ausgenommen 3 Fälle – vorzeitige Plazentalösung, Plazentainsuffizienz, hypoxische Dezellerationen in der Austreibungsphase – welche dann durch Sectio entbunden wurden.

Diskussion

Publikationen über die Anwendung der epiduralen Morphinapplikation in der Geburtshilfe liegen bislang von verschiedenen Arbeitsgruppen vor. So berichten Booker et al. [5] über eine komplette Analgesie bei 48% der Patienten und bei weiteren 16% über eine Schmerzminderung, wobei die Dauer der Analgesie zwischen $3^1/_2$ und 11 h bei einem Mittel von $5^1/_4$ h

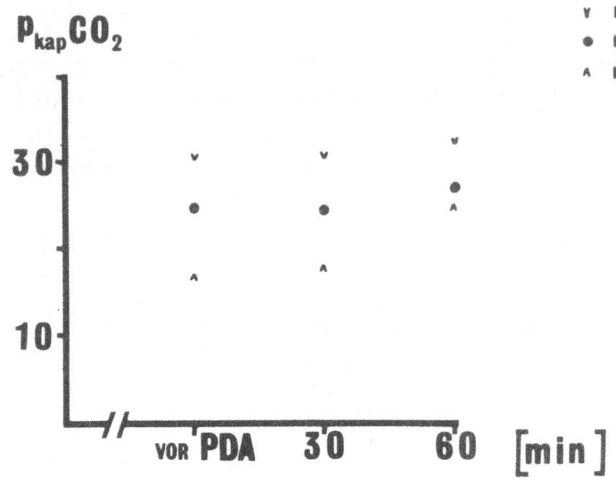

Abb. 2. paCO$_2$-Verlauf vor Morphin-PDA und nach Wirkungseintritt

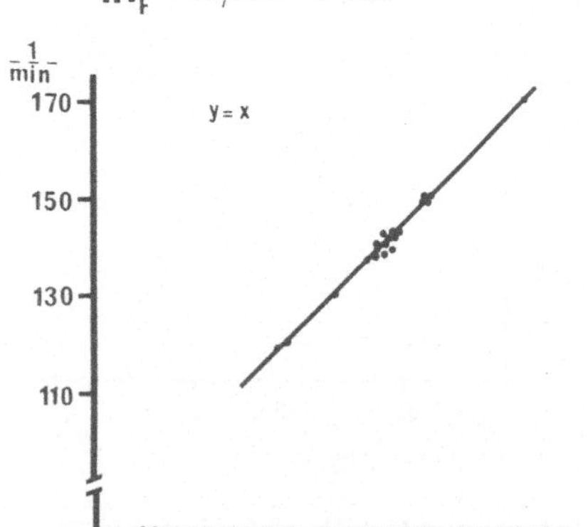

Abb. 3. Fötale Herzfrequenz wird durch die Morphin-PDA nicht verändert

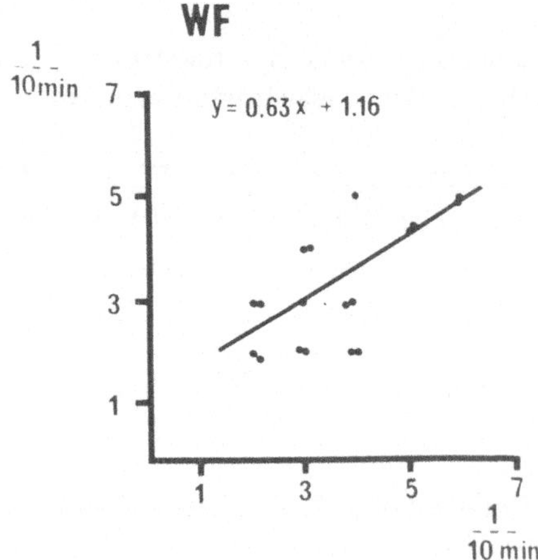

Abb. 4. Keine Beeinflussung der Wehenfrequenz

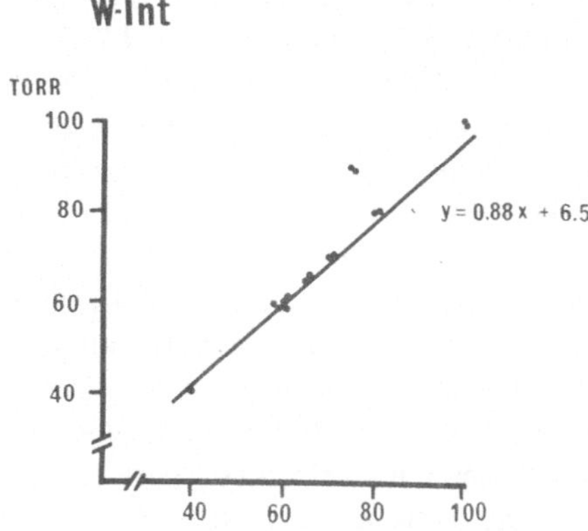

Abb. 5. Wehenintensität bleibt unverändert

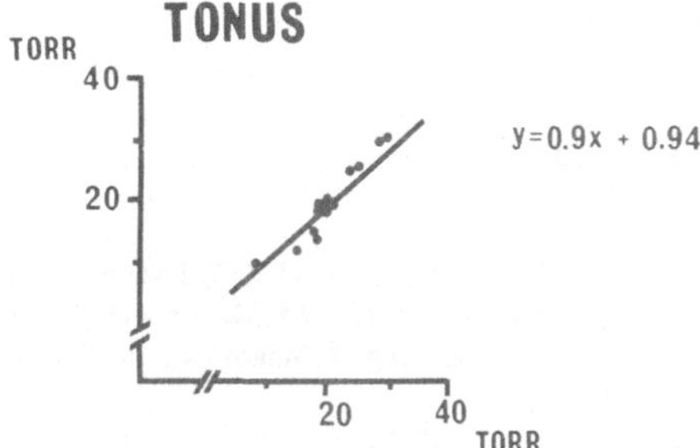

Abb. 6. Basaltonus vor und nach Morphin-PDA

Tabelle 4. Übersicht der Apgar-Scores; n = 42, p̄H: 7,255 (Minimum: 7,16, Maximum: 7,36)

4	5	6	7	8	9	10	t
1		1	1	7	32	–	t_1
		1	–	3	6	32	t_2
		1	–	1	4	36	t_3

variierte. Husemeyer et al. [14] konnten in 10 Fällen mit einer Dosis von 2 mg Morphin in 8 ml 0,9%iger Lösung keinen analgetischen Effekt erzielen. Magora et al. [16] berichteten bei Schwangeren am Termin über unbefriedigende Ergebnisse im Gegensatz zu Schwangerschaftsunterbrechungen im 2. Trimenon. Perris [17] fand nach epiduraler Pethidingabe gute analgetische Effekte bei bis zu 75% der Fälle. Er konnte dabei weiterhin zeigen, daß die Qualität der Analgesie sowie die Wirkungsdauer eindeutig dosisabhängig waren, wobei bis zu 100 mg Pethidin appliziert wurden.

Vergleiche mit den Ergebnissen anderer Arbeitsgruppen hinsichtlich der analgetischen Wirkung sind wegen nicht einheitlicher Methoden nur schwer möglich.

Mit Ausnahme von Perris [17] werden niedrigere Opiatdosen appliziert und eine nicht suffiziente analgetische Wirkung im Bereich der Geburtshilfe beobachtet. Unsere positiven

Erfahrungen sind möglicherweise durch eine relativ hohe Morphingabe bedingt, appliziert mit einem großen Volumen von 15 ml Trägerlösung.

Verschiedene Nebenwirkungen der Morphinepiduralanalgesie sind bislang beobachtet worden, so z. B. Übelkeit oder Erbrechen, Hautjucken, Urinretention und als ernstere Komplikation die respiratorische Depression [8, 10]. Reiz u. Westberg [18] berichteten in einer Serie von 1200 Patienten über einen Fall der Atemdepression. Weitere Fälle wurden von Christensen [7], Scott u. Clure [19] und Boas [4] veröffentlicht. Die dabei mitgeteilten Atemdepressionen konnten erfolgreich mit Naloxon behandelt werden, wobei der analgetische Effekt durch das systemisch applizierte Naloxon unbeeinflußt blieb. Da das Auftreten einer solchen ernsten Komplikation bislang keine Korrelation zur verabreichten Opiatmenge noch eine zeitliche Abhängigkeit erkennen ließ, ist eine sorgfältige Überwachung der Schwangeren über einen längeren Zeitraum unerläßlich.

Unsere eigenen Erfahrungen mit der morphininduzierten Epiduralanalgesie zeigten bislang keinerlei Nebenwirkungen am maternalen wie fötalen Organismus. Juckreiz oder Störungen der Blasendarmtätigkeit waren nicht vermehrt zu beobachten; in 2 Fällen trat Erbrechen ein.

Literatur

1. Allen PR, Johnson RW (1979) Extradural analgesia in labour. Anaesthesia 34:839
2. Bapat AR, Kshirsagar NA, Bapat RD (1980) Extradural pethidine. Br J Anaesth 52:637
3. Behar M, Olshwang D, Magora F, Davidson JT (1979) Epidural morphine treatment of pain. Lancet I:527
4. Boas RA (1980) Hazards of epidural morphine. Anaesth Intensive Care 8:377
5. Booker PD, Wilkes RG, Bryson THL, Beddard J (1980) Obstetric pain relief using epidural morphine. Anaesthesia 35:377
6. Bromage PR, Camporesi E, Chestnut D (1980) Epidural narcotics for postoperative analgesia. Anesth Analg (Cleve) 59:473
7. Christensen V (1980) Respiratory depression after extradural morphine. Br J Anaesth 52:841
8. Collier CB (1981) Epidural morphine. Anaesthesia 36:67
9. Cousins MJ, Glynn GJ, Wilson PR, Mather LE, Graham JR (1980) Epidural morphine. Anaesth Intensive Care 8:217
10. Duffy BL (1981) Itching aside-effect of epidural morphine. Anaesthesia 36:67
11. Graham JL, King R, McCaughey W (1980) Postoperative pain relief using epidural morphine. Anaesthesia 35:158
12. Howard RP, Milne LA, Williams NE (1981) Epidural morphine in terminal care. Anaesthesia 36:51
13. Husemeyer RR, Cousins MJ (1979) Aspects of epidural morphine. Lancet II:383
14. Husemeyer RP, O'Connor M, Davenport HT (1980) Failure of epidural morphine to relief pain in labour. Anaesthesia 35:161
15. Johnston JP, McCaughey W (1980) Epidural morphine. Anaesthesia 35:155
16. Magora F, Olshwang D, Einerl D, Shorr J (1980) Observations on extradural morphin analgesia. Br J Anaesth 52:247
17. Perris BW (1980) Epidural pethidine in labour. Anaesthesia 35:380
18. Reiz S, Westberg M (1980) Side-effects of epidural morphine. Lancet 26:203
19. Scott DB, Clure JMc (1979) Selective epidural analgesia. Lancet I:1410
20. Torda TA (1979) Epidural analgesia with morphine. A preliminary communications. Anesth Intensive Care 7:367
21. Wolfe MJ, Davies GK (1980) Analgesic action of extradural fentanyl. Br J Anaesth 52:3
22. Wright RMB, Goroszemink K (1980) Epidural fentanyl for pain of multiple fractures. Lancet 8:1033
23. Zenz M, Piepenbrock S, Otten B, Otten G (1980) Epidurale Morphin Injektion zur Schmerzbekämpfung. Fortschr Med 98:306

Epidural Morphine in Obstetrics

J. S. Crawford

We have injected morphine via a catheter into the epidural space in eight patients in an attempt to relieve the pain of labour. The morphine was supplied in sterile ampoules – 2 mg in 10 ml saline. In six cases the cannula was inserted through a lumbar vertebral interspace, and in two entry was through the space between the 10th and 11th thoracic vertebrae. Two patients received one dose each, four were given two doses and two received three doses of 2 mg morphine (Table 1). Only one of these patients claimed to have experienced some pain relief in response to the morphine, the remainder reported excellent analgesia when bupivacaine was substituted for morphine. Morphine failed to prevent the considerable pain experienced by two patients in the series who had a surgical induction of labour. There was no evidence of maternal drowsiness or of narcotic-induced neonatal depression in this series. One mother vomited copiously.

A double-blind study comparing the effectiveness of 2 mg morphine with saline injected into the epidural space during caesarean section did not demonstrate an impressive degree of post-operative pain relief to be associated with the use of morphine in this way. There were 60 patients in each group – with comparable numbers of elective and emergency section, and comparable numbers of section conducted under epidural and under general anaesthesia. The only noteworthy distinguishing feature was that only one (1.7%) of the patients who received saline vomited during the first 12 h post-operation, whereas 13 (21.7%) of those who were given morphine did so.

Table 1. Data referable to doses of morphine (2 mg in 10 ml saline) injected into the epidural space of eight patients in labour

No. of doses	Interval between successive doses (min)	Effectiveness
1	–	No relief
3	30,120	No relief
3	55,125	No relief
2	15	No relief
2	60	No relief
1	–	No relief
2	40	No apparent relief but patient satisfied
2	60	No relief

In summary we have been quite unimpressed by the effectiveness of epidural morphine in obstetrics. Furthermore, in view of other reports which have continued to appear regarding the associated incidence of delayed respiratory depression (and, in one report, of neonatal depression), I would be very reluctant to advocate the use of this technique in patients (such as post-natal patients) who are unlikely to be under close observation at all times throughout the first 12 h after the procedure.

Discussion

Lanz:
You said that the morphine acts on a central level. How do you explain the significant differences in effect between an epidural and an intramuscular injection of the same dose of morphine?

Crawford:
When you inject morphine intrathecally or epidurally, you get a considerable passage of morphine or the other narcotic into the cerebrol spinalfluid. You get a local action on the cerebrum rather than waiting for the blood-borne passage of intravenous or intramuscular morphine. I know that there are still claims made of the ability to identify segmental distribution, but I have yet to see any of these claims that I could really accept as being truthful or correct.

Lanz:
The spread up to the cerebrum is rather slow. In several studies it has been shown that the circulation of the CSF is unpredictable. According to the work of Di Chiro, it takes about 4 to 6 h until a substance which is injected into the lumbar space arrives at the fourth ventricle. If there should be a local cerebral action by diffusion through the CSF, the effect should then be a long away from the site of injection. How do you explain then the longer lasting effect of an epidural dose of morphine in comparison with the intramuscular injection?

Crawford:
I would question that it takes all that time for the diffusion of substances entering the lower part of the cerebrol spinal fluid to get up to the cerebrum. Even the results presented today have shown, for example, changes in the EEG very shortly after the injection of the narcotic. The vomiting and itching, which are central nervous effects, come on quite quickly. So if morphine provokes centrally induced vomiting, nausea, and itching, why should'nt it also produce analgesia quickly.

Stanton-Hicks:
We don't yet know the kinetics. The CSF circulation is dependent on the vascular status. The cardiovascular function may be changing all the time. This may well explain why in some instances there seems to be a sequestration of the narcotic, so that in 12 or even in as late as 14 hours, it can arrive in the cerebrum and cause central nervous depression. Furthermore, there may be other changes in kinetics which affect the release of morphine from the lumbar spine which then affects the medullary centers.

Clinical Survey of Spinal Anesthesia with Morphine

I Effects on Respiration and Pain Relief

C. B. Devaux, and C. Tessier

Introduction

Morphine which is intrathecally administered interferes with the spinal function by inhibiting the liberation of P substances in the substantia gelatinosa. The transmission of nociception is blocked at the spinal level [1–3, 7, 10, 11–13, 17, 20, 21, 22]. On the basis of this evidence, it was possible to give spinal anesthesia with morphine for operations followed by very painful postoperative periods [5], used in this manner, morphine gives produces exceptional pain relief [7, 17, 18]. During animal and human trials of intrathecal application of morphine, undesired side effects were not noticed in animals and no narcotics dependence was seen in cancer patients [15, 16, 18, 20, 23].

Patients and Methods

Twenty-four patients, classified as ASA 1 or AHA 0, who were to undergo hemorrhoidectomy gave their written consent to participate in the study. Patients were included in the study if they suffered from (1) intolerable or considerable pain during the immediate postoperative period and (2) experienced a period of relative disability exceeding 72 h. They were allocated three different doses of morphine. There were no differences between the groups with regard to age, weight, height, and hemoglobin (Table 1). Spinal anesthetization was carried out at the L3–L4 level with a 25 gunge needle with the patient in a sitting position without barbotage. Morphine hydrochloride diluted in equal volumes of 20% dextrose was injected in doses of 15, 30, and 50 μg/kg body weight in the different groups.

Arterial blood gases, tidal volume, and respiratory rate were recorded prior to and after the injection of the drugs for 24 h. At the same time, the pain scores were quantified by questioning the patient on the basis of the following scale: 0 = no pain; 2 = considerable pain; 3 = unbearable pain. The data obtained were tested using a protected Student's t test with regard to changes of respiration, $PaCO_2$, and the latency and duration of the sensitive block for the individual and between groups.

Table 1. Biometric data in the three groups

Doses (μg/kg^{-1})		Age (years)	Weight (kg)	Height (m)	Hb (9%)
15	Mean	32.2	69.5	1.67	13.1
	SD	8	13.5	0.07	0.2
	SEM	2.8	1.8	0.02	0.07
30	Mean	30	67.5	1.65	12.8
	SD	7.4	7.7	0.05	0.3
	SEM	2.6	2.7	0.01	0.1
50	Mean	31.6	67.3	1.67	12.5
	SD	7.5	13.5	0.08	0.4
	SEM	2.6	4.8	0.03	0.1

Table 2. Changes in tidal volume

Doses (μg/kg^{-1})		Time (min)								
		0	30	60	90	120	240	360	480	720
15	Mean	364	341	346	325	300	290	285	285	306
	SD	43	43	51	42	38	37	41	41	40
	SEM	15	15	18	15	13	13	15	14	14
	P<		0.01	0.01	0.01	0.01	0.01	0.01	0.01	NS
30	Mean	375	351	331	312	281	265	262	262	265
	SD	32	28	31	35	40	32	32	32	33
	SEM	16	10	11	12	11	11	11	11	11
	P<		0.01	0.01	0.01	0.01	0.01	0.01	0.01	0.01
50	Mean	343	315	293	268	237	237	237	237	237
	SD	42	32	41	43	35	35	35	35	35
	SEM	15	11	14	15	12	12	12	12	12
	P<		0.05	0.05	0.05	0.05	0.05	0.05	0.05	0.05

Results

Tidal Volume

Tidal volume decreased after the injection of the three different doses of morphine and reached a maximum after 15 and 30 μg/kg 6 h after the injection of the drug. The maximal effect of the 15 μg/kg dose of morphine was already seen after 120 min. Eight hours after the injection of the morphine, the tidal volume was significantly reduced in comparison with the preoperative control. The changes were 23% and 26% in the group receiving 15 and

Table 3. Changes in respiratory rate

Doses (μg/kg^{-1})		Time (min) 0	30	60	90	120	240	360	480	720
15	Mean	16	16	16.5	17.1	15.7	14.2	13.2	12.5	13.3
	SD	1.0	1.0	1.1	0.8	1.2	1.1	1.0	0.9	1.0
	SEM	0.3	0.3	0.4	0.2	0.4	0.4	0.3	0.3	0.3
	P<		NS	NS	NS	NS	NS	NS	NS	NS
30	Mean	15.6	15.8	16	17.1	16.3	14.2	12.6	11.6	11.5
	SD	1.4	1.3	1.3	1.5	1.9	1.1	1.1	0.7	0.7
	SEM	0.5	0.4	0.4	0.6	0.6	0.4	0.3	0.1	0.1
	P<		NS	NS	NS	NS	NS	NS	NS	NS
50	Mean	15.8	15.8	16.6	16.8	14.6	12.7	11.3	11.0	11.2
	SD	1.2	1.2	0.9	0.8	0.5	0.7	0.7	0.5	0.7
	SEM	0.4	0.4	0.3	0.2	0.1	0.2	0.2	0.2	0.2
	P<		0.01	0.01	0.01	0.01	0.01	0.01	0.01	NS

Table 4. Onset of hypoalgesia

Doses (μg/kg^{-1})		Time (min) 0	10	15	30	45	60
15	Mean	0	14.5	13.2	12.6	12.2	12
	SD	0	1.3	1.6	0.9	0.7	0
	SEM	0	0.4	0.5	0.3	0.2	0
	P<		0.01	0.01	0.01	0.01	0.01
30	Mean	0	13.2	12.5	11.7	11.5	11.1
	SD	0	1.5	1.0	1.0	0.5	0.3
	SEM	0	0.5	0.3	0.3	0.2	0.1
	P<		0.01	0.01	0.01	0.01	0.01
50	Mean	0	13.0	12.3	11.3	11	10.8
	SD	0	1.9	1.0	0.4	0.4	0.5
	SEM	0	0.6	0.3	0.1	0.1	0.2
	P<		0.02	0.02	0.02	0.02	0.02

30 μg/kg morphine, respectively, and 31% after the injection of 50 μg/kg morphine. In the group of patients who received 50 μg/kg morphine intrathecally, the tidal volume tended to normalize again after 12 h, while it still remained reduced in the two other groups (Table 2).

Respiratory Rate

After the application of 15 and 30 μg/kg morphine, respiratory rate decreased insignificantly; 50 μg/kg reduced respiratory rate significantly and the effect lasted for 8 h (Table 3).

Table 5. Upper limit of the sensory block tested with ice and upper extention of the block to the dermatome. $T_{10} = 10$, extention to $T_{12} = 12$, $L_1 = 13$, $L_5 = 17$

Doses (μg/kg^{-1})		Time (min)								
		0	30	60	90	120	240	360	480	720
15	Mean	12.6	12.2	12	12	11.5	10.8	10.7	11.5	17
	SD	0.9	0.7	0	0	0.7	0.8	0.7	0.5	0.3
	SEM	0.3	0.2	0	0	0.2	0.3	0.2	0.1	0.1
	P<		0.01	0.01	0.01	0.01	0.01	0.01	0.01	0.01
30	Mean	11.7	11.5	11.1	11	10.5	10.2	10.2	11.1	14.5
	SD	1.0	0.5	0.3	0.5	0.7	0.4	0.4	0.3	2.6
	SEM	0.3	0.2	0.1	0.1	0.2	0.1	0.1	0.1	0.9
	P<		0.01	0.01	0.01	0.01	0.01	0.01	0.01	0.01
50	Mean	11.3	11	10.8	10.6	10.2	10.2	10	11	14.5
	SD	0.5	0.5	0.5	0.7	0.5	0.4	0.4	0.5	2.6
	SEM	0.1	0.2	0.2	0.2	0.2	0.1	0.1	0.2	0.9
	P<		0.02	0.02	0.02	0.02	0.02	0.02	0.02	0.02

Table 6. Correlation between the extent of the block in overweight patients in all three groups

Height (m)	Weight (kg)	Time (min)					Equations
		10	15	30	45	60	
1.64	79.6	12.6	12.1	11.6	11.5	11.3	y = −0.362x + 4.600
0.08	8.5	0.3	0.5	0.5	0.5	0.5	r = 0.916
0.02	2.8	0.1	0.1	0.1	0.1	0.1	
P<		0.01	0.01	0.01	0.01	0.01	
1.68	63.5	13.8	12.7	12.1	11.8	11.8	y = −0.210x + 2.932
0.06	8.6	1.7	1.2	1.1	0.7	0.4	
0.01	2.2	0.4	0.3	0.2	0.2	0.1	
P<	0.02	0.02	0.02	0.02	0.02	0.02	

Extention of the Sensitive Block

Hypoalgesia was tested with ice and in all three groups rapid onset of the block was found (Table 4). For each dose, the T12 level was reached within 30 min (Tables 4 and 5). The analgesia continued to spread for 6 h and 24 h later a sensitive block of considerable magnitude remained. The upper limit of L5–S1 was reached in the group that received 15 μg/kg morphine and L2–L3 in the group that received 30 and 50 μg/kg. The extent of the block correlated closely with body weight in patients who were overweight (Table 6). Taken together, height and weight affected the extent of the block significantly in the entire series.

Discussion

These preliminary results showed dose-related effects of intrathecal morphine on respiration. Respiratory rate and tidal volume decrease, while the $PaCO_2$ in the arterial blood increases. There was no correlation between changes of respiration and changes of PCO_2 in the arterial blood. Glynn and co-workers [8] have suggested that this effect is related to the activation of chemoreceptors in the medulla induced by acid analgetic solutions. Like Haruka et al. [9] and Liolos et al. [14], we found a segmental distribution of the sensitive block.

References

1. Basbaum AI, Clanton CN, Fields HL (1976) Opiate and stimulus produced analgesia: functional anatomy of a medullo-spinal pathway. Proc Natl Acad Sci USA 73:4685
2. Besson JM, Wyon-Maillard MC, Benoist JM, Conseiller C, Hammannk F (1973) Effects of phenoperidine on lamina V cells in the cat dorsal horn. J Pharmacol Exp Ther 187:239
3. Besson JM (1977) Effets de la morphine sur la transmission des messages nociceptifs au niveau médullaire. Actual Pharmacol (Paris) 119
5. Devaux CB, Tessier C (1979) Clinical surgery and medullary opiate analgesia. Proceedings of 8th Belgian congress of anesthesiology
6. Devaux CB, Tessier C (to be published) Comparative hemodynamic studies of morphine anesthesia (sub-Arachnoïd-Epidural). In: Special topic Opiates. 7th World congress of anesthesiologists
7. Duggam AW, Hall JG, Headley PM (1976) Morphine, enkephalin and the substantia gelatinosa. Nature 264:456
8. Glynn CJ, Mather CE, Cousins MJ, Wilson ZR, Graham JR (1979) Spinal narcotics and respiratory depression. Lancet 8138:356
9. Haruka A, Kazujei I, Toshimari S, Takehisa S (1981) Segmental effects of morphine injected into epidural space in man. Anesthesiology 54:75
10. Kitahata LM, Collins JC (1981) Spinal action of narcotic analgesics. Anesthesiology 54:153
11. Lamotte C, Pert CB, Smyder SH (1976) Opiate receptor binding in primate spinal cord: distribution and changes after dorsal root section. Brain Res 112:407
12. Lebars D, Menetrey D, Conseiller C, Besson JM (1975) Depressive effects of morphine upon lamina V cells activities in the dorsal horn of the spinal cat. Brain Res 98:261
13. Le Bars D, Guilbaud G, Jurna I, Besson JM (1976) Differential affects of morphine on responses of dorsal horn lamina V type cells elicited by A and C fibre stimulation in the spinal cat. Brain Res 115:518
14. Liolos A, Hartmann A, Andersen F (1979) Selective spinal analgesia. Lancet 8138:357
15. Tung AS, Temicella R, Winter PM (1980) Opiate withdrawal syndrome following intrathecal administration of morphine. Anesthesiology 53:340
16. Ventafrida V (1980) Cervical. Sub-arachnoïdal morphine infusion (abstract). Second worlds congress on pain. Pain 1:199
17. Wang JK (1977) Analgesic effect of intrathecally administered morphine. Reg Anesth 2:3
18. Wang JK, Mauss IA, Thomas JE (1979) Pain relief by intrathecally applied morphine in man. Anesthesiology 50:149
20. Yaksh TL, Rudy TA (1976) Analgesia mediated by a direct spinal action of narcotics. Science 192:1357
21. Yaksh TL, Rudy TA (1977) Studies on the direct spinal action of narcotics in the production of analgesia in the rat. J Pharmacol Exp Ther 202:411
22. Yaksh TL (1978) Inhibition by etorphine of the discharge of dorsal horn neurons: effects on the neuronal response to both high and low threshold sensory input in the cerebral spinal cat. Exp Neurol 60:23
23. Zielgans Berger W, Bayerl H (1975) The mechanism of inhibition of neuronal activities by opiates in the spinal cord of cat. Brain Res 115:111

Clinical Survey of Spinal Anesthesia with Morphine

II Hemodynamic Effects of Morphine Anesthesia

C. B. Devaux, and C. Tessier

The aim of this study was to evaluate whether there were differences in the effect of 50 μg/kg morphine on cardiovascular function when administered either by epidural or subarachnoid routes.

Patients and Methods

Twenty patients suffering from chronic pain due to a metastatic carcinoma of the gastrointestinal tract, classified as ASA 1 or 2 and AHA 0, were included when their written consent to participate in the study was obtained. There were no statistically significant differences between the two routes of administration regarding the biometrical data (Table 1). The effect of 50 μg/kg morphine sulfate diluted in 20% dextrose applied either epidurally or intrathecally on the cardiovascular function was studied in these patients. After control measurements, the heart rate, arterial blood pressure, pulmonary artery pressure, pulmonary capillary wedge pressure, and cardiac output were monitored for 12 h. The changes within the group were evaluated using the paired Student's *t* test and the differences between the two groups were tested using Student's *t* test for unpaired data.

Table 1. Biometrical data

Analgesia	Values	Age (years)	Body area (m^2)	Hb (g %)
Epidural	Mean	61.6	1.69	12.08
n = 10	SD	10.4	0.14	2.75
	SEM	3.4	0.04	0.91
Spinal	Mean	63.5	1.68	13.19
n = 10	SD	12.4	0.16	1.71
	SEM	4.1	0.05	0.57

Table 2. Changes of heart rate

Analgesia	Heart rate (beat cm^{-1})	Control	Time (min) 15	30	60	90	120	240	360	720
Epidural	Mean	89.6	89.5	91.7	94.9	98.6	100.2	100.4	96.0	92.5
n = 10	SD	9.4	9.4	9.5	9.7	9.9	10.0	10.0	9.7	9.6
	SEM	3.1	3.1	3.1	3.2	3.3	3.3	3.3	3.2	3.2
	P<	–	0.05	0.05	0.05	0.05	0.05	0.05	NS	NS
Spinal	Mean	92.2	95.3	101.7	106.7	109.8	105.7	99.1	93.8	92.8
n = 10	SD	9.6	5.7	10.0	12.4	10.4	9.5	9.7	2.8	3.2
	SEM	3.2	1.9	3.3	4.1	3.4	3.1	3.2	0.9	1.0
	P<	–	0.05	0.05	0.05	0.05	NS	NS	NS	NS

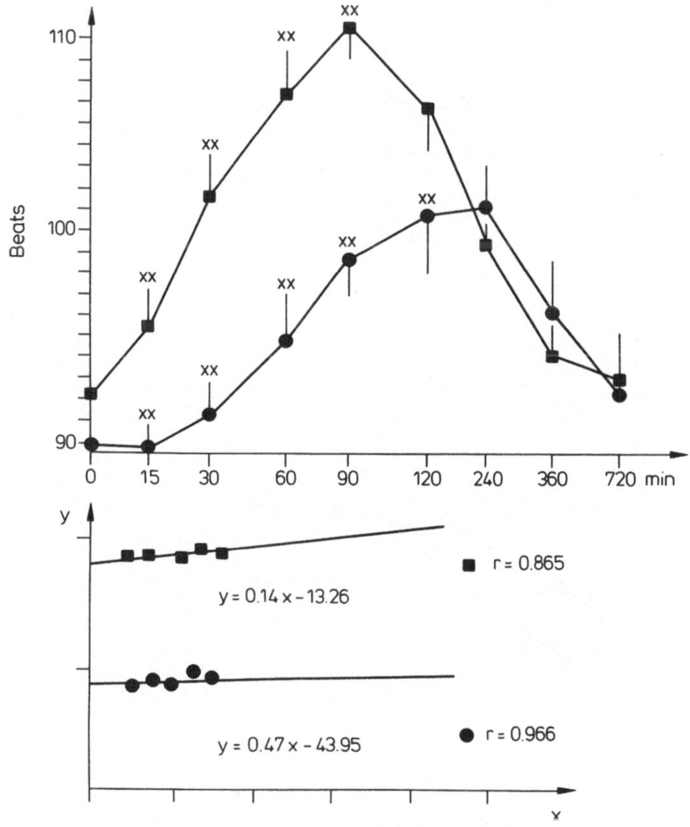

Fig. 1. Heart rate (*beats/min*) changes after epidural or intrathecal administration of morphine. The increase is more pronounced and shorter after intrathecal (■ —— ■) than after epidural (● —— ●) Administration

Table 3. Changes of the cardiac index in the two groups

Analgesia	Cardiac index lm^{-2}	Control	Time (min)							
			15	30	60	90	120	240	360	720
Epidural n = 10	Mean	2.79	2.83	2.88	2.89	2.88	2.86	2.84	2.85	2.83
	SD	0.27	0.22	0.20	0.19	0.17	0.17	0.17	0.16	0.16
	SEM	0.09	0.07	0.06	0.02	0.05	0.05	0.05	0.05	0.05
	$P<$	–	0.05	0.05	0.05	0.05	NS	NS	NS	NS
Spinal n = 10	Mean	2.84	2,90	2.96	2.99	3.03	3.02	3.01	2.98	2.97
	SD	0.12	0.13	0.12	0.12	0.11	0.12	0.13	0.10	0.11
	SEM	0.04	0.04	0.04	0.04	0.03	0.04	0.04	0.53	0.03
	$P<$	–	0.01	0.01	0.01	0.01	NS	NS	NS	NS

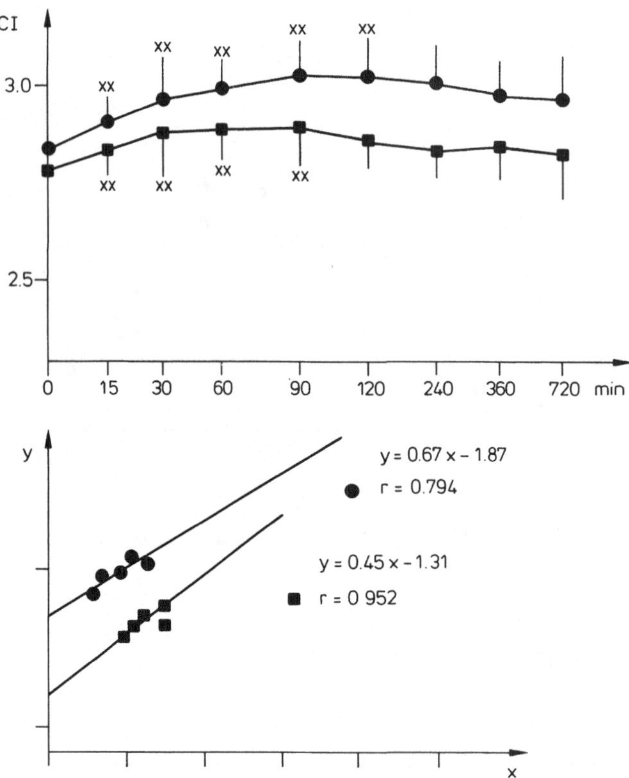

Fig. 2. Changes of cardiac index after intrathecal (■ —— ■) and epidural (● —— ●) injection of morphine. After injection of morphine, cardiac index (*CI*) increased in both groups. Following epidural injection of morphine, the changes were more pronounced and longer lasting than after intrathecal injection

Table 4. Total peripheral resistance

Analgesia	Total peripheral resistance dy s^{-1} cm^{-5}	Control	Time (min)							
			15	30	60	90	120	240	360	720
Epidural	Mean	1,098.2	1,096.5	1,093.2	1,081.2	1,068.00	1,045.7	1,040.5	1,044.3	1,074.3
n = 10	SD	70.56	70.88	69.87	64.83	66.26	62.40	58.87	60.13	61.18
	SEM	23.52	23.62	23.29	21.61	22.08	20.80	19.62	20.04	20.39
	$P<$	–	0.05	0.05	0.05	0.05	0.05	0.05	NS	NS
Spinal	Mean	1,055.8	1,044.3	1,034.9	1,025.1	1,014.1	1,011.5	919.0	1,028.9	1,039.2
n = 10	SD	63.42	59.94	58.65	55.29	59.85	63.56	288.7	66.59	71.40
	SEM	21.14	19.98	19.55	18.43	19.95	21.18	96.26	22.19	23.80
	$P<$	–	0.01	0.01	0.01	0.01	0.01	0.01	NS	NS

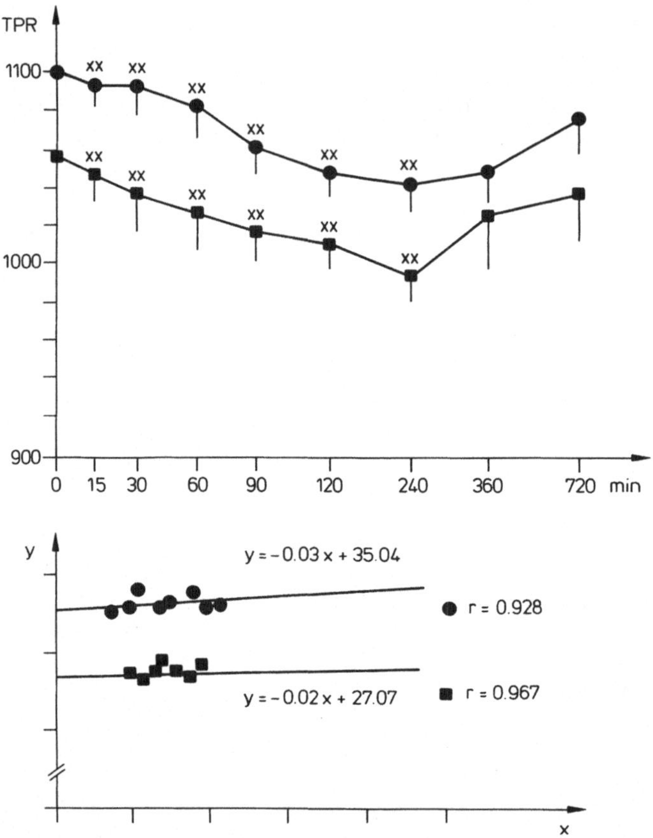

Fig. 3. Total peripheral resistance (*TPR*) decreased independent of the route of administration

Results

Heart Rate

Heart rate increased in both groups. In the epidural group, an 11% increase over the preoperative control group was seen after 240 min. After 6 h and 12 h, the heart rate decreased again in this group, while in the spinal group the heart rate increased to a maximum of 16% after 90 min before decreasing slowly again (Table 2, Fig. 1).

Cardiac Index

For both routes of administration the cardiac index increased only slightly, but significantly (Table 3, Fig. 2). After 90 min, the increase of cardiac output was more pronounced when morphine was injected intrathecally.

Total Peripheral Resistance

Total peripheral resistance decreased in both groups and was found to be lower up to 240 min (Table 4, Fig. 3). There were no differences between the two groups.

Table 5. Left ventricular stroke work in the two groups

Analgesia	Left ventricular stroke work gmM M^{-2}	Control	Time (min)							
			15	30	60	90	120	240	360	720
Epidural	Mean	57.16	57.72	58.37	58.82	59.21	59.73	60.11	59.75	57.83
n = 10	SD	2.40	2.27	2.06	1.91	1.87	1.54	1.39	1.18	1.48
	SEM	0.80	0.75	0.68	0.63	0.62	0.51	0.46	0.39	0.49
	P<	–	0.01	0.01	0.01	0.01	0.01	0.01	NS	NS
Spinal	Mean	57.46	58.0	58.22	58.51	58.72	58.71	58.68	58.37	58.02
n = 10	SD	2.99	2.87	2.89	2.88	2.84	2.75	2.62	2.54	2.59
	SEM	0.99	0.95	0.96	0.96	0.94	0.91	0.87	0.84	0.86
	P<	–	0.01	0.01	0.01	NS	NS	NS	NS	NS

Table 6. Correlation between the changes of heart rate and stroke work in the two groups

	Control	Time (min)							
		15	30	60	90	120	240	360	720
Epidural									
heart rate	89.60	89.50	91.70	94.90	98.60	100.2	100.4	96.00	92.5
Stroke work	57.16	57.72	58.37	58.82	59.21	59.73	60.11	59.75	57.83
Equation	$y = -0.212x + 38.577, r = 0.963, P < 0.01$								
Spinal									
heart rate	92.2	95.3	101.7	106.5	109.8	105.7	99.1	93.8	92.8
Left ventricular Stroke work	57.46	58.0	58.22	58.51	58.72	58.71	58.68	58.37	58.02
Equation	$y = -0.064x + 51.711, r = 0.968, P < 0.01$								

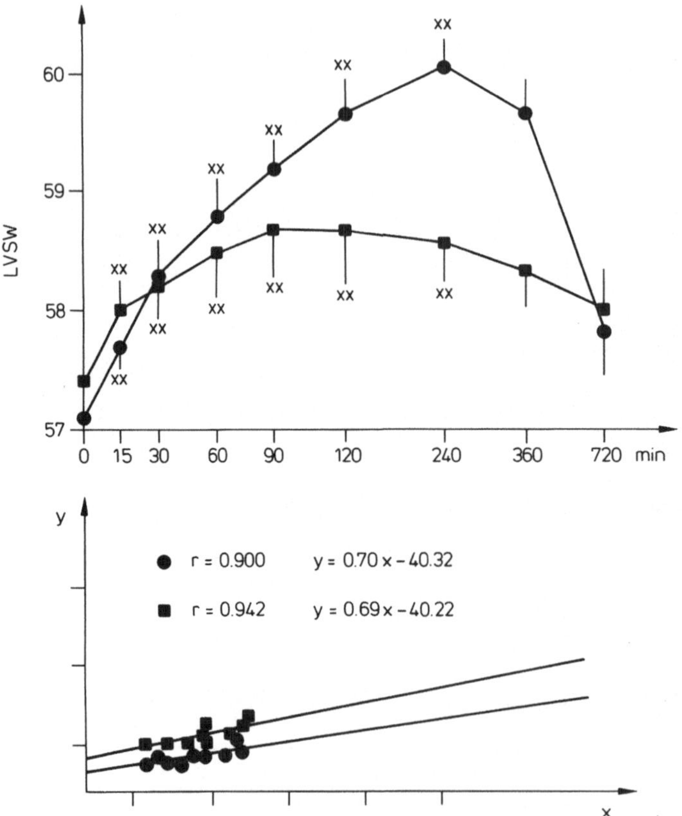

Fig. 4. Mean values of left ventricular stroke work (*LVSW*) following both routes of administration. The changes were more pronounced and longer lasting after epidural than after intrathecal morphine

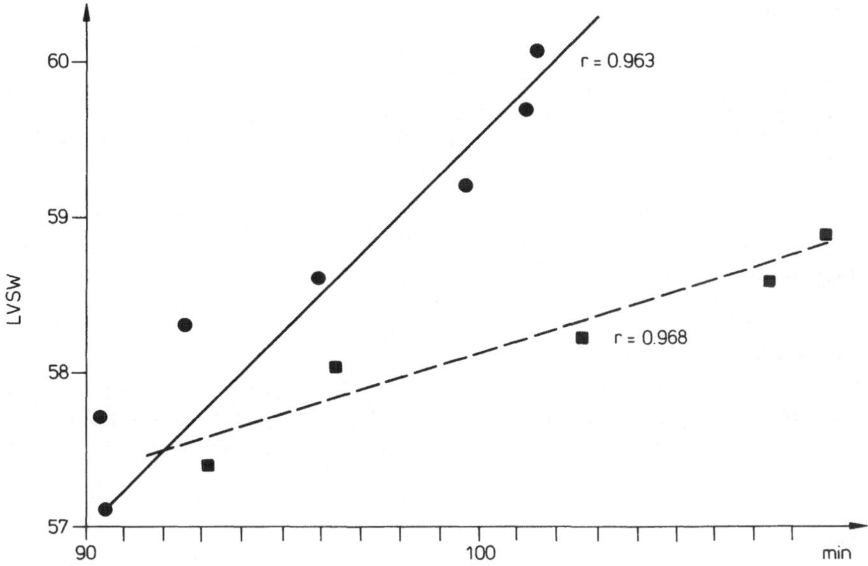

Fig. 5. Correlation between the changes of the heart rate (*HR*) and stroke work (*LVSW*) in the two groups. There is a close correlation between the changes of the heart rate and the stroke work indicating an impaired cardiac pump function. Independent of the route of administration

Left Ventricular Stroke Work

Left ventricular stroke work increased for a longer period (240 min) and the change was more pronounced when morphine was injected epidurally than when the injection was given intrathecally (Table 5, Fig. 4). The increase in stroke work was closely related to the increase in heart rate (Table 6, Fig. 5).

Discussion

The results of this study show, that heart rate and cardiac index changes are independent of the route of administration. The decrease in the total peripheral resistance is possibly caused by the increase in carbondioxide tension. Over all, these effects were moderate and less pronounced than the hemodynamic changes reported by Bonica et al. [1], when local anesthetics were used. This is in accordance with the reports of Writer and co-workers [2], who were able to show that morphine did not induce a vasomotor block.

Conclusions

The data presented show that morphine administered either epidurally or spinally influences respiration for many hours. These techniques provide a lasting sensory block that does not interfere with patient's mobility and cardiovascular function. These effects last longer when morphine is injected epidurally.

References

1. Bonica JJ, Kennedy WF, Ward RJ, Tocas AG (1966) A comparison of the effects of high subarachnoid and epidural anesthesia. Acta Anaesthesiol Scand [Suppl] 23:429
2. Writer WDR, James FM, Wheeler AS (1981) Double blind comparison of morphine and bupivacaine for continuous epidural analgesia in labor. Anesthesiology 54:215

Discussion

Stanton-Hicks:
In your study, you found almost the same duration of analgesia for buprenorphine as for morphine. Phenoperidine is a more lipid soluble drug, but the duration of action is not a function of lipid solubility, it is more a function of protein binding. How do you reconcile this paradox?

Devaux:
The duration of analgesia from morphine chloride, morphine sulfate, and buprenorphine is dependent on the pH of the solution and the strong binding to the opiate receptor.

Müller:
I have personal experience with epidural morphine. I tried everything to find a segmental spread both with ice and pin prick, but I was unable to find any.

Devaux:
In patients suffering from acute unbearable pain, e.g., multiple rib fractures, you will find a segmental spread in the ice test. In patients with chronic pain, however, it is different and sometimes you will not be able to demonstrate segmental spread. Until now we have treated acute pain by epidural morphine in 55 patients.

Haag:
Did you see any changes in the arterial blood gases 4, 6, or 12 h after the epidural injection of buprenorphine?

Devaux:
In all patients the arterial blood gases were in the normal range.

Question:
Isn't it very disturbing to find that the segmental nature of narcotic analgesia affects the cold sensation rather than nociception?

Devaux:
When you are using the cold test, you are testing the sensation for deep pressure and temperature, which are conducted in the more rapid fibers. These are more affected by narcotics.

Respiratory Depression Following Intrathecal Morphine (Abstract)

A. Harari, F. Clergue, F. Ghesquieres, and P. Viars

Profound respiratory depression has been reported by several authors after intrathecal morphine. To determine if these usually delayed accidents could be prevented, we investigated the CO_2-response curves in two groups of patients. Capnographic monitoring was carried out in group 1, which consisted of seven postoperative patients who each received 5 mg morphine intrathecally. These patients were held in a 30° head-up position until termination of analgesia. Group 2 consisted of six postoperative patients who received 2 mg morphine intrathecally. These patients were positioned with the head up at 30° for 3 h then lowered to the supine position for 1 h.

Results

In group 1, five out of seven patients did not show any respiratory depression throughout the study. Two patients in this group experienced a gradual decline of the slope of the CO_2-response curve. In group 2 all patients showed a marked depression of the CO_2-response curve following 1 h of lying in the supine position. The changes ranged from 22% to 58%.

Conclusion

The results of the first group show that respiratory depression occurs occasionally in some patients. The results of the second group show that the position of the patient is a major factor for the development of respiratory depression. To prevent this fatal complication, the supine position should be avoided and close clinical monitoring of the respiratory state is essential.

Discussion

Aldrete:
In your very nice study, when you injected 10 mg morphine in supine patients, you observed a respiratory depression which appears to be dose dependent and thus predictable. I wonder if it should occur in the other cases that have been reported this morning and where it was said nothing had happened.

Harari:
If you follow the patient closely, one out of every two patients will show a marked decrease of the CO_2 response. You therefore cannot say that nothing is happening, even if you say that you have not seen any respiratory depression in 100 patients. It just means you have not looked for it.

Aldrete:
The mechanism of respiration is changed by position, although apparently this mechanism does not play any significant role in this context. If you put a patient in the supine position, then the CSF will circulate more rapidly from the spinal canal to the respiratory center and therefore respiratory depression occurs more rapidly. In my opinion it is very difficult to keep a patient sitting for 48 h, especially, if he falls asleep.

Harari:
We have no problem keeping the patients in a position with the head up 20°.

Aldrete:
Did you look at the effect of position on analgesia? Did those patients, who were in a supine position, have faster and better analgesia than the patients who were sitting?

Harari:
This is a clinical impression in patients after laparatomy. We fear respiratory insufficiency and so put them in a 30° or 40° sitting position. In these patients, the lower part of the laparotomy is analgesic, while the patients complain of pain from the upper part of the wound. When these patients are then laid in a more supine position, we see after 2 or 3 h that the painfree area is extending upward.

Zindler:
How high was your naloxone dose? Since we know that the maximum effect is only 20 min, did you have to repeat it?

Harari:
We gave initially 0.4 mg naloxone, which was followed by 0.8 mg/h for to 7 h. This was a high dose that antagonized the respiratory depression but did not affect the analgesia.

Zindler:
Would it be sufficient to monitor the respiratory rate automatically? In a patient with normal lung function, the decrease in respiratory rate would not lead to a dangerous respiratory depression. But in a patient with impaired lung function you would see a respiratory depression by a rate which may decrease from 22 to 8. I think to monitor respiratory rate would be sufficient. Then the respiratory depression should be antagonized by naloxone.

Harari:
We agree with your opinion, that close monitoring (even clinically) of the respiratory rate is sufficient to detect any beginning of respiratory depression.

The Effect of Epidural Morphine and Postoperative Bladder and Stomach Function

P. Christensen, J. Asbjørn, V. Ø. Jensen, and M. R. Brandt

Introduction

Epidural morphine gives good and long-lasting relief from postoperative pain in comparison with parenteral morphine [3]. The epidural morphine causes a selective blockade of pain fibers in the spinal cord without affecting the autonomic or motor nerves or inducing general sedation [1]. The degree of bladder and stomach dysfunction in the postoperative period is influenced by systemically administered morphine, but the effect of epidural morphine has not been evaluated yet [4].

The aim of this study was to investigate the effect of epidural morphine per se on the bladder function. Furthermore, we investigated the bladder and stomach function after abdominal hysterectomy with systemic or epidural morphine used for pain relief during and after the operation.

Material and Methods

Ten otherwise healthy women scheduled for elective abdominal hysterectomy were randomized to recieve epidural or systemic morphine for the first 24 h after the operation. All patients gave informed consent to take part in the investigation. The epidural morphine was administered as 4 mg morphine chloride in 25 ml isotonic saline before the operation, 4 mg in 10 ml isotonic saline at skin closure, and, furthermore, postoperatively if the patient felt pain. After the first 24 h, epidural morphine analgesia was stopped and treatment continued with systemic morphine, which was administered as 10 mg nicomorphine IM on demand.

The patients were premedicated with 10 mg diazepam p.o. and anesthetized with thionembutal-halothane-N_2O-O_2 -pancuronium. No other analgetic was given during the operation. Isotonic saline was infused as 10–15 ml/kg/h for the first 2 h and 1–2 ml/kg/h thereafter. The bladder function was evaluated with a Lewis cystometer. The cystometry was done with the patient lying flat in her bed. We measured *the first sensation*, which was the bladder volume at which the patient had her first desire to urinate and *the maximal capacity*, which was the bladder volume causing irresistable need to urinate. The cystometry was done preoperatively and 24 h after the operation. Patients receiving epidural analgesia had an additional preoperative cystometry 15 min after epidural injection of morphine.

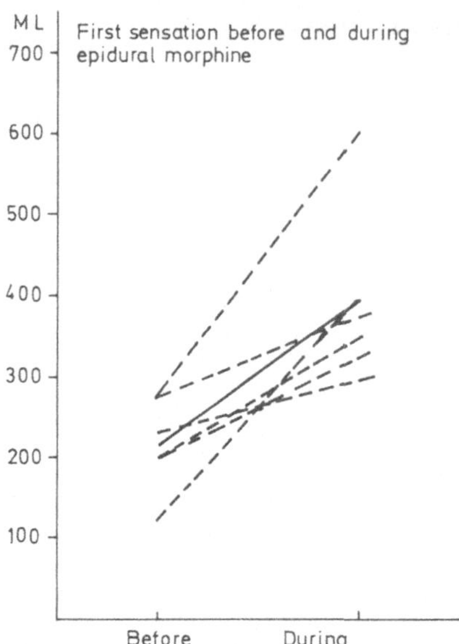

Fig. 1. First sensation before and during epidural morphine shown in each patient (– – –) and the mean value (——)

The stomach function was evaluated by an X-ray method used for gastrointestinal transit time measurement [2]. Twenty radiopaque markers 1 mm high and 3 mm wide were given to the patient as soon as she was fully awake after the operation. Four hours later an X ray was taken to locate the markers and their position was followed by daily X rays until all the markers had left the stomach.

Results

The groups were comparable with regard to age, weight, operation time, and blood loss. The epidural group consisted of six patients and the systemic group of four patients. The mean epidural morphine dose was 12 mg during the first 24 h and 50 mg nicomorphine in the systemic group. The first part of the study was concerned with the effect of epidural morphine per se on the bladder function. Figure 1 shows the changes in first sensation, where the volume increased in every patient from a mean of 218 ml to a mean of 392 ml, which was an increase of 80%. Figure 2 shows the changes in maximal capacity, which increased from a mean of 466 ml before to 620 ml after the epidural morphine, which was a relative increase of 33%.

The second part was concerned with the bladder function before the operation and 24 h later with either epidural morphine or systemic nicomorphine analgesia. Figure 3 shows the results in both groups. The first sensation declined equally – 43% in the epidural and 29% in the systemic group. The maximal capacity also declined equally – 51% in the epidural group and 39% in the systemic group.

The third part of the study was concerned with the stomach function after the operation during epdiural or systemic morphine for the first 24 h. One patient in both groups was excluded from this part on account of severe nausea. Figure 4 shows the results. There were great variations in both groups with a mean time of 3.6 days in the epidural and 3.3 days in the systemic group until all the markers had left the stomach.

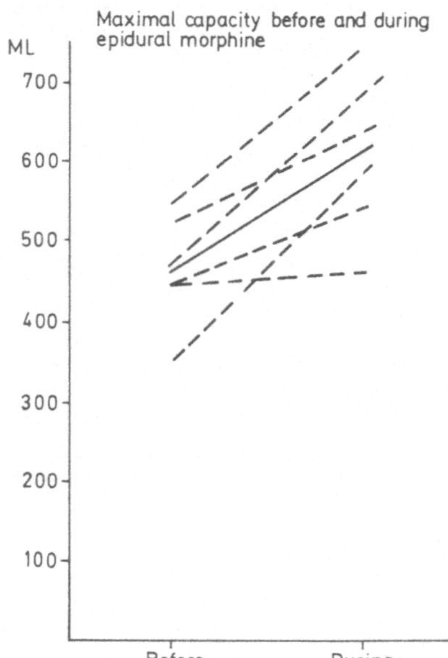

Fig. 2. Maximal capacity before and during epidural morphine shown in each patient (– – –) and the mean value (——)

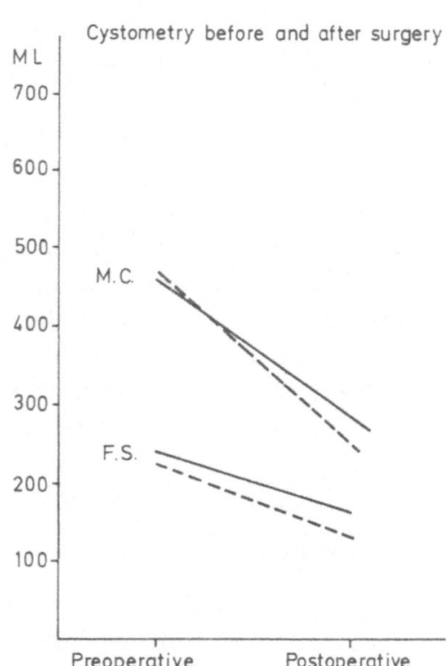

Fig. 3. First sensation (F.S.) and maximal capacity (M.C.) before operation and 24 h later with either epidural or systemic morphine. Epidural morphine, N = 6 (– – –); systemic morphine, N = 4 (——)

Discussion

In the postoperative period there is usually a depression of the bladder and stomach function leading to urinary retention and gastrointestinal paralysis. This dysfunction could be the effect of opiates used for postoperative pain-treatment [4]. Epidural morphine used for pain relief is effective in smaller doses than systemic morphine [3]. We therefore attempted to

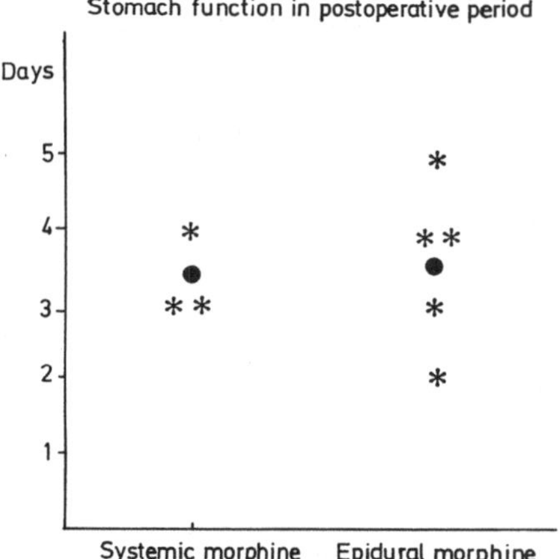

Fig. 4. Emptying time of ventricle in both groups. ⋆ individual value, • mean value

determine if it was possible to diminish the inhibition of bladder and stomach function using epidural morphine.

The first part of the study was concerned with the effect of epidural morphine per se on the bladder function. Depressed function was documented by an increase in both the first sensation and the maximal capacity. The first sensation showed the relatively greatest increase in volume.

The second part compared the bladder function before and after hysterectomy with epidural or systemic morphine for the first 24 h. The bladder function was equally changed with both methods.

The third part dealt with the stomach function, which was depressed equally with epidural and systemic opiates. Bladder function before surgery was depressed during epidural morphine, but postoperatively the bladder function was changed in the opposite direction – shown by a decrease in the first sensation and the maximal capacity – to the same degree with epidural as systemic morphine. Probably, therefore, the surgical trauma is the major mechanism of changes in the postoperative bladder function.

Conclusion

From the study we concluded that:

1. Epidural morphine inhibits impulses from the filling phase more than from the full badder.

2. The bladder function after hysterectomy is changed equally by epidural and systemic morphine analgesia.

3. The stomach function after hysterectomy is equally affected by epidural and systemic morphine analgeisa.

References

1. Behar M, Olshwang D, Magora F, Davidson JT (1979) Epidural morphine in treatment of pain. Lancet 1:527
2. Hinton JM, Lennard-Jones JE, Young AC (1969) A new method for studying gut transit times using radioopaque markers. Gut 10:842
3. Reiz S, Ahlin J, Ahrenfeldt B, Anderson M, Anderson S (1981) Epidural morphine for postoperative pain relief. Acta Anaesthesiol Scand 25:111
4. Vickers MD, Wood-Smith FG, Stewart HC (1978) Drugs in anaestetic practice, 5th edn. Butterworth, London, pp 188–194

Discussion

Stanton-Hicks:
It has been speculated for a long time what is the actual mechanism of bladder dysfunction following postoperative administration of intraspinal narcotics. From your study, it would certainly seem that epidural narcotics affect the afferent system. Parenteral narcotics may effect the bladder-function in a similar way and, particularly, just during the filling phase of the bladder.

Einfluß epiduraler Fentanylapplikation in der postoperativen Phase auf die Blutspiegel hypothalamischer Hormone

R. Dennhardt und B. von Bormann

Die somatischen und psychischen Belastungen des Patienten während der intra- und postoperativen Phase führen zu Reaktionen, die durch nervöse und humorale Regulationssysteme gesteuert werden. Die unmittelbare postoperative Phase ist durch eine im wesentlichen durch Schmerzen bedingte "Streßsituation" gekennzeichnet. Als weitere Stressoren kommen die Anaesthesie und das operative Trauma hinzu.

Der Organismus ist in der Lage, durch variationsreiche Möglichkeiten auf verschiedenen Ebenen den Schmerz zu verarbeiten. Entsprechend vielschichtig ist auch das Schmerzerlebnis und die sich daraus ergebenden Reaktionen. So ist es verständlich, daß Wege und Mittel der Schmerzausschaltung nur sehr schwer miteinander verglichen werden können. Die individuelle Variabilität der Patienten zeigen die Angaben von Jeffries (1970) [2], der angibt, daß nur die Hälfte der Patienten nach operativen Eingriffen nach einer Schmerzbehandlung verlangen. Nicht zuletzt wird die Qualität des Schmerzes durch den jeweiligen operativen Eingriff moduliert; das Ausmaß der postoperativen Schmerzen wird verständlicherweise durch die Art des Eingriffs, seiner Lokalisation und durch das Ausmaß der Traumatisierung bestimmt. Der Analgetikabedarf nach der Lokalisation des operativen Eingriffs kommt in den Angaben von Dundee (1977) [1] zum Ausdruck: 63% der Patienten mit Oberbaucheingriffen benötigen eine Analgesie, nach Unterbaucheingriffen sind es 51% und nach Extremitäteneingriffen nur noch 27%. Die übrigen allgemeinchirurgischen oder urologischen Operationen erfordern bei 49% der Patienten überhaupt keine postoperative Analgesie.

Das Schmerzempfinden kann durch verschiedenste Modalitäten beeinflußt werden. So ist es auch verständlich, daß von Patient zu Patient der zeitliche Abstand der benötigten Analgetikagaben wie auch der gesamte Verbrauch in der postoperativen Phase starken Schwankungen unterworfen ist. Besonders muß aber auch daran gedacht werden, daß das jeweilige Narkoseverfahren entscheidend das Verlangen nach postoperativer Schmerzausschaltung moduliert.

Wollen wir eine Methode zur postoperativen Schmerzausschaltung beurteilen, so bedarf es objektiver und vergleichbarer Kriterien. Da aber derartige Methoden nicht zur Verfügung stehen, sind sehr große Variationen in der Angabe über Erfolge, Mißerfolge, Wirkungen und Nebenwirkungen von Analgetika und Analgesieverfahren die Folge.

In früheren Untersuchungen wurden von uns deutliche Beziehungen zwischen den Blutspiegeln einiger hypothalamischer Hormone und perioperativen somatischen Belastungen gefunden. Besonders das antidiuretische Hormon (ADH) kann wegen seiner kurzen Halbwertszeit gut verfolgt werden. Voraussetzung ist jedoch, daß anderweitige Einflüsse ausge-

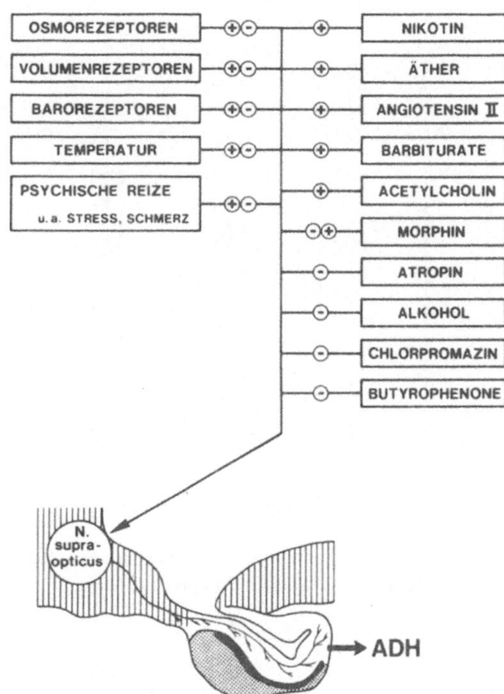

Abb. 1. Beeinflussung der ADH-Bildung bzw. Sektretion. (Mod. nach Hierholzer [2])

Tabelle 1. Verteilungskoeffizient Heptan–Wasser einiger Opiate als Maß ihrer Lipoidlöslichkeit

Morphium	<0,00001
Pethidin	3,4
Fentanyl	19,35
Methadon	44,9

schlossen werden können. Eine Vielzahl von Faktoren vermag die hypothalamische Ausschüttung von ADH zu beeinflussen; Abb. 1 vermittelt einen Überblick.

Für die intrathekale bzw. epidurale Opiatgabe kommen alle Substanzen in Frage, die in Wechselwirkung mit den Opiatrezeptoren treten. Der Wirkungseintritt der verschiedenen Opiate wird durch die jeweilige Lipoidlöslichkeit bestimmt (Tabelle 1). Es ist also nicht verwunderlich, daß Fentanyl wie auch die zur Erprobung anstehenden Weiterentwicklungen wie Lofentanil und Sufentanil eine rasche Anschlagszeit haben. Unabhängig von der Wirkungsqualität ist darauf zu achten, daß die Injektionslösung einen nicht zu sauren pH-Wert besitzt, da anderenfalls sehr schmerzhafte Sensationen beim Injizieren vom Patienten angegeben werden. Unterschiedliche Eigenschaften der zur Anwendung kommenden Pharmaka werden durch die jeweilige Pharmakodynamik aufgrund spezifischen Bindungsverhaltens an den Rezeptoren und durch Interaktionen mit anderen Pharmaka bedingt.

Ich möchte im folgenden die Erfahrungen und Ergebnisse ansprechen, die wir mit der epiduralen Fentanylapplikation intra- und postoperativ gemacht haben.

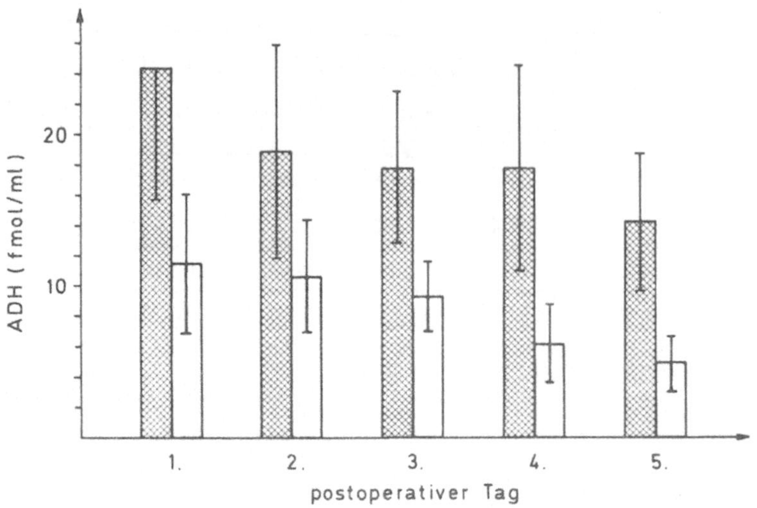

Abb. 2. ADH-Konzentrationen im Plasma nach intraabdominellen Eingriffen. *Säule I*: i.m.- bzw. i.v.-Analgesie mit Opiaten (Pethidin, Piritramid), *Säule II*: epidurale Fentanylanalgesierung

Gute Effekte konnten bei großflächigen, diffusen Schmerzen im abdominellen Bereich verzeichnet werden, besonders aber auch bei ischämischen Schmerzen bei Gefäßpatienten. Weniger erfolgreich war diese Methode bei akuten, lokalisierten Schmerzen sowie bei der Anwendung unter der Geburt, wo sie nur in Verbindung mit Lokalanaesthetika positiv zu beurteilen ist.

Bei insgesamt 116 Patienten überprüften wir die Wirkung von epidural appliziertem Fentanyl auf das subjektive Schmerzempfinden bei Patienten mit großen abdominellen Eingriffen. In Abhängigkeit von den jeweiligen Eingriffen variierte die Einzeldosis von Fentanyl zwischen 0,1–0,25 mg. Sie wurde zusammen mit 7 ml physiologischer NaCl-Lösung über einen periduralen Verweilkatheter gegeben. Der mittlere tägliche Verbrauch schwankte zwischen 0,006–0,02 mg/kg KG. Die Repetitionsintervalle unterschieden sich je nach Lokalisation und Ausmaß des operativen Eingriffs: bei Oberbaucheingriffen lag sie am 1. Tag im Mittel bei 5,5 h, am 2. Tag bei 8,2 h, am 3. Tag bei 10,8 h. Bei thorakalen Eingriffen betrug das Intervall am 1. Tag 4,6 h, am 2. Tag 5,3 h, am 3. Tag 7,5 h. Bei Gefäßoperationen mußte im Mittel am 1. Tag nach 6,9 h, am 2. Tag nach 10,3 h und am 3. Tag nach 15,0 h nachinjiziert werden. Wir beobachteten beim Fentanyl keinerlei Versager. Der Wirkungseintritt schwankte zwischen 5 und 15 min.

Die Objektivierung des analgetischen Effekts ist eingangs bereits angesprochen worden. Wir haben deshalb versucht, über die Analyse des antidiuretischen Hormons Anhaltspunkte für die Effektivität der jeweiligen Analgesierung zu erhalten. In Abb. 2 sind 2 Kollektive von Patienten gegenübergestellt, die sich bezüglich der Eingriffe und des mittleren Alters nicht voneinander unterschieden. Alle Patienten mußten sich großen intraabdominellen Eingriffen unterziehen. Die Gruppe 1 bekam über einen Periduralkatheter Fentanyl in den bereits erwähnten Dosierungen, die 2. Gruppe wurde herkömmlich mit intravenösen bzw. intramuskulären Gaben von Opiaten behandelt. Über 5 postoperative Tage wurde die Konzentration des antidiuretischen Hormons (ADH) verfolgt. Die 1. Säule der Abb. 2 gibt jeweils das mit intravenösen bzw. intramuskulären Opiaten behandelte Kollektiv an; die 2. Säule bezieht sich auf diejenigen Patienten, die mit Fentanyl epidural behandelt wurden. Um einen Vergleich ziehen zu können, sei darauf hingewiesen, daß die ADH-Spiegel bei Anwendung von Lokalanaesthetika zur Analgesierung stets im Normbereich lagen.

Die durch die epidurale Fentanylgabe erzielte Analgesie wird besonders nach Bauchoperationen von den Patienten als ausgezeichnet empfunden. Die subjektive Einschätzung der Schmerzqualität variiert allerdings von Patient zu Patient. Traten bei Patienten peritoneale Reize auf, so wurden diese stets prompt angegeben.

Das Verhalten der Prolaktinspiegel zeigt ein sehr variables Verhalten. Dies ist nicht verwunderlich, da einzelne Pharmaka, wie im besonderen Narkoseverfahren und perioperativer Streß, die Prolaktinsekretion anregen. Es ist bekannt, daß besonders die Opiate die Prolaktinausschüttung zu stimulieren vermögen.

Zusammenfassung

Die Wirksamkeit der epiduralen Applikation von Fentanyl konnte bei abdominalchirurgischen Patienten aufgezeigt werden. Fentanyl zeigte einen raschen und sicheren Wirkungseintritt, es wurden weder Versager noch Nebenwirkungen beobachtet. Die Wirkungsdauer variierte in Abhängigkeit von den operativen Eingriffen und dem postoperativen Zeitpunkt. Unter Verwendung der Plasma-ADH-Spiegel konnte gezeigt werden, daß die epidurale Opiatgabe herkömmlichen Verfahren zur Schmerzausschaltung durch intramuskuläre oder intravenöse Gabe überlegen ist.

Literatur

1. Dundee JW (1977) Problems associated with strong analgesics. In: Harcus AW, Smith RB, Whittle BA (eds) Pain. New Perspectives in measurement and management. Edinburgh, Churchill Livingstone, p 57
2. Jettries M (1970) Postoperative Analgesia. Amer Surg 36:296

Diskussion

Hack:
Welchen Stellenwert hat die epidurale Morphinapplikation bei oder nach gefäßchirurgischen Eingriffen? Es ist ja eigentlich offenkundig, daß durch die begleitende Sympathikusblockade bei Epiduralanaesthesien mit Lokalanaesthetika eine Vasodilatation im rekonstruierten Gefäßbereich und bei Rekonstruktionen im aortoiliakalen Bereich postoperativ eine Ileusprophylaxe erreicht wird.

Dennhardt:
Da die Bedürfnisse und auch die Reaktionen auf die Morphingabe gerade bei den älteren Patienten, um die es sich bei Gefäßpatienten in der Regel handelt, sehr unterschiedlich sind, schränkt dies die Bedeutung dieser Technik zur Schmerzbehandlung erheblich ein. Die post-

operative Schmerzbehandlung niedrig dosierter Lokalanaesthetika hingegen erscheint mir bei diesen Patienten die Methode der Wahl zu sein.

Stanton-Hicks:
When local anaesthetics are used for postoperative analgesia, the sympathetic blockade also introduces its own problems of management. With morphine you can obtain analgesia in the absence of any significant sympathetic effects, but this technique has of course a lot of side effects.

Lange:
Rupreht und Woraczyk in Rotterdam haben bei ca. 4000 Allgemein- und Regionalanaesthesien in 3–5% der Fälle ein zentral cholinerges Syndrom beobachtet. Könnte man Symptome bei Regionalanaesthesien, wie Übelkeit oder "shivering", nicht als Zeichen des Syndroms auffassen und mit Physostigmin behandeln?

Dennhardt:
Nach Lokalanaesthetika alleine habe ich diese typischen Zeichen des anticholinergen Syndroms nie beobachtet. Bei Kombinationen der Epiduralanaesthesie mit Psychopharmaka, Atropin u. a., sind die Symptome aufgetreten. Es war uns aber nicht immer möglich, durch Antagonisierung mit Physostigmin dieses Syndrom zu beweisen. Bei einigen Patienten konnten wir allerdings diese Symptome mit Physostigmin aufheben. Das Syndrom entsteht m.E. als Summationseffekt aus der Wirkung mehrerer Pharmaka, eingeschlossen der Prämedikation, die durchaus eine so lange Nachwirkung haben kann.

Comparative Effects of Epidural Morphine and Epidural Analgesia with Local Anesthetic on the Endocrine-metabolic Response to Surgery

P. Christensen, I. W. Møller, J. Rem, M. R. Brandt, and H. Kehlet

Introduction

Previous studies have shown that afferent neurogenic stimuli from the surgical area are a major release mechanism of the endocrine-metabolic response to surgery [4]. Thus, neurogenic blockade by epidural analgesia with a local anesthetic is effective in inhibiting the stress response to lower abdominal surgery [3], but no studies are available comparing the influence of different analgesic techniques on the surgical stress response. This study summarizes the comparative effects of epidural morphine [2], preoperative application of epidural analgesia with a local anesthetic, posttraumatic application of epidural analgesia [5], and general anesthesia with systemically administered opiates on the adrenocortical and hyperglycemic response to surgery.

Materials and Methods

Forty-eight otherwise healthy premenopausal women scheduled for elective abdominal hysterectomy were studied. The patients were divided into four groups of 12 patients. One group was operated under general anesthesia with halothane-N_2O-O_2 and received systemic opiates according to a standard regimen with 50–100 mg meperidine or 25–37.5 mg ketobemidone every 4 h in the postoperative period (group A). The second group was operated under continous epidural analgesia effective before skin incision with 0.5% bupivacaine and extending from T_4 to S_5 (group B). The third group was operated under general anesthesia with halothane-N_2O-O_2 and was given 4 mg epidural morphine in 25 ml isotonic saline before skin incision and 4 mg in 10 ml isotonic saline at skin closure (group C). The fourth group was operated under general anesthesia with halothane-N_2O-O_2 and had posttraumatic administration of epidural analgesia with 0.5% bupivacaine 30 min after skin incision, continued for postoperative pain relief, and extending from T_4 to S_5 (group D). The groups were comparable with regard to age, weight, blood loss, and duration of surgery (90 min).

The patients were premedicated with 1 mg/kg pethidine IM. Isotonic saline was infused at a rate of 10 15 ml/kg/h for the first 2 h and thereafter 1–2 ml/kg/h. Furthermore, blood loss was compensated by 2.5 ml isotonic saline per ml blood loss. Venous blood samples were taken from a central catheter 15 and 5 min before the induction of anesthesia, at skin incision and 0.5, 1, 2, 3, 4, 6, and 9 h later.

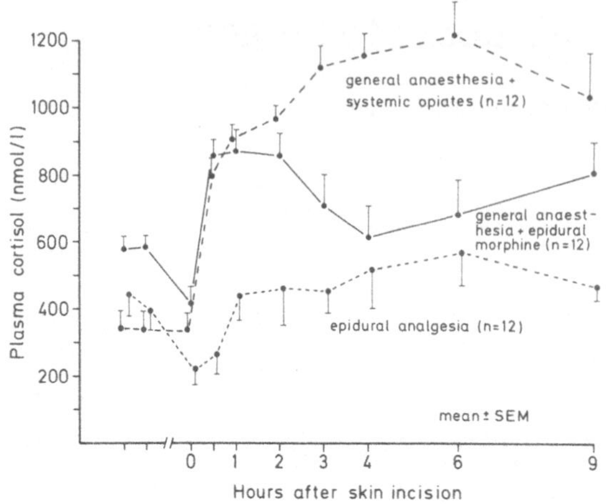

Fig. 1. Effect of different analgesic techniques on the cortisol response to surgery. Group A = general anesthesia with systemic opiates. Group B = epidural analgesia with bupivacaine. Group C = = general anesthesia with epidural opiate

Plasma cortisol was measured by a competitive protein-binding technique and plasma glucose by a routine glucose-oxidase method. Statistical analyses were made by the Kruskal-Wallis test for group comparison, the Mann-Whitney test for intergroup variation, and by Pratt's and Wilcoxon tests for intragroup variation. Statistical significant limits were p values less than 0.05.

Results

Comparison between plasma cortisol levels in the group operated under general anesthesia with epidural morphine (group C), the group operated under general anesthesia with systemic opiates (group A), and the group receiving continous epidural analgesia with bupivacaine (group B) are shown in Fig. 1. In group A, the plasma cortisol level increased from skin incision throughout the study. In group B, plasma cortisol showed no statistically significant change in relation to surgery. In group C, plasma cortisol increased from skin incision and remained elevated during surgery ($p < 0.05$), but decreased to preoperative values 3 h after skin incision and increased again 6 h later ($p < 0.05$). Plasma cortisol was significantly higher in group A from 30 min after skin incision and throughout the observation period compared with group B. In group C, plasma cortisol levels were significantly lower compared with group A 3, 4, and 6 h after skin incision. Cortisol levels were significantly higher in group C 0.5, 1, and 2 h and again 9 h after skin incision compared with group B. Comparison between plasma glucose changes in the same three groups are shown in Fig. 2.

In group A, plasma glucose increased from skin incision and remained elevated throughout the study. In group B, it showed no significant change. In group C, plasma glucose increased from skin incision and remained elevated throughout the observation period. In group C, it was significantly lower 3, 4, and 9 after skin incision compared with group A, but was significantly higher 1 and 3 h after skin incision compared with group B. Changes in

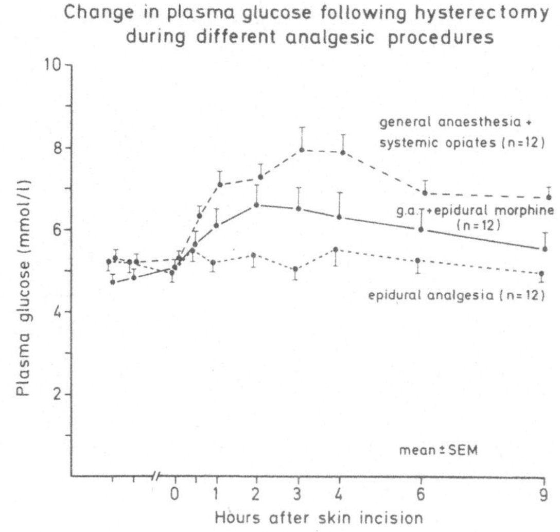

Change in plasma glucose following hysterectomy during different analgesic procedures

Plasma glucose (mmol/l)

general anaesthesia + systemic opiates (n=12)

g.a. + epidural morphine (n=12)

epidural analgesia (n=12)

mean ± SEM

Hours after skin incision

Fig. 2. Effect of different analgesic techniques on the glucose response to surgery. Group A = general anesthesia with systemic opiates. Group B = epidural analgesia with bupivacaine. Group C = general anesthesia with epidural opiate

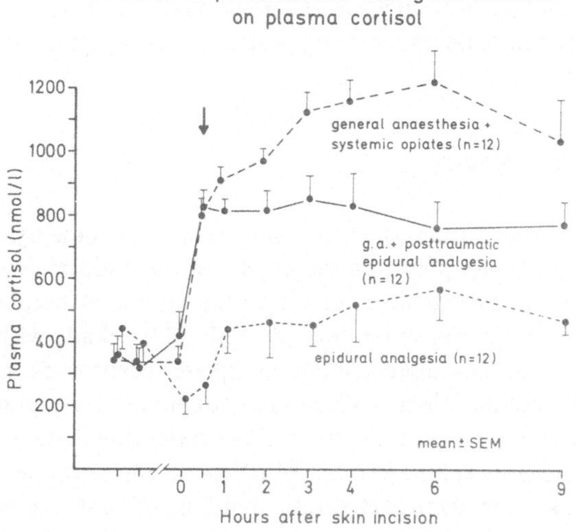

Fig. 3. Effect of different analgesic techniques on the cortisol response to surgery. Group A = general anesthesia with systemic opiates. Group B = epidural analgesia with bupivacaine. Group D = = general anesthesia plus posttraumatic epidural analgesia with bupivacaine

plasma cortisol in the group operated under general anesthesia with posttraumatic application of epidural analgesia with bupivacaine (group D) were compared with the changes in groups A and B in Fig. 3.

Plasma cortisol in group D increased from skin incision and remained increased in the observation period ($p < 0.05$). In group D, plasma cortisol levels were significantly lower 3, 4, and 9 h after skin incision compared with group A and significantly higher 3 and 9 h after skin incision compared with group B. Plasma glucose levels in the same groups are shown in Fig. 4. Plasma glucose in group D increased from skin incision and remained elevated throughout the study period. In group D, plasma glucose levels were significantly lower than in group A except at 0.5 h after skin incision and significantly higher than in group B 1 and

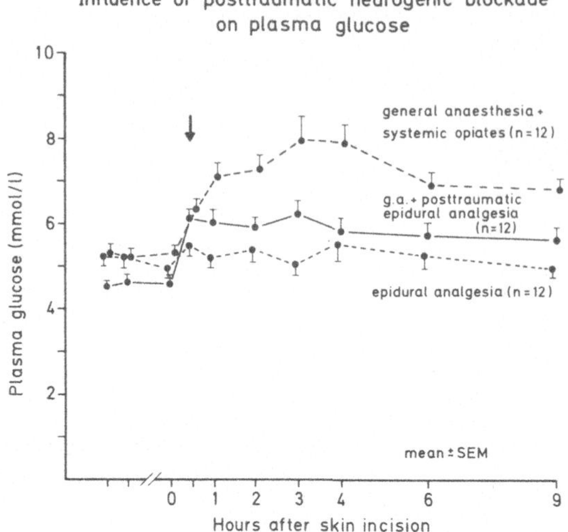

Fig. 4. Effect of different analgesic techniques on the glucose response to surgery. Group A = general anesthesia with systemic opiates. Group B = epidural analgesia with bupivacaine. Group D = general anesthesia plus posttraumatic epidural analgesia with bupivacaine

3 h after skin incision. There was no significant difference in plasma cortisol or glucose between patients receiving posttraumatic epidural analgesia and epidural morphine.

Discussion

It is well established that neurogenic blockade by epidural analgesia with a local anesthetic agent may prevent a major part of the endocrine-metabolic response to surgery [3, 4]. Epidural neurogenic blockade with a local anesthetic involves both motor, sensory, and autonomic nerves in contrast to epidural blockade with morphine, which causes a selective blockade of pain fibers containing opiate receptors in medulla spinalis [1]. Therefore, it is possible using this selective blockade with epidural morphine to study the importance of pain stimuli as a releasing mechanism of the endocrine-metabolic response to surgery. We found that epidural morphine had no influence on the *intra*operative stress response, but that opiate receptor-dependent pain stimuli had a significant role in releasing the *post*operative endocrine-metabolic response to surgery. This is in accordance with a previous study showing that autonomic blockade ($T_4 - S_5$) and not just pain relief ($T_{10-8} - S_5$) was necessary for blockade of the surgical stress response to hysterectomy [3].

The second part of the study considers whether *post*traumatic neutraumatic neurogenic blockade with a local anesthetic may abolish the stress response to surgery already released. The results show that the normal further increase in plasma cortisol and glucose is immediately interrupted when neurogenic blockade is produced 30 min after skin incision, but also that normal resting endocrine-metabolic activity is not restored. Comparison of patients receiving epidural morphine and posttraumatic epidural analgesia with a local anesthetic for pain relief showed similar levels in plasma cortisol and glucose during the postoperative period, but with higher levels than patients with epidural analgesia effective before skin incision, indicating that this latter technique is preferable if the aim is to preserve resting endocrine-metabolic activity during and after surgery.

Conclusion

From these studies we conclude:

1. Continuous epidural analgesia with a local anesthetic abolishes the cortisol and hyperglycemic response to lower abdominal surgery

2. Pain alleviation with epidural morphine inhibits, but does not prevent the stress response to surgery

3. Posttraumatic application of a neurogenic blockade interrupts the further amplification of the stress response, but does not reestablish resting endocrine-metabolic activity

4. The endocrine-metabolic response to surgery is primarily released by neurogenic stimuli other than pain stimuli involving opiate-receptor-dependent nociceptive pathways.

References

1. Behar M, Olshwang D, Magora F, Davidson JT (1979) Epidural morphine in treatment of pain. Lancet 1:527
2. Christensen P, Brandt MR, Rem J, Kehlet H (1982) Influence of epidural morphine on the adrenocortical and hyperglycemic response to surgery. Br J Anaesth 54:23
3. Engquist A, Brandt MR, Fernandes A, Kehlet H (1977) The blocking effect of epidural analgesia on the adrenocortical and hyperglycemic response to surgery Acta Anaesthesiol Scand 21:330
4. Kehlet H, Brandt MR, Rem J (1980) Role of neurogenic stimuli in mediating the endocrine-metabolic response to surgery. JPEN 4:152
5. Møller IW, Rem J, Brandt MR, Kehlet H (1982) The effect of posttraumatic epidural analgesia on the cortisol and hyperglycemic response to surgery. Acta Anaesthesiol Scand 26:56

Discussion

Hack:
If your upper normal limit for cortisol is 500 nmol per liter, your patients in the epidural morphine group have an elevated cortisol level.

Christensen:
We were forced to use different methods for premedication in our groups, which might explain these high levels. The patients receiving general anesthesia or epidural analgesia were premedicated with pethidine in the ward before going to the operating theater. The epidural morphine group, however, were premedicated after the placement of the epidural catheter. Their cortisol levels are elevated in the beginning because of the excitation before going to the theater and before the premedication was given, but then they dropped when the anesthesia was started. Therefore, we think that these groups are comparable.

Sachverzeichnis

Anaesthesiologie und Intensivmedizin

Anaesthesiology and Intensive Care Medicine

vormals „Anaesthesiologie und Wiederbelebung“
begründet von R. Frey, F. Kern und O. Mayrhofer

Herausgeber: H. Bergmann (Schriftleiter)
J. B. Brückner, M. Gemperle, W. F. Henschel,
O. Mayrhofer, K. Peter

Beiträge des Zentraleuropäischen Anaesthesiekongresses 1979
Band 139

Prae- und postoperativer Verlauf Allgemeinanaesthesie

Band 1
ZAK Innsbruck 1979: Begrüßungsansprachen, Festvortrag. Panel III: Präoperative Anaesthesieambulanz. Freie Themen: Allgemeinanaesthesie, Postoperative Nachsorge. Panel V: Anaesthesieletalität
Herausgeber: B. Haid, G. Mitterschiffthaler
1981. 106 Abbildungen, 86 Tabellen.
XXXIII, 225 Seiten (40 Seiten in Englisch)
DM 98,–. ISBN 3-540-10942-0

Band 140

Regionalanaesthesie Perinatologie Elektrostimulationsanalgesie

Band 2
ZAK Innsbruck 1979: Hauptthema I: Regionalanaesthesie. Freie Themen: Elektrostimulationsanalgesie. Panel II: Perinatalperiode
Herausgeber: B. Haid, G. Mitterschiffthaler
1981. 134 Abbildungen, 51 Tabellen. XI, 218 Seiten
DM 85,–. ISBN 3-540-10943-9

Band 141

Experimentelle Anaesthesie – Monitoring – Immunologie

Band 3
ZAK Innsbruck 1979: Freie Themen: Experimentelle und klinisch-experimentelle Anaesthesie, Technik und Monitoring, Anaesthesie und EEG. Panel I: Immunologische Aspekte. Freie Themen: Immunologie
Herausgeber: B. Haid, G. Mitterschiffthaler
1981. 183 Abbildungen, 32 Tabellen
XIII, 252 Seiten (7 Seiten in Englisch)
DM 98,–. ISBN 3-540-10944-7

Band 142

Herz Kreislauf Atmung

Band 4
ZAK Innsbruck 1979: Freie Themen: Kontrollierte Blutdrucksenkung, Anaesthesie bei Cardiochirurgie, Haemodynamik, Atmung
Herausgeber: B. Haid, G. Mitterschiffthaler
1981. 263 Abbildungen, 51 Tabellen. XIV, 335 Seiten
DM 128,–. ISBN 3-540-10945-5

Band 143

Intensivmedizin – Notfallmedizin

Band 5
ZAK Innsbruck 1979: Hauptthema II: Anaesthesie und Notfallmedizin. Hauptthema III: Grenzen der Intensivmedizin. Freie Themen: Intensivmedizin, Parenterale Ernährung und Volumenersatz, Säure-Basen-Haushalt
Herausgeber: B. Haid, G. Mitterschiffthaler
1981. 269 Abbildungen, 95 Tabellen. XV, 373 Seiten
(13 Seiten in Englisch)
DM 148,–. ISBN 3-540-10946-3

Band 144

Spinal Opiate Analgesia

Experimental and Clinical Studies
Editors: T. L. Yaksh, H. Müller
1982. 55 figures, 54 tables. XII, 147 pages
DM 68,–. ISBN 3-540-11036-4

Band 145
J. Beyer, K. Messmer

Organdurchblutung und Sauerstoffversorgung bei PEEP

Tierexperimentelle Untersuchungen zur regionalen Organdurchblutung und lokalen Sauerstoffversorgung bei Beatmung mit positiv-endexspiratorischem Druck
1982. 17 Abbildungen, 18 Tabellen. X, 84 Seiten
DM 54,–. ISBN 3-540-11220-0

Band 147
L. Tonczar

Kardiopulmonale Wiederbelebung

1982. 44 Abbildungen, 15 Tabellen. 160 Seiten
DM 58,–. ISBN 3-540-11760-1

Springer-Verlag
Berlin
Heidelberg
New York
Tokyo

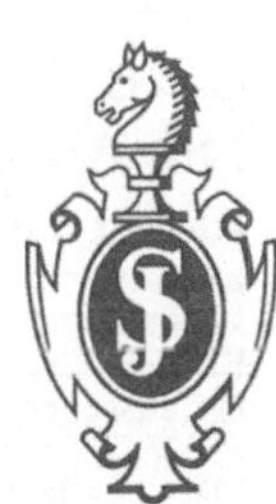

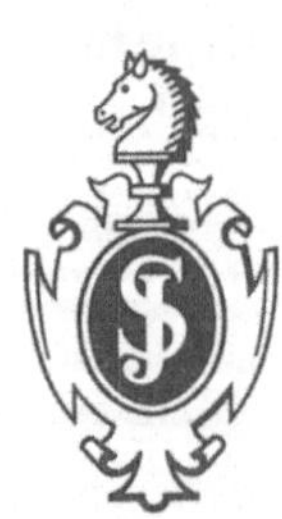